QUALITY IMPROVEMENT

Practical Applications for Medical Group Practice

by

Davis Balestracci, Jr., MS and Jeanine L. Barlow, MPH

Franciscan Health System

Center for Research in Ambulatory Health Care Administration
Englewood, Colorado

Center for Research in Ambulatory Health Care Administration (CRAHCA), the research and development arm of the Medical Group Management Association (MGMA), publications are intended to provide current and accurate information and are designed to assist readers in becoming more familiar with the subject matter covered. CRAHCA published *Quality Improvement: Practical Applications for Medical Group Practice* for a general audience as well as for MGMA members. Such publications are distributed with the understanding that CRAHCA and MGMA do not render any legal, accounting or other professional advice that may be construed as specifically applicable to individual situations. No representations or warranties are made concerning the application of legal or other principles discussed by the authors to any specific fact situation, nor is any prediction made concerning how any particular judge, government official or other person who will interpret or apply such principles. Specific factual situations should be discussed with professional advisors. In addition, the observations, opinions and conclusions in this text are those of the authors and do not necessarily represent the views of the Center for Research in Ambulatory Health Care Administration or the Medical Group Management Association.

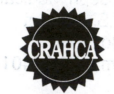

CENTER FOR RESEARCH
IN AMBULATORY
HEALTH CARE ADMINISTRATION

Center for Research in Ambulatory
Health Care Administration
104 Inverness Terrace East
Englewood, CO 80112-5306
(303) 799-1111
All rights reserved.

Library of Congress Catalog Card Number: 94-092370
ISBN: 1-56829-015-2

Printed in the United States of America

Dedication

To Stu and Rodney, true friends and colleagues on the journey, and Lynn, best friend and spouse: the three people who have never stopped believing in me regardless of the circumstances.

Thom's support has been particularly important.

We dedicate this book to our families, our friends and our colleagues and those working to improve healthcare quality and service. Without their support this work would not have been possible.

—Davis Balestracci, Jr.
and Jeanine Barlow

TABLE OF CONTENTS

ACKNOWLEDGEMENTS

The preparation of this book was truly a team effort. Experiences and insights from the organizations and individuals who participated in the demonstration site research were invaluable. Members of our advisory committee made numerous worthy contributions, from developing the coding project goals and measures to reviewing the entire manuscript. Other individuals helped by reacting to our ideas and research findings.

Foreword by James L. Reinertsen, MD

We greatly appreciate the considerate review of our publication by James L. Reinertsen, MD, Chief Executive Officer, HealthSystem Minnesota, Minneapolis. His comments in the "Foreword" provide an excellent introduction to our work by indicating its place in the dynamic, evolving world of healthcare quality improvement.

First Edition Review Team

CRAHCA/Medicode Total Quality Improvement Coding Project Demonstration Sites
We are indebted to the project teams and to the demonstration site leadership for their participation and whole-hearted support. The project demonstration sites were:

- Asheville Cardiology Associates, Asheville, North Carolina
- Northwestern Medical Faculty Foundation, Inc., Chicago, Illinois
- The Hitchcock Clinic, Keene Division (formerly Keene Clinic), Keene, New Hampshire

We thank these organizations for sharing their learning experiences with the MGMA membership and the health care community. They highlighted QI tools and principles that can be successfully applied in the dynamic environment in which we deliver health care.

Advisory Committee

The activities of this research project were guided by the Project Advisory Committee. The Committee provided excellent insight into the development of meaningful project goals and measures. Committee members were:

- *David J. Cooke, CPA, CMPE*, formerly Administrator/CEO, Keene Clinic, Keene, New Hampshire

- *Marilyn Haas, RN, PhD, AAN-C*, Director of Quality Improvement, Asheville Cardiology Associates, Asheville, North Carolina

- *Richard Nagengast*, Director, Professional Support Services, Northwestern Medical Faculty Foundation, Inc., Chicago, Illinois

- *Kevin Pearson*, Chief Financial Officer, Medicode, Salt Lake City, Utah

- *Margaret L. Stone, CMPE*, Vice President, Consulting Division, Cejka & Company, Norcross, Georgia

- *Tim Weddle*, Director, Decision Support Services, Loyola University Medical Center, Maywood, Illinois

- *Jeanine Barlow, MPH*, Research Project Manager, Center for Research in Ambulatory Health Care Administration, Englewood, Colorado

Numerous people at all levels at each site ensured that this project provided the desired learning experiences and contributions to the healthcare field. Medicode, led by Kevin Pearson, provided the financial resources for the QI research.

Reviewers

We would like to again thank our first-edition reviewers, who contributed thoughtful comments on the book's key concepts and structure:

- *Carleton T. Rider*, Continuous Improvement Officer, Mayo Foundation, Rochester, Minnesota

- *Sheryl D. Thies*, Vice President for Marketing, Dean Medical Center, Madison, Wisconsin

- *William Conway, MD*, Vice Chairman, Board of Governors, Henry Ford Medical Group, Detroit, Michigan, and *Louise Liang, MD*, Vice President of Clinical Operations and Chief Operating Officer, Straub Clinic and Hospital Inc., Honolulu, Hawaii

- *Carole V. Erickson*, Consultant, Healthcare Management, Marketing and Development, Missoula, Montana

- *Mary S. Mourar, MLS*, Librarian for MGMA's Library Resource Center

- *Victoria L. Melton*, former CRAHCA Research Associate and consultant, Zeneca Pharmaceuticals

Additional support was received from **Steven S. Lazarus, PhD; Anna Bergstrom, MSHA; Vivian Heggie** and **Joseph Burton.**

Second Edition Support

- *Stu Janis* provided essential, friendly technical and editorial support for both the first and second editions.

- *Cindy Kroeger* worked through many revisions to produce our final product.

- The authors would like to thank the following people, who supplied data for the chapter examples and exercises: American Group Practice Association; Christopher Bliersbach; Faith Broman, RN; Craig Davidson, MD; Joan Dearmin, RN; Carol Greenland; Debra Hanson; Robert Karasov, MD; Robert Knies, RN; Ardis Kunse; Elaine Massopust, RN; Joseph Mitlyng; Nancy Nelson; Sharon Reiter, RN; Laurie Ritz, RN; Steven Tarzynski, MD; Sara Taylor; Robert Welch, MD; David Wessner, Judith Wilson, RN. Their real data from everyday situations made this a better book.

   Davis Balestracci would also like to acknowledge Andrew Kirsch, who first suggested the idea for the Fundamentals of Variation. Also, a special thank you is due to Heero Hacquebord, whose 1988 seminar and subsequent interactions caused the big "AHA!" for Davis, and to the HealthSystem Minnesota employees, who create an atmosphere that makes one look forward to coming to work every day.

ABOUT THE AUTHORS

Davis Balestracci, MS is currently a Continuous Quality Improvement (CQI) Statistical Specialist for HealthSystem Minnesota, Minneapolis, Minnesota, which has adopted the management philosophy of W. Edwards Deming. He reports jointly to the Chief Operating Officer and medical director. Davis has a BS degree in chemical engineering and an MS degree in statistics.

In his fourteen-year career, Davis has developed a special interest in effective industrial statistical education and given talks and seminars on his unique approaches both at the local and national level. From 1985-1991, he worked for 3M during which time he won two corporate quality awards and two process technology awards for his innovative uses of statistical methods. Since 1989, his interests have evolved to adapting the manufacturing model for quality improvement to business management and service industries. He is a member of the American Statistical Association (ASA) and the American Society for Quality Control (ASQC), and was formerly president of the Twin Cities Deming Forum.

Davis has an avocation of classical music and has done graduate work in conducting. For relaxation, he plays the pipe organ and piano and studies symphonic scores (One never knows when the call will come!).

He is also an avid folk dancer and calls square dances and contradances in the Twin Cities. His favorite dancing partners are his wife, Lynn, and his three daughters, Julia, Andrea, and Susannah.

Jeanine Barlow, MPH is a Research Project Manager in the Center for Research in Ambulatory Health Care Administration (CRAHCA), research arm of MGMA. In that position, she has conducted two projects which applied quality improvement to medical group practice processes. She serves as a member of the Physician Profiling Project team, a multi-year grant from The Robert Wood Johnson Foundation. She is working to develop a comprehensive system to give practices comparative data about service cost-effectiveness and appropriateness.

Prior to coming to CRAHCA, Jeanine worked for seven years in a large Chicago-area network-model HMO, where she developed expertise in managed care contract negotiation, implementation, and system development. Previous experience in community education and geriatric social work have rounded out her healthcare experience.

She received a Master of Public Health degree with a Health Resource Management emphasis from the University of Illinois at Chicago in 1990. She is interested in making further contributions to the improvement of quality, access, and efficiency in the healthcare system. Her personal interests include hiking, skiing, music, and reading.

ABOUT THE PROJECT FUNDER

The research project featured in this text was funded by Medicode. Based in Salt Lake City, Medicode specializes in coding and reimbursement information systems for health care providers. It provides consulting support for system planning and implementation. Its clients include hospitals, medical group practices, HMOs, and other healthcare organizations nationwide.

ABOUT THE CENTER FOR RESEARCH IN AMBULATORY HEALTH CARE ADMINISTRATION AND THE MEDICAL GROUP MANAGEMENT ASSOCIATION

The Center for Research in Ambulatory Health Care Administration (CRAHCA) was founded in 1973 by the Medical Group Management Association (MGMA) to support the mission of MGMA/CRAHCA/ACMPE: "*advance the art and science of medical group practice management to improve the health of our communities*". The Center conducts its research and development projects through support from private foundations, corporate and government grants and self-funding. CRAHCA is a section 501(c)(3) tax-exempt charitable organization as defined by the IRS Code. CRAHCA activities are structured to benefit the general population as well as MGMA's membership. Its name reflects a broader mission to serve ambulatory care, including and beyond group practice.

CRAHCA focuses on development of:

- New management technologies and tools for effective and efficient administration of health care organizations;

- Databases, research, projects and surveys for research, information and education purposes;

- Publications, educational conferences, and other media covering issues for health care administrators and physician leaders; and

- Networks and avenues for collaboration with others in the health services research field.

With guidance from MGMA's Research Committee, CRAHCA is exploring new initiatives or expanding current activities to meet important needs in a number of research areas, including Financial and Clinical Performance Measures; Environmental Assessment of the Health Care Industry; Managed Care; Integration and Physician Profiling.

CRAHCA works closely with MGMA departments and the American College of Medical Practice Executives (ACMPE), both of which are located in MGMA's headquarters, Englewood, Colorado. The Library Resource Center, MGMA's comprehensive ambulatory care management library and information service, serves as a literature and information resource to CRAHCA. The MGMA Education and Conference departments provide consultation and assistance in educational programming and conference planning. Through MGMA's Government Relations department, CRAHCA has immediate access to information on pending legislation and regulation affecting group practice.

Founded in 1926, the Medical Group Management Association today is comprised of over 17,000 individual members and 6,300 medical groups representing over 144,000 physicians. It is the oldest and largest membership organization representing group practice administration. MGMA serves its individual and organizational members and their patients, and promotes the group practice of medicine as an effective form of health care delivery.

As an important contribution to the field of quality improvement, CRAHCA is pleased to publish the second edition of *Quality Improvement: Practical Applications For Medical Group Practice*. Through *Quality Improvement*, the reader is given a new perspective on the sets of conditions and skills critical to successful quality improvement implementation.

Funding for this edition was provided from the CRAHCA Research and Development Fund. These funds were utilized to support and provide additional resources to add to the value of this book.

FOREWORD

James L. Reinertsen, MD
Chief Executive Officer
HealthSystem Minnesota

For almost a decade, a growing number of health care organizations have been attempting to implement the management principles and methods articulated by Juran, Deming and others. There have been some successes. There have been a lot of enthusiastic starts which have bogged down. There have been organizations which have given up in disgust, saying, "This stuff may be okay for manufacturing, but it doesn't apply to us in health care." And there are many organizations which are simply sitting on the sidelines, waiting to see if it works for others.

Wherever your organization fits on this spectrum, this book will be very helpful to you for a number of reasons. First and foremost, the authors are not external observers of the health care scene. Balestracci, particularly, is personally immersed in the service/quality transformations of his own organization. They have experienced how difficult these changes are. They have seen first-hand the warts of flawed team process, inadequate data and measurement skills, and uncertain system support for improvement. And so they do not bring to you only the sanitized versions of their best projects. They have had the courage also to describe their failures. This book clearly demonstrates how much we can learn from these experiences.

Another reason for this book's value is its approach to data skills and statistical thinking. How many of your teams have failed to measure key process variables, or key quality characteristics of real meaning to customers? How many of your projects have floundered as the team waded through mounds of computer-generated data of uncertain relevance to the process and customers in question? After the team's work was done, how did you know that the process was really better? Stayed better? Did the team's data activities require a small army of quality staffers and programmers, or did the team plan, do, and analyze their own data? Did your team's measurement activities take on the characteristic of a major research trial, with large data sets available six to twelve months later, or was useful data about your processes available to your teams in hours, days, or weeks? If any of this sounds familiar, and you'd like to learn how to address these data problems, you should read this book.

This book is even valuable to those of you who have been sitting on the sidelines, waiting for this quality fad to pass, because the evidence is clear: whatever management method you are using now, it isn't working. Our purchasers, patients, and legislators aren't happy with our service, our costs, and our quality of outcomes. We need a new approach to the way we manage. We need a new way of thinking. If you want to make your group practice more successful and yourself a better administrator, you should learn and apply the principles and methods taught in this book.

Some parts of this book will be unsettling, particularly the chapter which deals with the statistical illiteracy which is embedded in our usual reporting formats. Finance staff, in particular, need to take a deep breath before reading the section on the havoc we wreak on truth and on management's ability to take intelligent action, when we create reports such as this month versus same month last year, this month versus budget, this month versus last month, and the rolling 12-month average.

This book does not deal in depth with the leadership issues involved in creating an organizational environment for quality and in managing change. The authors refer the reader to excellent texts on these important issues and touch on them repeatedly in their case examples. While the strength of the book lies in its extremely effective explanation of process-focused statistical thinking, this new set of skills is not enough to achieve sustained improvement. The major barriers to improvement in health care organizations are compartmental thinking, turf wars, and information policies, and compensation systems which punish innovation and reward optimization of one's own compartment at the expense of the whole system. Although we must certainly have process-oriented statistical thinking if we're going to improve, we must also depend on leadership to deal with these barriers to improvement if we are going to achieve the dramatic transformation seen in many other industries.

Balestracci and Barlow have made a major contribution to the literature on transformation of health care organizations. Combining their book with the texts cited in their introduction will provide a powerful core library for continuous improvement learning.

Minneapolis, August 15, 1996

Chapter One
Introductory Ideas

> *If I had to reduce my message for management to just a few words, I'd say that it all had to do with reducing variation.*
> —*W. Edwards Deming*

Such a simple statement, yet the implications are profound and revolutionary. In it lies the key to quality improvement (QI).

Has your organization already tried initiatives in the name of rightsizing, productivity enhancement, or just plain old-fashioned cost-cutting? Did anything really change, except perhaps making the organization more cynical? Is it any surprise that, despite management's best intentions, the common reaction to QI is, "Here comes another one!" QI is not simply reading a couple of books, going to some seminars, and putting a plan down on paper. One could observe, "A plan and $1 will get you a cup of coffee." What was missing from these earlier initiatives that is needed to succeed?

This book is about a new approach to management. Our message is: *the only way to significantly improve your organization is to reduce process variation through the application of statistical thinking.*

The fundamental ideas behind **statistical thinking** are:

- **All work is a series of interconnected, measurable processes.**

- **All processes exhibit variation, which impairs their predictability.**

- **Improvements are made through the understanding and reduction of inappropriate and unintended variation.**

This approach is markedly different from what is traditionally taught in statistics courses. They generally focus on statistical methods and techniques without the process perspective necessary for QI. The new approach is not intended to make people statisticians. Neither does it aim to develop Deming quality disciples.

Deming, Juran, and others have shown statistics to be invaluable to quality improvement, yet many people believe that its manufacturing roots limit its applicability to service environments like health care. Others want

to treat statistics as a panacea and expect massive training in statistical methods to cure all their quality woes. Especially in a service environment such as medicine, people do not need statistics—they need to solve problems.

Another common misconception holds that QI is achieved simply through the development of project teams, followed by results that hit the "bottom line." While this approach is not inherently wrong, there is a complicating factor: your organization's people are already doing jobs they perceive to take more than 100 percent of their time. Where are people supposed to find time for these projects?

Projects, teams, and training in statistical tools are necessary but not sufficient for lasting, significant improvement. Statistical methods and tools are just facets of a complex, synergistic quality improvement process completely framed by the broader concepts of statistical thinking. Ultimately, improvement does not exist in addition to one's everyday job; it must *become* everyone's job.

The Role of Data

True understanding of a process requires data, and using data through a scientific approach is an essential element of quality improvement. Data can provide an objective view of a situation, removing destructive emotions that sometimes lead to inappropriate actions.

True understanding of variation and the use of data requires both knowledge and a change in perspective. The transformation from a crisis-driven to a data-driven organization can be inhibited by initial perceptions of statistical thinking as contrary to "common sense." The proper response to data may not agree with first instincts.

This book will demonstrate that data skills can act as a conduit for the transformation process. Statistical thinking involves simple skills that can be applied immediately by anyone to create an atmosphere of continuous improvement. This allows people to:

1) view **variation** from a different, expanded perspective

2) use a **process-oriented** approach to define and analyze improvement opportunities

3) routinely use a variety of **charts to display and analyze data**

4) observe and interpret variation without **tampering** (taking inappropriate action)

5) ask better question to get to deeper improvements

6) understand that the goal is not just improvement but **transformation** of the organization

7) understand that the **psychology of change** is not trivial, and requires time

Whether they realize it or not, people make decisions in their jobs every day by reacting to observed variation in data. Whether the data are numerical, perceptual, or anecdotal, these decisions are in essence predictions. Actions based on these predictions have consequences. Any decision implicitly carries the risk of:

1) acting on a perceived difference when none really exists, or

2) failing to detect a real change and consequently taking no action

Statistical knowledge and skills are needed to minimize these errors. However, the appropriate knowledge is not part of a typical education, even if it includes statistics courses. As a result, most people have very minimal statistical skills and experience a lack of comfort with numbers. Since the success of QI depends on the appropriate organization-wide development of these skills, a commitment to the integration of proper data skills into all aspects of an organization's culture will accelerate and improve the improvement process.

Other Quality Resources

Books about quality have become quite prolific in the last few years, especially in health care. There are a lot of good materials out there and we do not wish to reinvent the wheel. We believe that this book provides a healthcare-specific introduction to QI, with a strong emphasis on the concept of variation.

We recognize that no single book can do it all. If we succeed in sparking your interest to learn more, you may wish to include the following books in your library. These books have been found to be virtually indispensable by people continuing their quality journeys. We unabashedly, unashamedly, and effusively recommend them:

The Deming Dimension by Henry Neave

Regardless of your opinion of Deming, this is by far the most complete perspective available describing improvement through organizational transformation. Whether you agree with Neave's theory or not, you cannot help but re-examine your own philosophy and extract key ideas to integrate into your organization's improvement process.

Understanding Variation by Donald Wheeler

Probably the most understandable book written on the practical use of statistics. It is written for managers and all examples are taken from managerial data. Each example is thoroughly discussed in a statistical thinking framework which does not bog down in the minutiae of techniques. Wheeler shows how to understand, analyze, interpret, and discuss common data situations for future action based on sound statistical theory.

Firing On All Cylinders by Jim Clemmer

This is the most comprehensive book on service quality available. It goes beyond theory and gives a practical framework which you must then adapt to your unique organization. It is not a cookbook. It is not healthcare-specific nor does it deal with statistics.

To fully understand Clemmer's ideas and motivation you should have a good grasp of quality improvement theory before reading this book. Be forewarned: the message is that if you are not prepared to implement the process as he states, you may as well do nothing, because other implementations will actually do more damage. (Good food for thought!)

The TEAM Handbook by Peter Scholtes

This is the essential book on teams and all cultural aspects of project-oriented improvement. Extremely practical, thorough, and well thought-out.

Fourth Generation Management: The New Business Consciousness, by Brian Joiner

One of the best books currently available to demonstrate how quality as a management philosophy can be integrated into *all aspects* of daily work. It is geared more toward the "traditional" American corporation, yet the case studies are eye-opening for those based in health care as well. There is a good balance of tools and philosophy. It is used as a core text for the course outlined in Appendix A.

Hidden Dynamics, by Faith Ralston

An outstanding recent find that treats *all* aspects of human emotion in a working environment. It gives actual techniques to address issues, e.g., "hidden agendas," and has well thought-out exercises for honest assessment of individuals and work teams. Three excellent chapters deal with change, "corporate craziness," and the manager's new role as leader/coach/facilitator.

Deming, Juran, and Others

Some of you may ask, "Deming and Juran who?" Deming and Juran provide the two predominant quality philosophies followed by most organizations that implement the QI model. The late Dr. W. Edwards Deming was an American statistician who became an internationally known consultant. He originally established modern sampling methods for the U.S. Census, and served as an advisor to the Japanese census in post-World War II Japan.

During that time, he also took part in the education of Japanese scientists and engineers on methods of quality control. While unsuccessful with similar quality training efforts in post-war America, he found a very willing audience in Japan. Japan's subsequent quality improvement successes are well-known.

Transformation is fundamental to Deming's approach. It applies to management practices as well as the structure of management and work processes. Their alignment is crucial and must be accomplished via a well-understood, broadly-communicated strategy. Deming's ideas are grounded on a theory relying on the synergistic interaction of four elements:

- Appreciation of a system,

- Psychology of intrinsic motivation,

- Understanding of variation, and

- Use of planned data collection to test improvement theories.

Another American, Dr. Joseph Juran, also took part in post-war Japanese industrial education. Juran was an electrical engineer who also obtained a law degree and established an internationally known quality consulting corporation—The Juran Institute. Juran's approach is heavily based in projects, planning, tools, and implementation that minimize disruption to current structures.

In deference to an organization's existing management structure, the Juran approach adds additional structure and a relatively formal approach to identifying, solving, and implementing improvement efforts. It is an empirically-derived strategy developed from judicious, keen observation of work cultures for over 50 years.

Based in Wilton, Connecticut, the Juran Institute is an excellent source of quality improvement materials. Juran's philosophy provides enormous help in understanding the human psychology of a work environment. Juran always reminds those having difficulty with implementing "textbook QI" to ask, "Yes, it didn't work; but did you think about...?" The Institute has especially good materials explaining the tools of quality improvement. They are also the major source for information addressing the resistance to change that naturally occurs during any individual or organizational change process.

The Institute for Healthcare Improvement (IHI) in Brookline, Massachusetts, provides excellent educational and networking opportunities. Formerly known as the National Demonstration Project in Healthcare Improvement, IHI is led by Donald M. Berwick, M.D. Dr. Berwick, a practicing pediatrician, is an internationally known speaker and writer on QI in health care. He is widely cited in our text. Numerous other leaders and texts are also cited in our work. These are fully listed in the bibliography.

Your Journey Continues

The authors of this book have combined their own QI experiences with those of their work environments as well as the experiences of the demonstration sites participating in CRAHCA research. The truths found in those experiences have practical applications regardless of practice size or specialty.

Quality improvement is extremely hard work. We hope to minimize the growing pains you are about to experience. We wish we could give you THE recipe, but you will have to educate yourself and join us in the kitchen so we can learn from each other. While we don't have all the answers, this book provides a framework for some of the major questions each organization must answer. It is an unending journey.

Welcome...

Quality in Medical Group Practice

Quality can be an elusive goal. The traditional approach to healthcare service quality has perhaps focused more on activities required to satisfy regulators and identify outliers than on continuous efforts to meet customer needs. But now, faced with increasingly sophisticated consumers making renewed demands for quality, medical groups and other providers are seeking effective ways to serve and retain patients within the realities of resource constraints.

Much has been written about defining, measuring, and evaluating quality in health care delivery. A variety of philosophies and approaches greets the manager who asks, "How can our practice improve quality?" Further complicating the issue are questions such as, "Can we afford a quality improvement program?" and "Will the physicians and other clinical staff accept further demands on their time and decision-making power?"

Leaders from all parts of the health care spectrum have come to believe that an efficient system resulting in demonstrable quality constitutes the key to continued provider survival. Private and publicly-funded projects are providing productive responses to these questions.

Entities such as the Institute for Healthcare Improvement have further developed the QI approach in the healthcare setting. However, most projects have focused on hospital settings. Much remains to be learned about translating earlier QI principles to medical group practice.

A growing number of medical group practice providers have adopted the QI approach as a model for significant administrative and clinical improvements. Numerous MGMA member groups continue to implement their own programs focusing on a wide variety of practice management concerns.

Several management models contain elements of quantitative quality measurements or of team decision-making. These include concepts like:

- quality control (quality by inspection)

- quality assurance (quality by preventing recurrence of outliers found by inspection)

- quality circles (quality by forming teams closest to the work), and

- motivation and awareness (zero defects; quality is free)

These approaches rely heavily on either the objectives or the people, without a system for incorporating true synergy between the two. The strength of the QI model developed by Deming, Juran, and others lies in its focus on three key concepts:

- customer needs must be met

- most inefficiencies are the result of measurable variations in a process, and

- a team approach is often the most effective means of identifying process problems and improving the process to meet customer needs

QI combines quantitative quality measurements and team efforts in an ongoing, systematically monitored process. As interdisciplinary practice staff seek to coordinate the complex clinical and administrative processes involved in patient service, QI becomes a logical model for improving medical group practice.

In addition to organizing improvement and ensuring that it lasts beyond initial implementation, QI involves people from all disciplines relevant to a process. Processes extend across departmental and traditional lines and the people needed to improve them will cross departmental lines as well. Key to this cross-functional effort is the support of both upper management and clinical leaders. While QI can improve specific areas without a guiding vision and proactive leaders, a reworked and transformed organization cannot occur without them.

The CRAHCA/Medicode Quality Improvement Coding Project

In 1991, MGMA/CRAHCA and project grantor Medicode selected the coding process as an excellent testing ground for the application of QI in group practice. Translation of services provided to patients into a variety of coding systems is a major activity in any practice, involving both clinical and non-clinical staff in a complex series of checks and balances.

MGMA/CRAHCA and Medicode believed coding must be managed as an integrated process, rather than simply a function within an organization. In the short-term, effective coding achieves greater regulatory compliance and maximizes reimbursement. In the long-term, it can be used to aid in competitive positioning for the practice's future because of its relation to measurable quality outcomes, standardized clinical protocols, and reduced costs. Effective, efficient processes result in streamlined practices able to respond swiftly and appropriately to the rapid pace of healthcare change.

Project Design, Development and Methods

Work soon began to address the two main project objectives:

- identify and evaluate issues which drive coding accuracy and compliance across a spectrum of practice management environments

- develop a specific QI approach as well as tools and guidelines for effective management of coding, for reimbursement and other key practice needs.

To identify the three demonstration sites, MGMA member practices interested in participation were evaluated on a number of variables, including:

- Practice size, based on number of full-time equivalent (FTE) physicians serving the group. Demonstration sites were sought to represent small, mid-sized, and large group settings.

- Practice setting. Demonstration sites were sought which reflected academic, single specialty, and community-based multispecialty group settings.

- Familiarity with QI concepts. It was felt that one site should have significant QI experience so it could serve as a leader for the other sites. The other two sites were required to have some degree of familiarity with QI concepts, but were not required to have previously implemented any QI projects.

- Geographic location. A mix of urban and rural locations was desired, as well as different regions of the country.

The following three demonstration sites were selected:

- The Keene Clinic (now the Hitchcock Clinic, Keene Division). Located in Keene, New Hampshire, this multispecialty group currently employs 50 FTE physicians

- Asheville Cardiology Associates, P.A. of Asheville, North Carolina, a single specialty group currently employing 16 FTE physicians

- Northwestern Medical Faculty Foundation, Inc., Chicago, Illinois, a 400+ FTE physician academic practice.

Following site selection, the Project Advisory Committee (PAC) was formed. The PAC included representatives from each of the demonstration sites, Medicode, and CRAHCA, as well as from the MGMA/CRAHCA Research Committee and other outside experts. (Please see the *Acknowledgments* chapter for a complete list of the PAC members.)

The PAC's mission was to guide and provide feedback to the demonstration sites. Topics addressed by the PAC ranged from the development of goals and measurement tools to "troubleshooting" of QI implementation issues as they arose.

The project flowchart (Figure 1.1) illustrates the study's structure. At the left appears the main project goal as developed by the PAC:

To achieve compliance with the coding requirements of the practice's internal and external publics, by accurately coding services provided.

This goal reflects QI's customer focus orientation as well as the committee's intent to consider the scope of coding activities beyond reimbursement.

Figure 1.1: CRAHCA/Medicode QI Coding Project Flowchart

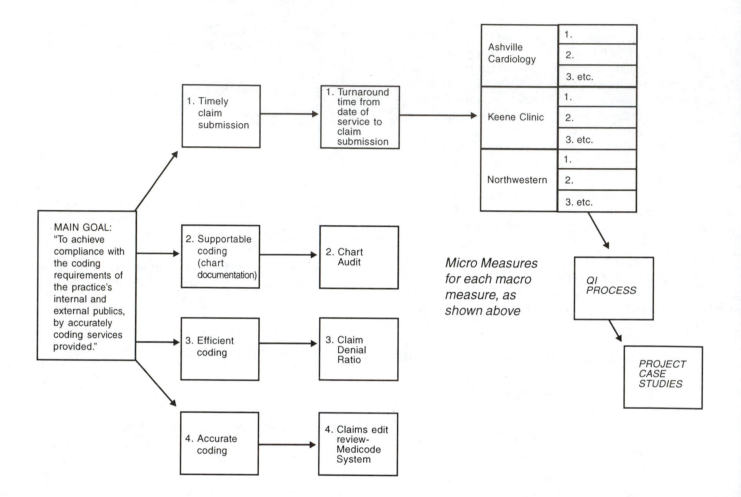

Project Macro Measures

The PAC recognized early on that to be valid, the project must measure global issues across sites. Measures applicable to all sites were determined, including operational definitions. The measures were:

- *Timely* claim submission, as measured by turnaround time from date of service to claims submission

- *Supportable* coding, as evidenced by information supporting the chosen coding (e.g., information in the medical record, invoices, etc.)

- *Efficient* coding, as shown by the ratio of claims denied to claims submitted

- *Accurate* coding, as measured using the Medicode Claims Manager System and other tools

Medicode's Claims Manager system provided proactive review of coding based on standardized coding rules as promulgated by Medicare and other payors.

These **macro goals** were measured by all three sites.

Micro measures grew from the macro goals and measures. They reflect those issues unique to each practice setting. As each site learned more about its unique processes, barriers, and strengths, the micro measures became the detailed level of study conducted to address their own process variations and nuances.

Sample sizes varied among the sites, but were consistent within each site from baseline to final measurements.

QI experience levels varied among the sites, with Keene having had the most experience with improvement teams. Asheville had some formal training and structure in place but no project experience, while Northwestern was in the very early stages of learning about QI.

Full descriptions and evaluations of the site experiences are found in Chapters 11 and 12.

Chapter Two
Introduction to Quality Improvement

Key Ideas

*   Quality improvement can be thought of as a progression from Symptom to Cause to Remedy. The first stage, "Symptom to Cause," is the Diagnostic Journey. The second stage, from "Cause to Remedy," is the Remedial Journey.

*   Quality assurance (QA) traditionally collects data to identify perceived individual negative variation and to correct outliers.

*   QI collects data to expose process variation, discuss it, and reduce that which is unintended and inappropriate.

*   All work is a process. Waste as well as improvement opportunities occur when current work processes break down or a consistent work process does not exist.

*   Successful change and QI require a customer orientation; modeling of QI skills and behavior at all staff levels; and reduction of inappropriate variation.

*   Both clinical and administrative people must be meaningfully involved from the beginning for an improvement project to be successful. False distinctions between clinical and administrative projects can create confusion and waste.

Introduction

No one is against quality. Yet the word "quality" can bring to mind negative associations from experiences with monitoring programs like QA and compliance audits, motivation programs, or managed care standards. When these perceptions of quality are considered in conjunction with statistics, another word often associated with negative academic experiences, it is not surprising that the current emphasis on QI is perceived as a passing fad—"Here we go again! What's so different? Isn't this all common sense, just everyone doing his or her best and doing work right the first time?"

Let us just say that if quality were just common sense we'd already be doing it. (Deming was fond of saying that common sense is our ruination!)

With QI, **a mission**—a business and social purpose for the work unit—is established. From the point at which the practice's mission is established, the QI measurement, feedback, analysis, and process reengineering cycle is used. This cycle is often referred to as the **P**lan-**D**o-**C**heck-**A**ct cycle It is also sometimes referred to as the Shewhart cycle or the Deming cycle. Later in his career, Deming began calling it the Plan-Do-Study-Act cycle.

Some Wisdom From Juran

Juran's writings demonstrate the wisdom of someone who has "been around the block." He considers the approach to improvement to be two separate journeys: a **Diagnostic Journey** from symptom to cause, followed by a **Remedial Journey** from cause to remedy (See Figure 2.1).

Figure 2.1
Diagnostic and Remedial Journeys

Symptom ————>Cause ————>Remedy
Diagnostic   **Remedial**
Journey   **Journey**

In the diagnostic journey, improvement efforts result when we react to variation, i.e., a result different than what we expect. Variation indicates an underlying problem or opportunity. To find root problem causes, the diagnostic journey requires asking many different questions to understand the variation. A team formed of diverse staff with varying experiences and skills is necessary.

Data collection within the context of the diagnostic journey (to be discussed in Chapter 6) is required to identify the significant improvement opportunities within the observed process. This requires theories about the root causes, study of work-in-progress, analysis, and resulting action. The diagnostic journey includes a lot of uncertainty and depends largely on technical expertise about the process to identify a root problem cause. Next, a potentially viable solution is developed. This solution is usually tested and evaluated on a pilot scale. If deemed unfeasible, the solution is discarded or revised and the QI process begins again. Figure 2.2 outlines the journey.

Figure 2.2: Diagnostic Journey—A Breakthrough in Knowledge

- **Choose a problem**

- **Understand the process**

- **Fix obvious problems I**

- **Establish stability/baselines**

- **Fix obvious problems II**

- **Generate theories for causation**

- **Localize a major opportunity**

- **Identify proposed solution**

- **Pilot and evaluate proposed solution**

After obtaining a viable solution, the remedial journey begins. There aren't as many technical unknowns and questions in this journey as in the diagnostic journey. The solution is now known and the appropriate areas can be targeted for change. The remedial journey's focus is more specific.

The issues surrounding the remedial journey involve more psychology than technology. The new solution must overcome people's natural resistance to change. Once the change is made, the QI process requires standardization of the new work process and proof that the theorized gains are made and held. Figure 2.3 outlines the remedial journey.

The diagnostic and remedial journeys are different in purpose, skills, and people involved. Juran deems their sequence a universal, natural progression for proper quality improvement.

Figure 2.3: Remedial Journey—A Breakthrough in Behavior

- **Overcome resistance to change**
- **Standardization**
- **Hold gains**

It is useful to look at process improvement as this natural progression for two reasons. First, there can be a tendency to jump from "symptom" directly to "remedy". This could add complexity to a process if the

remedy does not address the true root causes. Second, most project teams underestimate, if not totally ignore, the implications of the remedial journey. Planning the remedial journey is not trivial, but often minimal consideration is given to its key aspects. A solution's impact on the work culture should always be evaluated *prior* to its implementation. Data from a well-designed pilot is a start for providing objective proof, but does not necessarily address the sometimes mysterious reasons for resistance. Resistance to change is covered thoroughly in Chapter 5.

QA vs. QI

How do QA and QI fit into the concepts of the diagnostic and remedial journeys? Quality measurement and improvement have been part of practice activities for years through QA departments, peer review, etc. While both QA and QI follow diagnostic and remedial journeys, they differ in their approaches. The difference lies in the contexts in which they operate.

The key distinction between QI and QA is process-oriented thinking versus results-oriented thinking. Typically, QA is a peer review process that concentrates solely on observed outcomes and uses traditional statistical analysis of these results to identify alleged non-conforming outliers. QA's goal is to *maintain* a current standard of medical performance by sorting so-called "bad" performers from "good." In this context, improvement takes place by revising individual performances to meet the standards set by external organizations.

QI takes a more fundamental approach:

Health care is a **process** which leads to an output.

QI acknowledges that results vary, but considers variation to be the result of process breakdowns or unwitting lack of knowledge rather than outright failures by individuals. Attributing blame or sorting out poor performers is not the focus. QI looks closely at data from the processes to identify significant sources of variation and *prevent* similar occurrences. Improvement comes not only from outside research approved by external organizations. It comes from finding hidden **improvement opportunities** (i.e., "positive" variation) in current work processes, and from the development of robust practices.

Figure 2.4 uses traditional statistical normal (or bell-shaped) curves to illustrate the contrast between QA and QI. The area under the curves represents the

2

range of results. The QA "Before" curve shows a distribution of results obtained, both good and bad. A predetermined number, commonly one to five percent, are identified as "significant outliers." Attention is focused on the outliers, and those seen as responsible are told to correct the outlying behavior — not so simple, especially where human psychology is involved.

As shown in the "After" curve, the action attempts to chop off the left end of the distribution. At best, this leads to only a small increase in overall average quality. This seemingly arbitrary selection and judgment is usually not based in sound statistical theory. While such analyses are well-intended, many are in essence lotteries; this will be clarified in the remainder of the book. This tends to lead to a climate of defensiveness and lack of cooperation, particularly among physicians. In traditional QA, the potential of the high achievers to influence the other processes is not recognized and therefore lost.

Figure 2.4: Quality Assurance vs. Quality Improvement: Traditional Statistical Normal Curves

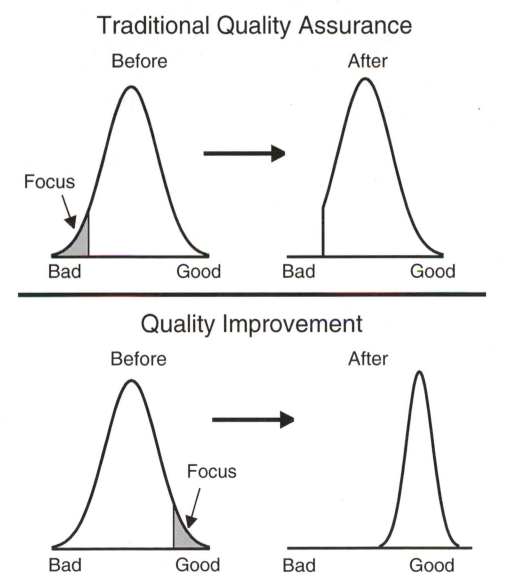

Traditional QA focuses on removing the poor performers, while QI focuses on the top performers to improve the work of all employees.

In QI, the focus shifts from the "negative" end of performance to the other, "positive performance" end of the curve. QI identifies the one to five percent of people who consistently achieve superior results, including those who do not realize they are doing so! This identification is often referred to as **best practices** or **benchmarking**. Thus, QI's shift in focus can identify practices from which *all* can learn and benefit, resulting in not only higher, but also more consistent quality.

What about those who truly may be poor performers? These persons are still identifiable with QI. They sort themselves out if and when they do not cooperate in the improvement implementation.

QA certainly has a role in QI[1]. Its energies are redirected to a positive application rather than the outlier or "bad apple" mentality. QA's purpose changes to one of expanding and providing the underlying measurement system used to monitor process performance. Data from the QA system currently used to rank people or departments can be used either to make immediate adjustments to the process or identify QI opportunities.

The role of statistics also changes between the two contexts. In QI, statistical thinking becomes more important than statistical tools. Instead of being a set of tools for analyzing results, statistical thinking becomes an umbrella to encompass the entire improvement process.

In summary, there are two quality dimensions in healthcare. The first is the quality of the healthcare outcomes themselves (the traditional focus of QA). However, QI adds a second aspect: the study of process quality. Processes must work together as a system to deliver care. QI results are measured in terms of customer needs and experiences. Examples of customer needs include diagnosis, access, and treatment as well as operational and financial services like medical record transportation, dictation, and patient billing. Figure 2.5 is a comparison of the two facets.

Figure 2.5: Comparison of Peer Review (Quality Assurance) and Quality Improvement[2]

Characteristic	Peer Review (Quality Assurance)	Quality Improvement
Object of Study	Physicians	Processes
Types of flaws studied	Special	Common and special
Goal	Control	Breakthrough
Performance referent	Standard	Capability/need
Source of knowledge	Peers	All
Review method	Summative (Enumerative)	Analytic
Functions involved	Few	Many
Amount of activity	Some	Lots
Linkage of design, operations, and business plan	Loose	Tight
Tampering	Common	Rare

Significant improvement opportunities arise because *quality fails when any one of these processes fails, even in the case of excellent outcomes*. For example, a practice's excellent clinical results can be negated by poor processes that cause significant delays, unnecessary visits, or poor communication that causes unnecessary duplication. When examined in this context, traditional healthcare delivery and healthcare management can be seen as two virtually parallel processes whose independence has created much waste and inefficiency.

The core business of medical practice is to deliver health care to customers and to meet obligations to insurance payors and the overall community. The entire system must be studied and optimized as a whole instead of separating healthcare delivery and healthcare management. This separation unknowingly optimizes separate processes to meet separate specific goals while the organization suffers.

A primary benefit of using QI is the potential for discovering waste in a process. Variation creates waste, such as work done more than once with no value added or a process involving more steps or staff than are required to meet customer needs. By focusing on the whole spectrum of variation rather than simply the negative end, inefficiencies can be found in processes throughout the system. Waste reduction, of course, equals improved resource allocation, with time, energy, and money used more appropriately.

All Work is a Process

All clinicians and their patients are involved in processes, from local ones in private offices to the mammoth processes of national health care. Many of us have been victims of a lost test result, misinterpreted order, cumbersome paperwork, or an unreliable on-call system. However, some clinicians do not recognize the key role that they play in improving the processes (patient scheduling, patient instruction, or claims management) that lie behind these errors.

Both clinicians and those with more administrative roles should consider five questions posed by Berwick[3]:

1) Do you ever waste time waiting, when you should not have to?

2) Do you ever redo your work because something failed the first time?

3) Do the procedures you use waste steps, duplicate efforts, or frustrate you through their unpredictability?

4) Is information that you need ever lost?

5) Does communication ever fail?

Think of how each question affects a patient's perception of quality. How about payors' perceptions when such events are related to them? Can financial losses caused by these events ever truly be quantified? What about employee turnover and loss of morale?

Why do these things happen and keep happening? They represent breakdowns in current work processes or they occur due to lack of a consistent work process. *These breakdowns are generally not the fault of the people doing their jobs, but of the processes themselves.* Assigning blame and responsibility to the individual perceived to be "at fault" will not fix the problems. The work environmental odds are against them 85 to 15, as established empirically by Deming and Juran.

The **85/15 rule** states that individuals have direct control over only approximately 15 percent of their work problems. The other 85 percent are controlled by the processes in their working environment. Only their management can change these processes. In fact, by the end of his life, Deming had come to the conclusion that the workers themselves can directly control only 3 to 6 percent of their work environment, so the odds against the workers could be as high as 97 to 3! Thus, the problems alluded to by Berwick will not go away unless the processes in which the people operate are improved. Please note that the 85/15 rule is a completely different concept than the 80/20 phenomenon also known as the Pareto Principle (see Chapter 6).

What Does QI Take?

A look at quality in this broader context reveals QI as a potentially powerful strategic weapon that begs for strong executive response and involvement. When managers and leaders begin their organizations' QI work, they can be confused by the many quality theories which have evolved. Where should one start?

While there is no single right way, a surprisingly cohesive set of principles has evolved[4]:

*   Customer-first orientation

*   Top management leadership of the quality improvement process

*   Continuous improvement as a way of everyone's work life

*   Respect for employees and their knowledge, resulting in their active involvement in the improvement process

*   Reduction of product (e.g., outcomes) and process variation

*   Provision of ongoing education and training of employees

*   Familiarity with a statistical way of thinking and the use of statistical methods throughout the organization

- Emphasis on prevention rather than detection
- View of vendors as long-term partners
- Performance measures that are consistent with the goals of the organization
- Standardization: the development and adherence to the best known ways to perform a given task
- Emphasis on product and service quality in design
- Cooperation and involvement of all functions within an organization

- Awareness of the needs of internal customers
- Substantial culture change

The concept of quality improvement inherently makes common sense, but if it were only common sense there would be no need for this book. It is the implementation of QI and the associated transformation that require more. Figure 2.6 presents a conceptual model showing four major steps in this long-term transition.

Figure 2.6: Conceptual Model Showing Major Steps to World-Class Status[5]

Top management awareness and education	Building a critical mass	Achieving total quality	World-class quality/ world-class competitor

• Understand needs and benefits
• Learn and apply:
  • Quality improvement processes
  • Problem-solving tools
  • Statistical thinking
• Develop vision, change strategy, plans
• Form steering committee
	• 25-50% of management committed to quality
	• Pilot projects (limited scope)
	• Education in quality concepts/philosophy (20-30% of organization)
	• Training in basic tools (10-20% of organization)
	• Facilitation training (employee involvement, team process)
	• Education in advanced tools (1-2% of organization)
		• All employees in all departments introduced to basic tools/philosophy of total quality (TQ)
		• Organization-wide commitment
		• Many cross-functional improvement efforts
		• Suppliers heavily involved
		• QI promotion organization/upper management audits
		• Ways of life
		  • Customer orientation
		  • Continuous improvement
		  • Elimination of waste
		  • Prevention, not detection
		  • Reduction of variation
		  • Statistical thinking/ use of data
		  • Adherence to best known methods
		  • Respect for people and their knowledge
		  • Use of best available tools
			• Design quality dominates efforts
			• Reorganization around key products/services, markets
			• Process institutionalized and self-sustaining
			• Totally consistent management practices
			• 50% + trained in advanced tools

Many question the time required for full transformation of an organization to statistical thinking. Deming has said that a good company will take five years to reach full transformation and that most will take ten.

Why so long? Everyone knows that things need to change or improve. Why can't we set some goals, give everybody training, and start benefiting *now*?

Everyone needs to change and, in their hearts, most want to change. However, an organization must remain in business, and though current methods may not be perfect, the organization knows only one way to stay in business: the current way. Change requires a lot of resources, but if all of its resources —time, staff, capital—are consumed by operating with the current methods, where do people find time to improve?

Joiner Associates[6] defines the following laws of organizational change:

1) Things are the way they are because they got that way.

2) Unless things change, they will likely remain the same.

3) Change would be easy if it weren't for all the people.

4) People don't resist change, they just resist being changed.

The psychological manifestations inherent with change are not trivial. The QI process must be prepared to deal with change. In addition to overall cultural change, the incremental changes tied to various projects have their own psychology. People *are* the organization. Mysterious resistance is often encountered even when implementing a change that is obviously beneficial to a specific area.

In spite of the fact that many opportunities for improvement lie behind daily frustrations, people find a strange comfort in the predictability of a daily work situation. Any change is a potential threat to this predictability and, possibly, to people's jobs. Without proper communication, those who perceive themselves as losing will find a way to win. They may even sabotage quality improvement efforts in their attempts to win.

Dealing with change can be frustrating. Even Juran[7], with his excellent framework for dealing with the phenomenon of natural resistance, allows a last rule:

"When all else fails, forget it!" We can't always solve all resistance. Strategies for overcoming resistance to change will be discussed in Chapter 5.

Does this mean there is little value in the five-to-ten-year transition required for complete QI transformation? Not at all. It is an investment in the future. QI can provide results with a project-level approach but, especially in the first three years, major, instant, bottom-line results cannot be expected. There is no such thing as "improvement in general."

Again, the inertia of operating the business at the current level cannot be overestimated. Change is very difficult, with its own majestic, deliberate pace that cannot be hurried. However, just because the journey is long does not mean it should not begin. Developing project team members' enthusiasm for statistical thinking and the team process approach is an important step on the learning curve to full transformation. While complete change does take time, awareness of the data-driven QI approach will provide increasing value, and people will gain experience with statistical thinking and tools as they develop, analyze, revise, implement, and evaluate various improvements.

The CRAHCA research demonstration sites approached QI with a less-than-full transformation. As is common in many organizations, managers were more willing to devote time and energy to QI projects on a pilot level than to lead full QI rollout and training throughout the organization. The project approach did provide some positive financial, morale, communication, and process efficiency results for the groups.

However, the research results support the theory that significant improvement throughout the organization requires ongoing involvement from the leadership throughout all levels. Further discussion of the impact of this is found in Chapters 11 and 12. The significance of improvements is largely related to the use and scope of QI throughout the practice.

Lessons Learned

Transformation to a QI framework is at best an awkward adolescence. Many organizations have made many mistakes along the way, and you should expect to make some too. The coding project case studies illustrate many of the bumps and realities in the transformation. The following discussion is intended to caution readers about the traps awaiting them. None of the mistakes or traps are inherently bad. The problems occur when the organization attempts to implement part of the QI philosophy without embracing the entire concept of transformation.

It is much easier to begin than to keep going. Experience shows that the initial enthusiasm, which can almost border on the intoxicating, is often followed by a nasty hangover. The initial flurry of training and team creation generates a lot of heat, but probably not much light, and improvements do not necessarily last long after project completion.

In a typical first attempt at implementation, the initial outburst of enthusiasm can lead management to create projects with scopes that are too wide, in essence, designed "to solve world hunger." People's jobs already take up 100% of their time. Now, in addition to performing their daily job responsibilities, staff are trying to improve their work processes using new concepts and tools that have been poured into their heads, generally in a stimulus-response "short course" format. People are out of their normal comfort zones. And these are good people doing their best and trying to do it right the first time. Training issues are not trivial, and are discussed further in Chapter 10.

Appointment of a "QI coordinator," usually someone who seems to like this quality "stuff" and may have had a course or two in college or a past job, also does not guarantee success. This appointment should not be made lightly. Without management's commitment to QI, this only means a new arm, known as "quality," has now crept into the organization. Everyone proudly points to this unit and defers to it at the earliest opportunity—"That's quality's job."

Unfortunately, "quality's" prime directive often becomes developing the aforementioned short courses. People take them and count them like notches on a belt. At any time, one can report how many people have been through how many courses and what percent of people have participated on a team. Yet, "the big payoff" does not seem to appear.

For QI to succeed, everyone must use at least basic QI skills in their jobs. However, best intentions and training do not necessarily translate to expected behaviors, especially with adult learners. Quality is more than just training, teams, and projects. These are necessary, but not sufficient. The QI coordination function is necessary, but its role must be one of directing a transformation of organizational behavior. This will be addressed in the "QI vs. Transformation" table in Chapter 9.

In spite of the 85/15 rule the front-line workers are often the ones mandated to take in-depth training while management gets enough abbreviated training to "know what's going on." While hiring the best people and putting them through quality training may be a good policy, even the best people are up against 85 to 15 odds—at best, they have direct control over only 15 percent of their work problems. The 15 percent certainly need attention, but generally do not address issues vital to business survival. Instead, they should fall into a more focused category known as "task teams," which will be discussed in Chapters 6 and 9.

The 85/15 rule is also manifested when employees are trained and subsequently "empowered" to choose a project. Unfortunately, the problems chosen and presented directly to managers usually tend to be "obvious," related to the 15 percent, and do not represent "deep fixes" (see Chapter 3). *The important problems are the opportunities that no one is aware of.* In essence, management has charged 85 percent of the work force to provide less than optimal solutions for 15 percent of available improvement opportunities. Is this a sensible deployment of resources?

Another common initial error is to initiate projects that are really just implementations of "known" solutions to long-standing, vague problems. Joiner warns, "vague solutions to vague problems yield vague results." Unless a solution directly addresses a root cause and can be backed by data, chances are that these solutions will only add yet another layer of complexity (with no added value) to already frustrating situations. Complexity will be discussed further in Chapter 3.

Again, quality is not so simple as "everyone doing his or her best" or "doing work right the first time." Everyone is already doing their best—the best their given work processes and practices and environment will allow. People's behaviors are a result of the organization's management process. In terms of "doing work right the first time," do the people have the proper work methods, machines, materials, data, and work environment to allow them to consistently do it right the first time? If not, what should they be doing differently? Chapter 3 will describe some answers to these questions.

To quote Clemmer from *Firing On All Cylinders*[8]:

> *Only about 15 percent of the [problems] can be traced to someone who didn't care or wasn't conscientious enough. But the last person to touch the process, pass the product, or deliver the service may have*

been burned out by ceaseless [problem solving]; overwhelmed with the volume of work or problems; turned off by a "snoopervising" manager; out of touch with who his or her team's customers are and what they value; unrewarded and unrecognized for efforts to improve things; poorly trained; given shoddy materials, tools, or information to work with; not given feedback on when and how products or services went wrong; measured (and rewarded or punished) by management for results conflicting with his or her immediate customer's needs; unsure of how to resolve issues and jointly fix a process with other functions; trying to protect himself or herself or the team from searches for the guilty; unaware of where to go for help. All this lies within the system, processes, structure, or practices of the organization.

Part of the change to QI is a change in focus from the 15% to the 85%. To cover the broader scope of the latter problems, projects will be fewer but at a higher level in the organization. Upper management should be brought directly into the improvement process and integrate this focus into business strategy. Future significant opportunities for improvement will then be aligned to and based on customer needs.

Physician Involvement

Some practices begin improvement efforts with processes that seem purely administrative. The team membership is confined to administrative personnel, with a plan to involve physicians at a later time. However, this almost always results in slow going and inevitable rework. As illustrated in the project case studies (Chapter 11), physician leadership at the beginning of the project had a significant impact on improvement success.

Physicians have a major impact on virtually every practice process. By involving the physicians from the beginning, their concerns, ideas, and perceptions are addressed. Their impact on the process is included in the data collection and analysis process. This is essential to improvement.

Another common QI development error is the creation of separate, parallel clinical teams (consisting of only physicians and medical support staff) and administrative teams. Unless physicians are properly trained in improvement theory, the clinical teams tend

to function as clinical research teams rather than QI teams. These teams have a tendency to attempt either controlled studies in a chaotic, variation-filled practice environment, or to blindly implement practices suggested by literature review. Such teams can be continually frustrated by the 85 percent variation beyond their control in a non-research environment. It is no surprise to find results that differ from those stated in the literature. The purpose of quality improvement is *not* to do clinical research but to standardize processes as they currently exist and to expose "positive" variation. QI has an entirely different set of objectives from clinical research via clinical trials. This will be discussed more thoroughly in Chapter 4.

As one continues into quality management, the barrier often erected between clinical and administrative issues becomes false. *Identical* processes and thinking are used for both. As previously noted, very few processes are purely clinical, i.e., involving only doctors and patients, or purely administrative, i.e., not involving doctors at all. Almost all important healthcare processes touch physicians as either customers, suppliers, or processors. Physicians in formal administrative roles and informal physician opinion leaders must be involved from the beginning in efforts to use quality improvement as a strategy. This will be discussed further in Chapter 10.

Illustrating one source of this division from the physician perspective, Berwick states[9]:

> *For many physicians, the central notion of "process, not people" as the most powerful cause of both quality and flaws contradicts long-standing assumptions about individual responsibility and the shouldering of blame in medical care. Process thinking challenges strongly held views—enshrined in medical rituals and lore—that the quality of care rests fundamentally on the shoulders of the individual physician.*

> *Of course, that challenge is illusory; QI counsels not an abandonment of individual responsibility, but rather that individuals, through systematic methods, take on even deeper responsibility to help develop and improve the interdependent processes of the work in which they are inextricably bound. Teamwork and individual responsibility are not opposites; indeed, the former implies the latter.*

More Thoughts for Managers

1) The literature is virtually unanimous: top management cannot merely be committed to quality improvement (who isn't?), but must provide leadership in the quality improvement process.

   How is this accomplished? Learn the philosophy of continuous improvement. Use its language and exhibit its behavior. Educate, educate, educate your culture through your daily interactions. This goes far beyond mere training classes and short courses. Education and awareness are never finished. Don't let *one* opportunity go by to comment on quality. Reprioritize your objectives and work style accordingly.

   Transition is painful. Participants want to know, What's in it for me? Remember, people who perceive they are losing will find a way to win. Justify the reason for emphasis on quality and constantly repeat it. Assure them that they will have jobs, although their individual roles may change in the transformed culture.

   Empathize with all involved. Acknowledge that the rules of the healthcare game are changing, but let people know, "You are smart human beings. You need to help each other do it, but you can do it."

2) Develop an almost fanatical obsession with customer needs.

   This means recognizing one's internal customers as well as more obvious external customers. Constantly be aware of your external customers' needs. At the same time, realize that you cannot even begin to satisfactorily meet their needs until your work force truly understands its job. Your work force must understand its relationship to and needs of its internal customers. While internal customer awareness is extremely difficult to develop, it is a vital concept in service quality improvement.

3) Empower your employees to act at "moments of truth."

   A "moment of truth" is *any* interaction with a customer, external or internal. All promises to customers must be kept. Give your employees a vision to use as a guideline in making decisions when the customer's perception of quality is at stake.

4) Incorporate the use of "statistical thinking" routinely throughout the organization.

   The most compact summary of quality improvement available is Deming's statement, "If I had to reduce my message to management to just a few words, I'd say it all has to do with reducing variation."

   Statistical thinking means looking at *everything* the organization does as a series of processes that have the goal of consistently providing the results your customers desire. *All* processes exhibit variation, which must be studied via data to take the appropriate improvement actions.

   Thinking in terms of processes is perhaps the most profound change needed for continuous improvement. One must blame processes, not people, for undesirable results, as previously alluded to in the "85/15" rule.

5. Address "demotivators".

   Demotivators are performance inhibitors that insidiously creep into organizational environments. The issue of culture change and top management leadership of the transformation can no longer be treated in traditional ad hoc fashion. This may have been adequate in the past, but the current unrelenting, unprecedented change forced onto medicine by external environmental factors must be addressed with more formality.

   The whole psychology of the workplace is in upheaval, and the ever-present danger of demotivators is magnified by this new source of stress. Traditional structures and rewards must be redesigned both for the future (which is now) and for leading people into the future. Figure 2.7 lists 21 demotivators identified by Dean Spitzer in his book, *SuperMotivation: A Blueprint for Energizing Your Organization from Top to Bottom.*

Figure 2.7: 21 Workplace Demotivators that Breed Fear and Anger[10]

• Politics • Unclear expectations • Unnecessary rules • Poorly designed work • Unproductive meetings • Lack of follow-up • Constant change • Internal competition	• Dishonesty, feeling "lied to" • Hypocrisy, not "walking the talk" • Withholding information • Unfairness, preferential treatment • Discouraging responses to ideas • Atmosphere of criticism • Capacity underutilization of individuals	• Tolerating poor performance • Being taken for granted • Management invisibility • Overcontrol • Takeaways of past privileges • Being forced to do poor-quality work

Figure 2.8: The Three Sides of the Joiner Triangle[11]

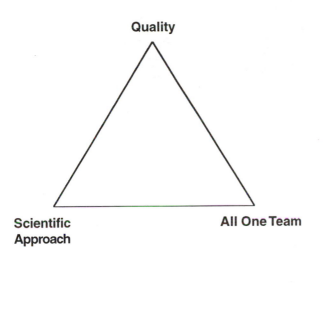

Quality	Scientific Approach	All One Team
• Develop a passion for delighting customers	• Use data to speed up learning and improvement	• Treat everyone as if we are all in the same boat together
• Develop a passion for eliminating waste	• Develop process and system thinking	• Practice win-win
	• Optimize the system as a whole	• Believe in people
	• Learn to hear the signal through the noise—variation	• Focus on releasing people's intrinsic motivation

The Joiner Triangle (Figure 2.8) provides a simple yet essential summary of what is needed for a successful transformation to quality improvement management strategy.

The three elements of the Joiner Triangle must be practiced together to produce rapid, sustained improvement. To accelerate improvement we must move away from rewarding individual heroic efforts, and focus on building smooth effective processes and teamwork throughout the organization.

The short-term challenge is to create a work culture which has:

• the **will** to change

• the **belief** that the organization is capable of change

• the **wherewithal** to undo old habits by constant re-education in quality philosophy and techniques

• the ability to take continual action toward change and improvement. Rather than just talking and complaining about QI, the organization just **does** it.

The long-term goal is to create a culture where the words "quality" and "statistical" are dropped as adjectives from programs because they are givens.

Summary

It takes nothing less than an **obsession with quality** to overcome the current inertia created by daily existence of the organization. This is done by using a **scientific approach** to study the relationships in and variation of processes through the objective use of data. The methods of improvement are as important as results. An **all one team** atmosphere improves processes by involving the people who are closest to the customers and actually doing the work. This ensures that the whole system is optimized. Management's new role on this "one" team is to understand and improve processes and customer relationships. Managers must facilitate the improvement process because they are responsible for at least 85 percent of the improvement opportunity, and they must lead efforts to break down barriers between departments and other customer groups. Addressing the demotivators of the current culture is necessary to transition to the new culture of continuous change.

Notes to Chapter Two

1.   Berwick DM. "Peer Review and Quality Management: Are They Compatible?"

2.   *Ibid.*

3.   Berwick DM. "Sounding Board: Continuous Improvement as an Ideal in Health Care."

4.   Huge EC. *Total Quality: An Executive's Guide for the 1990's.*

5.   *Ibid.*

6.   Scholtes PR. *The TEAM Handbook.*

7.   Juran JM. *Managerial Breakthrough.*

8.   Clemmer J. *Firing On All Cylinders.*

9.   Berwick DM. "The Clinical Process and the Quality Process."

10.   Spitzer D. *SuperMotivation: A Blueprint for Energizing Your Organization from Top to Bottom.*

11.   Joiner BL. *Fourth Generation Management: The New Business Consciousness.*

Chapter Three
Process-Oriented Thinking

Key Ideas

- While service outputs may seem more difficult to define than manufacturing outputs, all processes in both settings have measurable outputs.

- Significant quality improvements result only when data collection and analysis are used to establish work processes and to identify elements of work processes that do not provide value.

- All work is a process, including the unique interactions between clinicians and patients.

- All processes exhibit variation and have measurable values associated with them.

- Inputs to a process include people, methods, machines, materials, measurements, and environment. All inputs carry variation.

- Outputs are those quantifiable things e.g., tests, reports, examinations, or bills, which go to internal and external customers.

- Data collection is itself a process made up of inputs, outputs, and variation.

- Common errors in QI which result when process-oriented thinking is not used include action based on anecdotes and the addition of unnecessary complexity to a process.

- Operational definitions can prevent inappropriate actions based on anecdotes.

- Flowcharts reduce problems created by disagreement and variation in perceptions about how processes currently operate.

Process-Oriented Thinking: Manufacturing Concepts in a Service Environment

Much of the statistical emphasis in current quality improvement training originated from quality control efforts developed in American manufacturing around World War II. They achieved widespread popularity in Japan after the war through the efforts of Deming and Juran. Because manufacturing uses an observable, physical process to produce an actual measurable product, data and statistical analysis have been used for quality improvement in manufacturing for almost 50 years. The emphasis in that environment has been primarily on product improvement.

The concept of measuring a work process within a service environment may appear harder to define. Processes are perceived to be intangible and difficult to define numerically. Observed events tend to be anecdotal and reflect perceptions rather than data.

It can be difficult to see how techniques for improving machines are related to services. It may also be difficult to understand how statistics can be helpful other than for summarizing a company's financial performance. Derived indices and aggregated financial figures presented in tabular form are common examples of the service organization's standard approach to using statistics. An example is shown in Figure 3.1.

3

Figure 3.1: Traditional Tabular Presentation of Data
XYZ MEDICAL CENTER
LINES OF BUSINESS ANALYSIS
FOR THE PERIODS ENDED DECEMBER 31, 1995
(in thousands)

	1995 ACTUAL				1995 BUDGET			
	TOTAL	UNDER 65	SENIORS & GOV'T	OTHER	TOTAL	UNDER 65	SENIORS & GOV'T	OTHER
Total Bookings	$179,177	$140,307	$38,870		$197,550	$153,457	$44,093	
Patient Revenue	$149,645	$125,763	$23,882		$159,804	$134,213	$25,591	
Medical Retail Sales	17,054			17,054	17,036			17,036
Other Revenue	3,932			3,932	2,773			2,773
TOTAL REVENUE	170,631	125,763	23,882	20,986	179,613	134,213	25,591	19,809
Expenses:								16,907
Operating	108,921	71,882	19,914	17,125	112,157	73,990	21,260	
Professional	62,315	48,797	13,518		63,594	49,400	14,194	
TOTAL EXPENSES	171,236	120,679	33,432	17,125	175,751	123,390	35,454	16,907
INCOME (LOSS)	(605)	5,084	(9,550)	3,861	3,862	10,823	(9,863)	2,902
Hospital Fund	2,854	2,995	(141)		380	380	0	
OPERATING INCOME (LOSS)	2,249	8,079	(9,691)	3,861	4,242	11,203	(9,863)	2,902
NON OPERATING INCOME	928			928	1,123			1,123
REVENUES IN EXCESS (DEFICIT) OF EXPENSES	$3,177	$8,079	$(9,691)	$4,789	$5,365	$11,203	$(9,863)	$4,025
Prior Year Adjustments	2,929	1,845	1,084					
TOTAL	$6,106	$9,924	$(8,607)	$4,789				
1994	$5,539	$7,976	$(6,440)	$4,001				

	95 Actual	95 Budget	94 Actual
Breakeven	86.0%	80.4%	82.1%
Average unit fee increase	5.7%	6.0%	7.5%
Average unit cost increase	10.7%	3.8%	7.6%

Other income consists of:	Actual	Budget
Medical Retail	$689	$760
AMED Sale and Interest	1,415	1,415
Net Rental Income and Other	2,685	1,850
Total	$4,789	$4,025

For this schedule, bad debt expense is reclassed from operating expense to patient revenue.

Healthcare professionals in particular feel that their field is unique and quite different from manufacturing. They often espouse concepts like:

- Medicine is an art.

- People are not "widgets," e.g., healthcare professionals and patients are unique individuals who cannot be consistently measured or categorized.

- Statistics' role is a narrow, rigorous one defined by clinical trial research and quality assurance.

- Individuals' statistical needs involve a basic knowledge of descriptive statistics with an occasional hypothesis test or regression.

- Individual accountability is the bottom line.

These perceptions have led people to believe that only huge, random data sets external to the process can provide the information needed for improvement. Berwick points out that this is the misconception behind the traditional QA process of identifying the "bad apples" in a "sort and shoot" mindset.[1] The uniqueness of patient cases and provider skills can seem too individualized to measure.

However, the processes in which both patients and providers participate are quantifiable and, to a large extent, predictable. Collecting data on the processes themselves is the key to identifying and eliminating the problems that people experience. Studying the number of lost medical records tells us how many records are lost. Studying the process of creating, transporting, and filing the records may tell us where and why they were lost as well as give us information necessary to permanently reduce the number of lost records.

Despite perceptions, it makes no difference whether the improvements are being made in a manufacturing or service environment. The quality improvement process is *identical*. It is only the emphasis on individual components of the process that differs greatly between them.

The primary challenges for non-manufacturing organizations are to recognize both the existence of processes and the need to standardize those processes to eliminate tasks that do not add value for the customer.

Everything Is a Process

Thinking in terms of processes is perhaps the most profound change needed to shift to continuous quality improvement. What is a process? All work is a process! Personal experience has shown that concentrating on the process inherent in any improvement situation leads to:

- higher quality work results

- an atmosphere of cooperation due to depersonalization of problems and elimination of "blame"

- simpler and more effective solutions to the problems presented

- happier and more educated customers with more willingness to learn the QI process

Processes are sequences of tasks aimed at accomplishing a particular outcome. Everyone involved in a process has a role of **supplier**, **processor**, or **customer**. A group of related processes is called a **system.** The key concepts of process are:

- A **process** is any sequence of tasks that has **inputs** which undergo some type of **conversion action** to produce **outputs**

- The inputs come from both internal and external **suppliers**

- Outputs go to both internal and external **customers**

Process-oriented thinking is built on the premise of:

- understanding that **all** work is accomplished through a series of one or more processes

- using data collection and analysis to establish consistent, predictable work processes

- recognizing and eliminating work procedures that do not add value (i.e., only add cost with no payback to customers)

Understanding interactions between systems and establishing predictable systems is crucial to achieving superior healthcare quality. The simple yet powerful concept of process is shown in Figure 3.2.

Figure 3.2: Concept of Process

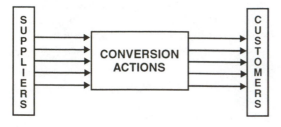

A full understanding of process-oriented thinking recognizes that:

* all processes exhibit variation

* some variation can be controlled and some cannot

* all processes have measurable values associated with them

Because all processes produce measurable data (outputs), it is as valid to apply statistical methods to healthcare processes as to manufacturing processes. Chapter 4 discusses statistical needs at both individual and organizational levels.

The interactions between an organization's processes and systems can be understood by collecting data on key business outputs. Studying patterns of variation allows more predictable processes and systems to be established.

A short list of service process outputs is shown in Figure 3.3. Are some entries surprising?

Figure 3.3: Some Service Process Outputs

* Patient length of stay
* Cost variances
* Lost time from accidents
* Percent patient "no shows"
* Absenteeism
* Lab tests ordered
* Complaints
* Meetings
* Telephone calls
* Days per 1000
* Patient satisfaction scores
* Medication error rate
* Time from order to shipment
* Data entry errors
* Percent of meetings rescheduled
* Percent of meetings missed
* Number of referrals to x specialty
* Percent of junk mail
* Percent waste
* Time to retype documents
* Accounts receivable by payor

One of the best ways to reduce variation in process outputs is by studying the inputs to the process. Any process has six types of inputs (Figure 3.4):

* People
* Methods
* Machines
* Materials
* Measurements
* Environment

Each input can be considered a potential source of variation and barrier to quality. All data collected about a process exhibit the *aggregated* effects of the variation from these six inputs. When brainstorming problems about a process, any theory can be categorized into at least one of those six sources.

It is worth noting that the "Measurements" source can have two interpretations. Obviously, measurements can affect our perception of process outputs, but measurements can be inputs to the process, too. In fact, many processes have a resulting measurement as a primary output, which is in turn an input to another process. Examples include a laboratory result used by physician to decide the course of action for a patient, and an accounting system, the numerical output of which is used by management to evaluate the state of the organization.

Figure 3.4: Concept of Process

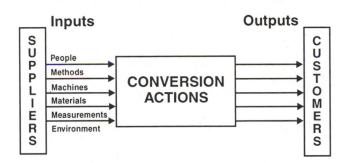

Many quality programs focus only on people, their attitudes, and simply "doing it right the first time." While well-intentioned, these motivational programs address only one of six inputs to an organizational process—people. Each of the six inputs contributes variation that must be addressed. One-day "smile training" (usually "smile or else!") customer service courses are not effective because they reinforce a "you're the problem" message rather than address the underlying problems in the processes. Why don't people want to smile?

The process-oriented context cannot be emphasized enough:

Blame the process, not the people.

A process can sabotage one's thinking into the tendency to blame people in many subtle ways. People are visible. The processes, systems, and organizational culture which shape their behavior are not as easily seen. Yes, people do make mistakes (the "15 percent" controllable by the individual in the 85/15 rule), but who hires, trains, coaches, measures, and rewards them? Do the processes allow the people to perform to expectations?

Clemmer's comments from Chapter 2 are worth revisiting.[2] When something goes wrong, it is easy to find the last person who touched it and lay the blame there. But many service breakdowns are due to process issues: systems, procedures, policies, rules, and regulations. Process-oriented questions to ask when something fails are, Was this a unique event or an event waiting to happen? or Could this just as easily have happened to another person? If we fired and replaced *everyone*, not just this person, could this happen again? Often people claim to just "know" that a specific person is the problem. In this case an interesting question is, What kind of process (hiring, promotion, etc.) allowed a "person like that" to get into that position? A surprising revelation to most people

is: Your current processes are perfectly designed to get the results you already observe.

Variation and Process Analysis: A Cornerstone of the Improvement Process

Variation in inputs and outputs of a process is just one type of problem. When studying a process, be aware of the six key sources of problems shown in Figure 3.5:

Figure 3.5: Sources of Problems in a Process[3]

1. Inadequate knowledge of how a process currently works

2. Inadequate knowledge of how a process <u>should</u> work

3. Errors and mistakes in executing the procedures

4. Current practices that fail to recognize the need for preventive measures

5. Unnecessary steps, rework, wasteful data collection, inventory / time buffers

6. Variation in inputs and outputs

While the last four are self-explanatory, the first two may need some clarification. While they both are related to knowledge of the process, the first deals with variation in people's behavior. This can be due to variation in their training, individual variation while performing the process, or undocumented reactions to unforeseen inputs or situations. Inadequate knowledge of how a process should work is related more to consistent problems experienced by everyone. It can be caused by naïve design, outdated procedures, a poor training program, or expansion beyond the process's initial needs and capacity.

The authors have found this thinking process to be the most useful piece of information in educating people about process analysis and problem-solving. These problem sources provide a useful roadmap for those poised to improve a process. Many of the examples in later chapters demonstrate the effects of these sources.

A common initial reaction to a problem is to immediately and feverishly collect data solely on the output. This is inefficient, and will be horribly contaminated by the first five sources. Immediate data collection could be an initial strategy whose objective is to establish a baseline for the current extent of the problem, but ultimately, the problem types cannot be accurately exposed and separated by looking merely at outputs. Each of the six problems can introduce multiple sources of variation into the process output. Each problem needs its own uniquely designed data collection process which addresses variation of the **inputs** as well as outputs.

Further complications arise when poorly planned output data are combined with previously collected data that have been stored in a computer "just in case." The usefulness of the "just in case" data is further diminished because they were not collected with the process improvement objective in mind. It is easy to draw false conclusions about cause-and-effect relationships when looking at data that were not intended to study those relationships. Deeper insight into the sources of variation is needed to identify the true causes. Data collected without any clear purpose will eventually prove someone's hidden agenda.

Much of a typical organization's work efforts are devoted to problem containment rather than discovering a problem's root cause. It always seems easier to shout, "Don't just stand there; do something!" Many times root problem causes are buried deep in procedures and processes. One coding project site found that its coding problems were intertwined with larger issues of billing and claims follow-up. Several of the common errors made in improvement efforts can result from taking a problem-containment approach. For example, people often try to improve a process by adding or rearranging steps instead of learning how to prevent the problem. This can make a process more complicated without necessarily adding any value.

Another common error is the recommendation to implement an anecdotal solution, generally considered the "known" solution to a long-standing problem. This ad hoc problem solving can result in unforeseen distortion of other parts of the process and further unexpected consequences. Implementing solutions does not necessarily address root causes.

Processes become complex as extra steps are added to work around root causes. As other problems appear resulting from this distortion, more and more steps are added elsewhere to compensate. The effects of the distortions often multiply and cause problems with other processes, which in turn are solved with extra steps adding still more complexity. Studying the reasons the steps were added can often bring true root causes to the surface.

Complexity is often the first problem identified when teams begin to study problems with a process. There are at least four kinds of complexity:

1) Mistakes and defects.

   These cause repeated work, take extra steps to correct, and require damage control to repair customer relationships. Could this have been *prevented* by proper design of earlier process steps? The sole focus of many QI efforts is here. This is inefficient because it addresses symptoms and not root causes. The same problems end up being solved repeatedly.

2) Breakdowns and delays.

   These interrupt the work flow and cause waiting time. Waiting times are sometimes designed into work processes because of the prevalence of breakdowns and delays. Good questions to ask are:

   • Which input is the major cause?

   • Are internal customer needs fully understood?

   • How do these affect the external customer?

   • Could it be eliminated?

   • What would the process look like if it were one continuous flow?

   These can become so accepted as a natural part of work that people become blind to them as sources of waste.

3) Inefficiencies.

   These are either the result of the design of work processes or of physical space. Why was the process *originally* designed this way?

4) Variation.

   A wide range of unintended, unplanned results forces workers to react. They individually add steps to compensate for unpredictability, thus increasing variation in a naïve "standard" process.

- Why aren't results consistent?

- What scenarios caused the added steps?

- Can the process be designed more robustly?

- Are people doing the right things?

- Are they doing the right things right?

Each of these factors causes rework. **Rework** is:

- handling products more often than is necessary

- fixing an existing product (scraping burnt toast)

- redelivering a service.

Rework introduces unnecessary costs to the organization and compromises customer satisfaction. While some of the procedures tied to rework are ingrained into the work culture, they must be recognized as opportunities for improvement. A much deeper understanding of the implications of waste must be developed.

Before further discussion of statistical thinking, the authors wish to re-emphasize an important implication of process-oriented thinking on the "scientific approach" of the Joiner Triangle (Figure 2.8)—the use of data. Data-based decisions and statistical skills should not be reserved exclusively for the formal teams that develop during the course of the QI process. It is an important element of QI that *all staff levels should have the skills to collect, manage, understand, analyze, and interpret data* in the simplest, most efficient manner possible.

Part of management's transformation should be a serious re-evaluation of the way data are used throughout the organization. A data inventory process is suggested in Chapter 4. This parallel effort is necessary to establish the self-empowered work teams inherent in the QI philosophy.

A Complicating Factor: Information Gathering as a Process

The more you know what is wrong with a figure, the more useful it becomes.
—*John Tukey*[4]

Recall that:

- A process has six types of inputs: people, methods, machines, materials, measurements, and environment

- All work is a measurable process

- While it may not be clear initially how to measure a process, any process has outputs which can somehow be captured

Think of a typical process and its six inputs. If it is desired to quantify the output, a measurement process is used to produce an actual piece of data. These individual measurements undergo a **collection** (or formal accumulation) process. After collection, the data are input into an **analysis** process whose output then goes through an **interpretation** process. The interpretations usually result in a management **action**. This action then feeds back as an input into the process being studied. The concept of data collection as a process is summarized in Figure 3.6.

3

Figure 3.6 Information Gathering as a Process—Input/Output Flowchart

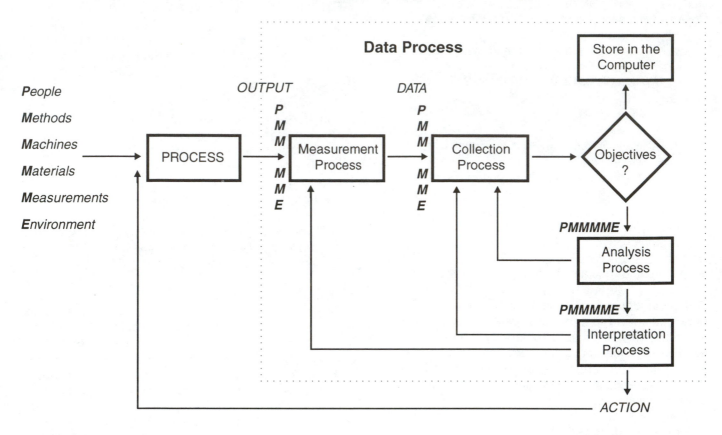

Each process–measurement, collection, analysis, and interpretation–has inputs of people, methods, machines, materials, measurements, and environment. Each input is also a potential source of variation. The data-gathering process itself contains multiple sources of variation in addition to the true, underlying variation of the process under study. Variation from all of these processes aggregates into the decision-making process. If ignored, the aggregated variation of the data process can further cloud, sometimes hopelessly, an already serious situation requiring meaningful action. The importance of studying the data-gathering process along with the work process can never be overestimated. Implications of this will be discussed in Chapter 6.

A Key Emphasis in a Service Culture: Operational Definitions

> *Words have no meaning unless they are translated into action, agreed upon by everyone. An operational definition puts communicable meaning into a concept... There is no true value of anything.*
> *—W. Edwards Deming[5]*

Quality problems often persist due to different perceptions of the meaning of words. All meaning begins with concepts–thoughts, notions, images in the mind. These perceptions bring the element of human, non-quantifiable variation into data processes. Human variation complicates the interpretation of a process's true variation by (unknowingly) invalidating the statistical analysis. Several people assessing the same situation can come up with conflicting sets of data if operational definitions are not clarified upfront. Operational definitions of all key process terms are critical for data to be comparable across individuals, departments, or organizations.

An operational definition is not open to interpretation, but instead quantitatively interprets a concept by describing what something is and how it is measured. It defines a procedure which yields consistent results regardless of who measures the process.

While people may not fully agree on an operational definition, the definition provides at least some consensus so that regardless of who measures a given situation, virtually the same number is obtained. If an operationally defined measurement procedure is replaced with a different operationally defined procedure, the same situation will likely yield a different number. Neither procedure would be right or wrong, but the effects of changing the procedure would be clear. However, if the procedure is <u>not</u> operationally defined, latitude taken by individuals practically guarantees different numbers even with supposedly the same procedure.

This was recently demonstrated at a meeting where three health centers presented mammography data to a customer. After viewing the presentation the customer had two comments: "The way you've each defined your data, I can't compare you," and "You've each defined your data in a way that was [unintentionally] self-serving." The definitions were appropriate for each organization's internal objective, but not for a customer's objective of comparing of the health centers' results.

As an exercise in identifying terms that require operational definitions, consider what is meant by the following terms: grossly contaminated, late, clean, careful, satisfactory, attached, correct, level, secure, fresh, user-friendly, too many, complete, uniform, significant improvement, on-time, majority, large majority, Rush, RUSH!!, STAT, unemployed, accident, denied, error. When creating an operational definition, the team should not view the procedure as "right" or "wrong," but should instead ask, Does the measurement satisfy the current objectives of the data collection and analysis?

In the absence of operational definitions, people often resort to anecdotal data, i.e., stories about the seriousness of a problem and the solution to it, which are influenced by the perspective of the person telling them. To prevent inappropriate action based on anecdotal information, the following process is recommended:

1) Ask further questions about the anecdote to clarify exactly what is meant by the terms it includes. Develop an operational definition of key terms like the ones in the above exercise. Collect data on the number and types of occurrences, or

2) Recognize the anecdote as a breakdown of a process. Ask whether there is adequate knowledge of how the process works or how it should work. Clarify this human variation in perception by facilitating a session to develop a map, i.e., flowchart, of the situation. Talk to customers to get their needs and then operationally define them.

Project teams should be careful not to rush into data collection. As will be discussed in Chapter 6, current in-house data should first be exhausted. If a team collects data and later decides they are not useful, their credibility will be destroyed with the people whose jobs were interrupted for the purposes of the data collection. Objectives for improving a process must be clearly identified and operational definitions established before data collection begins.

Flowcharts: Describing the Current Process

Perhaps the most serious problems in service processes result from variation caused by a lack of agreed-upon processes. These are similar to the problems that result from lack of operational definitions. Inappropriate and unnecessary variations seen by customers stem from excessive, unintended variation in individual work processes and from variation in management's perceptions of these processes. Flowcharts provide an opportunity for those involved in a process to describe its current operation in a concise, visual way. Flowcharts provide everyone involved with new perspectives on process complexity and variation.

To quote Henry Neave in *The Deming Dimension*[6]:

> ...systems are unlikely to be defined in practice unless they are both suitable and adequate for the jobs for which they are intended, *and are written down in a way comprehensible to all involved*... One or more forms of flowchart may be helpful, or the definition may be purely textual—but the system does need to be documented in some way.

> Yet again, there can be big differences between what is written down—the way the system is intended, or thought, to operate—and what actually happens. Incidentally, the acquisition of this latter information can be difficult if not impossible in an unfriendly work environment...But, even in a constructive environment, it may still turn out to be almost impossibly difficult to complete a flowchart or other description because what is going on is so *un*systematic.

> To be blunt, if a system cannot be written down, it probably doesn't exist: that is to say it probably functions more on the basis of whim and "gut-feel" rather than on any definable procedure. This surely implies that the variation being generated is some scale of magnitude higher than really necessary,

with the resulting well-known effect on quality.

The preliminary work of flowcharting creates a common team understanding and terminology. It exposes and helps eliminate process inconsistencies often rooted in a lack of process documentation and inadequate training.

There are three basic types of flowcharts:

1)   Top-Down flowchart

This is a macro view of the basic processes, showing their natural relationships to each other as well as supplier/customer relationships. Simple descriptions of each subprocess are listed under each basic process. The top-down flowchart describes what work is supposed to be done, but does not show how the work actually is done.

2)   Detailed flowchart

This provides a more detailed version of a major process identified in the top-down flowchart. It shows the actual processes that transform the inputs into outputs. Parts of this chart include:

*   Beginning and ending boundaries of the process, designated by ovals

*   Key process steps, designated by rectangles (the description usually includes a verb)

*   Decision steps containing a "Yes/No" question, designated by diamonds, and showing the result of each path

An example of a detailed flowchart from the coding project is shown in Figure 3.7. Notice that the group did not use the standard symbols (diamonds, rectangles, etc.). The use of symbols other than ovals, rectangles, and diamonds does not invalidate a flowchart. But the use of standard symbols does provide a common language, thus reducing variation for all those using these tools.

Illustrating Neave's comment are the three flowcharts shown in Figure 3.8. The first is typical of many

processes in their "official" documented form— documented as they are *supposed* to work. As shown in the second flowchart, many times the perception never matches the reality. (A simple data collection suggested by the chart would be to answer the question, Does part A, B, or C tend to be missing from the kit most often or is it evenly distributed?) This, in turn, creates a third, unnecessary process that becomes a routine part of the manager's job (if not the entire job). Processes must be understood in their current actual form if they are to be improved.

Figure 3.7: Office Visit Charge Submission Process-Detailed Flowchart

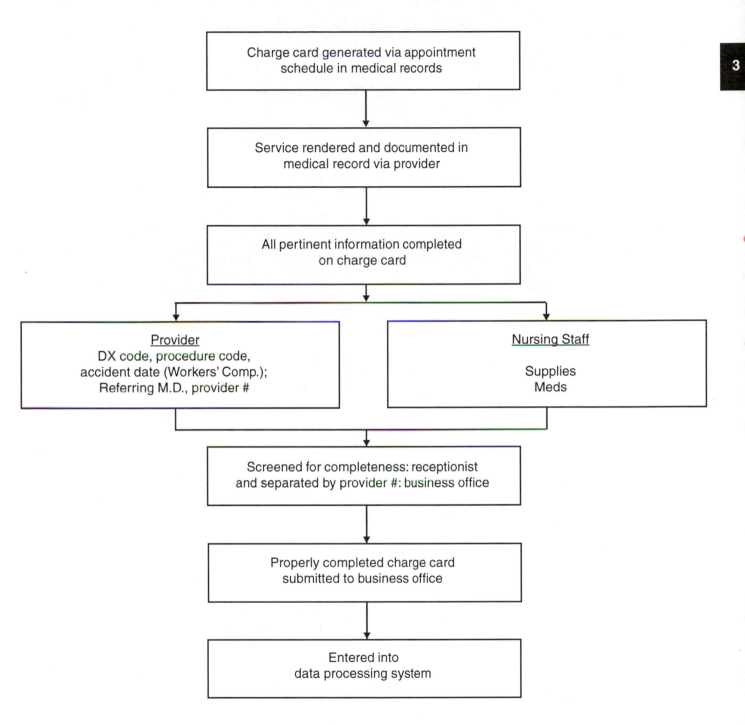

Figure 3.8: Examples of Detailed System Flowcharts[7]

A. System With No Errors

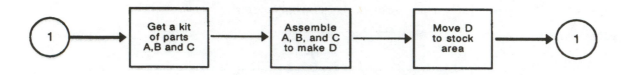

B. What Really Happens

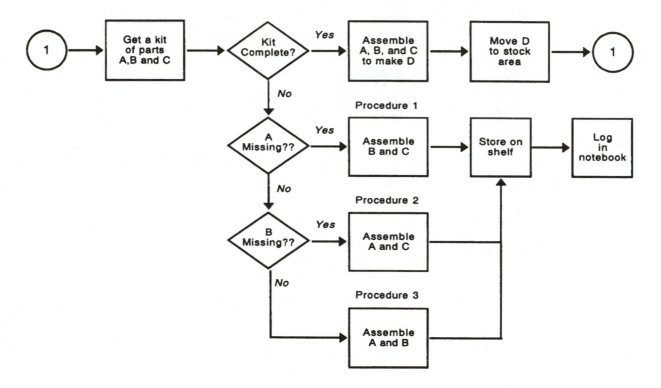

C. Manager's or Supervisor's Current Job

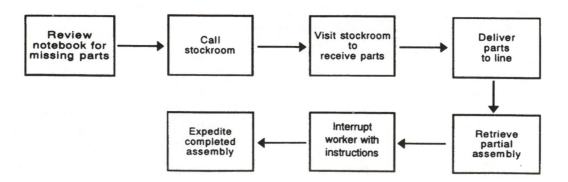

3) Deployment flowchart

This can be used with either of the above two flowcharts, or in combination with them. The deployment flowchart adds another dimension to the previous charts: space.

Departments involved in the process are listed horizontally across the top of the chart. The process flow is drawn from top to bottom, indicating the passage of time. At the same time, each specific process activity is placed in the vertical column below the department responsible for it. Obscure relationships requiring other departments' consultation and participation are indicated by horizontal lines extending from the primary department.

The deployment flowchart can be useful for indicating time bottlenecks due to too many parallel approval steps. It can also show inefficiency created by too much "back and forth" work between departments. This is a very useful chart in medicine's multiple supplier/ customer/ processor environment. A deployment flowchart of an automated telephone system is shown in Figure 3.9.

Figure 3.9: Deployment Flowchart - Automated Telephone System

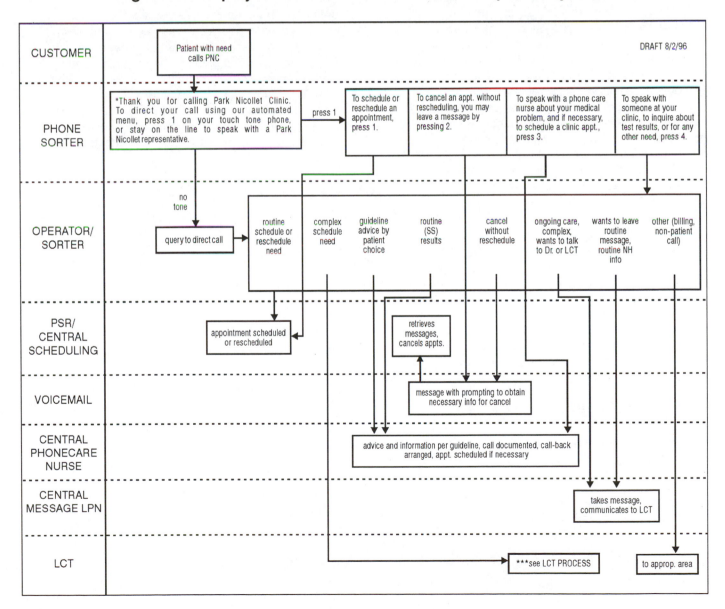

To find a problem's true root cause, exposure of individual variations in what was thought to be standard is crucial. The flowcharting process helps to establish not only that people are doing the best job possible with the current process, but that the process can be further improved and standardized. Sometimes obvious problems are exposed during flowcharting that can be fixed using minimal data. Flowcharts can establish agreement on:

- what the current process actually is

- what the best current process might be

- the need to collect data.

Flowcharting provides motivation and identifies the most effective leverage points for data collection. The questions from Figure 3.5, How does the process currently work? and How should the process work? will have been answered. Goals and objectives for the rest of the improvement project can be set based on the answers. This allows for the most efficient data collection because human variation based on perception has been minimized and more specific objectives have been defined. In addition, flowcharts can be used for current process documentation, which could be useful for future employee training. A very useful paper on flowcharting, "Quality Improvement In the Office," is available from Joiner Associates. It explains a quality process for administrative/service teams, describes the importance of using flowcharts in early project stages, and provides additional detail about the various types of flowcharts and their uses.

In the early stages of a project, it is common to concentrate too much on flowcharting the specific details of the process. It is best to narrow the scope of by:

- getting a macro view of the problem by using a top-down flowchart.

- discovering where data may be available.

- collecting data to localize which process represents a major opportunity within the larger system.

Localizing major opportunities within larger systems will be further discussed in Chapter 6.

It is also a common error in the early stages of a project to skip flowcharting because "Everyone already knows what goes on" or "We already have the answer." In the authors' and in the case study experiences, it always takes the team far longer to flowchart and understand the current process than they anticipated. "Oh, my gosh! We do that?!" is a common remark during flowcharting.

Flowcharts, while not numerical, meet the authors' definition of data: "any physical piece of information that aids in understanding variation." Flowcharts provide critical data in any improvement effort by reducing human variation in perceptions of the process and by improving the subsequent quality of the team process. The goal in the early stages of a project is to understand the existing process and the supplier / customer relationships it contains, not necessarily to understand all microprocesses required to get the work done.

Before any numerical data are collected, the questions, How does this process currently work? and How should this process work? must be answered. Joiner Associates provides guidance in the area of studying a process prior to collecting numerical data. Figures 3.10, 3.11, and 3.12 contain methods and questions a team can use to collect non-numerical data about a process. The answers can significantly narrow their focus and provide direction for future efforts.

Figure 3.10: Observation Form

Instructions: When you first arrive at your assigned area simply watch what is going on. Before you leave, jot down your thoughts and reactions to the questions below.

1. How would this area look to someone who hadn't seen it before?

2. Rate this area on the following characteristics (circle one number for each characteristic).

						Notes
Messy	1	2	3	4	Neat	
Chaotic	1	2	3	4	Orderly	
Ugly	1	2	3	4	Attractive	
Bland	1	2	3	4	Colorful	
Noisy	1	2	3	4	Peaceful	

3. What evidence do you see of a concern for quality or customers?

4. What types of improvement opportunities do you see?

5. What kind of atmosphere is there? Are people friendly? Informal? Do they seem to work together, or is there little interaction?

Figure 3.11: Interview Questions

Instructions: After you have completed your observations, randomly select an employee in your target area. Introduce yourself, explain that you belong to a team trying to better understand what happens in that work area, and ask if the employee would take a few minutes to answer a few questions. Assure the employee that all responses will be kept confidential within the team. If the person says no, thank them for their time and try someone else.

Questions

1. What do you like best about working here?

2. If you could improve one thing, what would it be?

3. What happens to improvement suggestions you or your co-workers come up with?

4. What do you know about improvement efforts going on in your area? In other departments?

Figure 3.12: Questions to Ask About a Process

Instructions: Working with your team, select several questions you think are most relevant to the project. Divide those questions among individuals or small groups, decide whether you want to use a standard reporting format, and set a (reasonable!) deadline for reporting back to the team. Between meetings, gather whatever available data you can, talk to process operators, etc. Repeat this process until all relevant questions have been answered.

The process being studied is _____

1. Who are its external customers? What individuals, groups, or systems outside our organization rely on or could benefit from this process? Who has (or could have) expectations about this process?

2. How do we know what the external customers like or don't like about this process? What satisfies or dissatisfies them?

3. Who are its internal customers? Describe those within our organization who do (or could) rely on the successful operation of this process or the resulting product or service.

4. How do we determine what the internal customers like or don't like about this process? What satisfies or dissatisfies them?

5. What are the operational definitions of quality in this process? What specifically determines whether the process is working well or poorly?

6. What records are kept regarding quality? Who uses this information? How do they use it? Are these record formats suited to how they are used?

7. What are the most common mistakes or defects that occur? What is the operational definition for each mistake or defect? What proportion of these is commonly assumed to be a worker's fault? What proportion do we usually attribute to the system? How do people arrive at these conclusions?

8. By what process do we inspect, evaluate, and report problems regarding:
    A. Planning required for this process.
    B. Incoming materials, supplies, and information critical to this process.
    C. The process itself.
    D. The final product or service received by the external or internal customer.

9. List the critical elements of this process: materials, ingredients, components, parts, information, etc.

10. List the suppliers or vendors of each critical element.

11. Describe the company's procedures for purchasing materials or ingredients brought in from outside the facility (plant office, company, etc.). To what extent is "low bid" a governing factor in our purchasing decisions?

12. Describe the impact of the most common mistakes or defects in this process. What do they cost in time, money, customer loyalty, or worker pride?

13. Who is responsible for quality in this process? Who is responsible for detecting mistakes/defects? Who is responsible for identifying and correcting the causes of mistakes or defects?

Summary

Any application of statistics to a quality improvement opportunity must be preceded by:

- a systems understanding of the observed problem

- an assessment of critical inputs and outputs from an internal supplier/customer perspective of the system

- agreement on numerical (not anecdotal) measures of these indicators through operational definitions.

Even though it is sometimes not perceived as formal statistics, the statistical perspective is inherent in process-oriented thinking. It creates essential readiness for subsequent efficient use of statistical methods.

Notes to Chapter Three

1. Berwick DM. "Sounding Board: Continuous Improvement as an Ideal in Health Care."

2. Clemmer, J. *Firing on All Cylinders.*

3. Scholtes PR. *The Team Handbook.*

4. Neave HR. *The Deming Dimension.*

5. Neave HR. *The Deming Dimension.*

6. Neave HR. *The Deming Dimension.*

7. Fuller FT. "Eliminating Complexity from Work: Improving Productivity by Enhancing Quality."

Chapter Four
Statistical Thinking and the Use of Data

Key Ideas

- To create significant lasting improvement, appropriately-collected data must be used for decision-making.

- Statistics can provide a unified language to break down barriers created by varied perceptions of how a process works.

- All data collection must have a specific agreed-upon objective and measurement process in order to prevent excessive variation.

- Processes represent repeatable actions occurring over time and must be studied that way.

- Most people are taught enumerative statistical methods. However, only analytic statistical methods can accurately analyze a process and its variation in a way that allows predictive actions to be taken.

- Clinical trial research methods control variation in ways that cannot be replicated in the unstable environment of the real world, making them less suitable for QI.

- Special causes merely indicate differences in processes. Many times the differences are unintended; sometimes they are appropriate and even desirable.

"In God We Trust, All Others Bring Data"

While vague anecdotal descriptions of quality problems abound, these do not provide objective data that can be statistically analyzed. Many times, an anecdote provides management with a catalyst to "rally the troops" and do something about the described situation "once and for all." This usually results in formation of a task force, followed by several meetings in which the task force brainstorms solutions. After much mental arm-wrestling, someone's solution wins and a team is formed to implement it. The previous chapter described how vague solutions that do not address root causes actually add layers of complexity to already frustrating situations. Sound familiar?

A scientific approach and the proper use of data can prevent much of this inefficient activity. **Valid data, collected appropriately, are critical to understanding processes and therefore, to quality improvement**. A motto of the scientific approach is, "In God we trust, all others bring data." Additionally, Berwick has said, "Do you know what the plural of 'anecdote' is? NOT DATA!" To create significant, lasting improvement, an organization's culture must erase:

- anecdotal data

- "shooting from the hip" or "instant answers"

- guesswork without data

- any debate that leads directly to "known" solutions

- arbitrary numerical goals.

The creativity that can be harnessed by a team is unbounded. However, the psychology implicit in a team atmosphere can present quite a formidable barrier to improvement. Various team members bring with them a wide variety of process perceptions. Everyone should approach problem-solving from a unified perspective, especially when data collection will be involved.

By providing a unifying language, statistics can serve to break down barriers created by varying perceptions. Good data strip the emotion out of a situation and depersonalize issues. While data inevitably contain variation, they must be used with an agreed-upon theory (statistical) to make objective decisions in conjunction with the team members' knowledge of the process. Data-based decisions that help teams to understand variation and enhance prediction are key elements in quality improvement.

When a team uses statistics to appreciate a system and understand its variation, significant quality improvements can occur. Understanding root causes of variation through planned data collection aided by statistical methods and theory leads to appropriate action.

Are You "Measuring Envelopes?"

As an example of the hidden dangers of data collection, Figure 4.1 shows an actual data set one of the authors obtained while teaching a class. Quantities of envelopes and various types of rulers were distributed. The class was asked to find the thickness of an envelope and record it on a flipchart. Those present were told to apply a "moderate" amount of physical pressure to the stacked envelopes when they measured. There were no other instructions. Very few clarifying questions were asked by the class.

Figure 4.1: Initial Envelope Thickness Measurements

.25" (top corner)	1.02 mm
.019" Bottom corner	.0125"
.017" Bottom corner	.0106
12.600 mils	.0106
0.01875"	.015625 (Blue)
1.02 mm	.01219 (Green)
.018"	.02
.01875"	.01
	.017"

Isn't it interesting? The numbers are different!

The class was asked to brainstorm why so much variation was present, which resulted in approximately thirty reasons. Significant differences in measurement techniques, calculation of the number, and location of the measurements became evident. The lack of an objective for the data collection resulted in a variety of perceptions regarding what problem was being addressed and therefore, how to measure it. Some people had perceived the exercise as a total waste of time (Sound familiar with some of your routine processes?) and gave it a half-hearted effort. All these factors resulted in a poor quality data set.

Think of this exercise as a process and ask yourself why the numbers might be different. Can you classify the reasons for variation into people, methods, machines, materials, measurements, or environment?

What should be done with these data? Often, the response is "Put them in the computer!" Seriously, do these data have any use?

In fact, they are quite useful because they show there is neither an agreed-upon objective nor measurement process. However, if this same collection process were followed with data taken in a similar manner day after day, month after month, it would immediately cease to

be useful. Consistent, repeated collection would just institutionalize the lack of objective and process.

In effect, variation in human perceptions became non-quantifiable variation that could not be understood through a formal statistical analysis. Suppose the data had been sent to a computer center to be keyed into the database just as it was—a list of numbers. Any formal statistical analysis would have been ludicrous.

The numbers would have been different even if there was agreement on the objective and measurement process. However, they would have exhibited less variation and statistical analysis could be legitimately attempted. Can you see that less variation translates into a higher quality data set?

Think back to Professor Tukey's comment in the previous chapter:

> ***The more you know what is wrong with a figure, the more useful it becomes.***

A seemingly trivial exercise became quite complicated, generating much confusion and chaos. Aren't daily work processes more complicated than measuring envelopes?

Two major points can be made with this exercise:

- a good statistical analysis of a bad set of data is worthless

- if we can agree on what to measure, but cannot agree on how to measure it, any data generated will essentially be worthless.

In the authors' experience: never underestimate how much people can affect data. When instructions go through someone's personal "filter" (or hidden agenda), they are often unintentionally altered, thus adding variation to the process.

Conflicting mental models about data (Figure 4.2) also contribute significant human variation. A measured result could change depending on someone's belief about the objective of the data. Even more likely, the presentation, analysis, and interpretation of the data will differ from one mental model to another. In truth, the first and last models in Figure 4.2 are the only two of value. The others are statistically dysfunctional manifestations of the improvement model, and are contaminated by human psychology. They rely heavily on faulty assumptions in their data processes as designed (collection, analysis/display, interpretation).

They result in much inappropriate, though well-meaning, action. Non-quantifiable, human variation in a data set will render statistical analysis virtually meaningless.

Figure 4.2 : Conflicting Mental Models About Data

- Research
- Inspection (comparison/finger pointing)
- Micromanagement (from "on high")
- Results (compared to arbitrary goals)
- Outcomes (for bragging)
- Improvement

Improvement of data quality occurs as both quantifiable and non-quantifiable sources of variation are reduced. That is, prediction capability is enhanced by understanding, controlling, and reducing variation through study of the measurement process that produced these numbers. Confidence is thereby built into the system, and the data can be used for their true objective. As shown in Figure 3.6, objectives drive the measurement, collection, and analysis of the data, and statistical theory drives the interpretation of the variation to lead to appropriate action.

How Are You Using Data?

What data are routinely collected in your organization? Is there an objective? There is a tendency to routinely amass numerical data on various perceived key process outputs and business indicators and produce monthly reports at incredible rates. One could say (with apologies to Samuel Coleridge and the Ancient Mariner), "Data, data everywhere, and not a thought to think."

An interesting clinical perspective comes from Heero Hacquebord[1], who notes in an article about a recent hospital stay, "While the health care professionals that I came in contact with collected and recorded a great deal of data about me during my stay, it is not clear to me that this information was fully utilized to improve my care, or the care of future patients…Vital signs on a patient's condition should not be just simply recorded; it is necessary to interpret such data effectively so that correct remedies and actions are taken…I believe this problem of data overload comes about in health care because there is often no explicit theory that one is testing that could then be used to drive data collection and the identification of key information."

Unless a process has been analyzed using the six process problems (Figure 3.5), any data collection will be significantly contaminated with excessive variation. **Data with excessive variation that are used for business or clinical decisions could have a serious negative impact**.

Think about how your organization measures itself. Mark Graham Brown lists seven categories of organizational metrics[2]:

1. Customer satisfaction
2. Employee satisfaction
3. Financial performance
4. Operational performance (e.g., cycle time, productivity, etc.)
5. Product/service quality
6. Supplier performance
7. Safety/environmental/public responsibility

In his original article, Brown includes a survey that describes the characteristics of an effective measurement system and allows an organization to assess its own (Fig. 4.3). The 50 questions are divided into three categories and address the overall approach to measurement, specific types of measures, and how to analyze and use the data to improve the organization.

Following an assessment with Brown's survey, a process can be developed to define goals and critical success factors, after which one redefines the measures. This process must start from the top and cascade down to all levels in the organization with the net result being that each employee has a balanced set of measures covering the seven categories. Another good reference is chapter 11 of *Improving Performance*, by Rummler and Brache.[3]

Are your data collections truly adding value to your organization? As mentioned earlier, data collected without any clear purpose can eventually be used to prove virtually any hidden agenda. Does today's constantly changing business environment have time for such nonsense?

What implications does this have if you are collecting process outputs in the absence of clear objectives communicated to the people involved in the measurement, collection, analysis, and interpretation processes?

4

Figure 4.3: Is Your Measurement System Well-Balanced?[4]

Taking measure of your measurement system

Questionnaire directions — The questionnaire is divided into three sections, each addressing an aspect of your measurement system.

- Part I (questions 1-5) is about your overall approach to measurement.
- Part II (questions 6-41) questions ask specific types of measures.
- Part III (questions 41-51) is about how you analyze and use the data to improve your organization.

Read each statement and check the appropriate box, depending on the extent to which you strongly agree (5) or strongly disagree (1) with the statement. Answer every question even if you have to guess.

The scope of the questionnaire should pertain to your entire organization, or at least a large enough portion of the company or organization that could be a stand-alone business/organization. For example, you could do a business unit rather than the whole company, or one hospital in a chain of hospitals. You could and should not use the questionnaire to apply to a single department such as radiology, or human resources.

Part I: Overall approach to measurement

1. Our organization has developed a specific set of criteria for screening out extraneous measures from our data base.
   ___ ⑤ Strongly agree ④ Agree ③ Somewhat ② Disagree ① Strongly disagree

2. Our data base was built with a plan, rather than something that just evolved over time.
   ___ ⑤ Strongly agree ④ Agree ③ Somewhat ② Disagree ① Strongly disagree

3. Our CEO or President looks at no more than 20 measures every month to evaluate the overall organization's performance.
   ___ ⑤ Strongly agree ④ Agree ③ Somewhat ② Disagree ① Strongly disagree

4. Measures of performance are mostly consistent across our business units/locations.
   ___ ⑤ Strongly agree ④ Agree ③ Somewhat ② Disagree ① Strongly disagree

5. We have a well balanced set of measures, with about equal amounts of measures/data in each of the following categories: financial performance, operational performance, customer satisfaction, employee satisfaction, product/service quality, supplier performance, and safety/environmental performance.
   ___ ⑤ Strongly agree ④ Agree ③ Somewhat ② Disagree ① Strongly disagree

Part II: Specific types of measures on your scorecard

Customer related measures

6. Our data base includes good hard measures of customer satisfaction such as repeat/lost business, returns, etc.
   ___ ⑤ Strongly agree ④ Agree ③ Somewhat ② Disagree ① Strongly disagree

7. Our organization collects data on customer feelings/ satisfaction levels using a variety of techniques such as telephone surveys, mail surveys, and focus groups.
   ___ ⑤ Strongly agree ④ Agree ③ Somewhat ② Disagree ① Strongly disagree

8. Our scales for measuring customer satisfaction focus on delighting customers rather than just satisfying them.
   ___ ⑤ Strongly agree ④ Agree ③ Somewhat ② Disagree ① Strongly disagree

9. What we ask customers in our satisfaction surveys or discussions is based upon thorough research to identify customers' most important requirements.
   ___ ⑤ Strongly agree ④ Agree ③ Somewhat ② Disagree ① Strongly disagree

10. We combine various hard and soft measures of customer satisfaction into an overall Customer Satisfaction index.
    ___ ⑤ Strongly agree ④ Agree ③ Somewhat ② Disagree ① Strongly disagree

Employee related measures

11. We survey our employees at least once a year to determine their satisfaction levels with various aspects of how the organization is run.
    ___ ⑤ Strongly agree ④ Agree ③ Somewhat ② Disagree ① Strongly disagree

12. Employee surveys are anonymous and more than 75 percent are returned each year.
    ___ ⑤ Strongly agree ④ Agree ③ Somewhat ② Disagree ① Strongly disagree

13. Research is done to determine what is important to employees before putting together or buying a survey with standard questions.
    ___ ⑤ Strongly agree ④ Agree ③ Somewhat ② Disagree ① Strongly disagree

14. Our organization collects data on other metrics that relate to employee satisfaction such as voluntary turnover, absenteeism hours worked per week, requests for transfers, et cetera.
    ___ ⑤ Strongly agree ④ Agree ③ Somewhat ② Disagree ① Strongly disagree

15. Individual measures of employee satisfaction are aggregated into an overall employee satisfaction index, similar to the customer satisfaction index.
    ___ ⑤ Strongly agree ④ Agree ③ Somewhat ② Disagree ① Strongly disagree

Financial measures

16. We have identified a few (e.g. 4-6) key measures of our overall financial performance.
   ___ ⑤ Strongly agree ④ Agree ③ Somewhat ② Disagree ① Strongly disagree

17. Financial measures are a good mix of short and long-term measures of financial success
   ___ ⑤ Strongly agree ④ Agree ③ Somewhat ② Disagree ① Strongly disagree

18. Financial measures are consistent across different units/locations.
   ___ ⑤ Strongly agree ④ Agree ③ Somewhat ② Disagree ① Strongly disagree

19. We collect financial data on our major competitors to use in evaluating our own performance and in setting goals.
   ___ ⑤ Strongly agree ④ Agree ③ Somewhat ② Disagree ① Strongly disagree

20. The organization aggregates financial data into one or two summary statistics that reflect overall performance, such as economic value added (EVA) or return on assets (ROA).
   ___ ⑤ Strongly agree ④ Agree ③ Somewhat ② Disagree ① Strongly disagree

Operational measures

21. The organization has developed a set of 4-6 common operational measures such as value-added per employee that are used in all locations/functions.
   ___ ⑤ Strongly agree ④ Agree ③ Somewhat ② Disagree ① Strongly disagree

22. Any process measures that are collected are directly related to key product/service characteristics that customers care about.
   ___ ⑤ Strongly agree ④ Agree ③ Somewhat ② Disagree ① Strongly disagree

23. Cycle time is used as a key operational measure throughout the organization.
   ___ ⑤ Strongly agree ④ Agree ③ Somewhat ② Disagree ① Strongly disagree

24. Operational measures allow you to prevent problems rather than just identify them.
   ___ ⑤ Strongly agree ④ Agree ③ Somewhat ② Disagree ① Strongly disagree

25. The organization has established measurable standards for all key process measures.
   ___ ⑤ Strongly agree ④ Agree ③ Somewhat ② Disagree ① Strongly disagree

Supplier measures

26. The organization has a rating system for evaluating supplier performance.
   ___ ⑤ Strongly agree ④ Agree ③ Somewhat ② Disagree ① Strongly disagree

27. Our supplier rating system is a mix of hard data such as products returned/shipments rejected, and soft measures such as our satisfaction levels with suppliers' responsiveness.
   ___ ⑤ Strongly agree ④ Agree ③ Somewhat ② Disagree ① Strongly disagree

28. The quality of goods and services purchased from suppliers is measured on a regular basis.
   ___ ⑤ Strongly agree ④ Agree ③ Somewhat ② Disagree ① Strongly disagree

29. Our organization asks suppliers for process data and encourages self-inspection.
   ___ ⑤ Strongly agree ④ Agree ③ Somewhat ② Disagree ① Strongly disagree

30. Staying within our price guidelines is only one of many measures used to evaluate and select suppliers.
   ___ ⑤ Strongly agree ④ Agree ③ Somewhat ② Disagree ① Strongly disagree

Product/service quality measures

31. Characteristics of products/services that are measured are those that are most important to customers.
   ___ ⑤ Strongly agree ④ Agree ③ Somewhat ② Disagree ① Strongly disagree

32. If 100 percent of products/services are not checked, then large enough sample sizes are used to ensure that all products/services meet standards.
   ___ ⑤ Strongly agree ④ Agree ③ Somewhat ② Disagree ① Strongly disagree

33. Automated measurement devices are used wherever possible to avoid errors caused by poor human judgement.
   ___ ⑤ Strongly agree ④ Agree ③ Somewhat ② Disagree ① Strongly disagree

34. Measures for services are related to accomplishments rather than behaviors (e.g. percent of correct orders filled, or percent of flights that take off on-time versus smiling when greeting customer).
   ___ ⑤ Strongly agree ④ Agree ③ Somewhat ② Disagree ① Strongly disagree

35. Measures of product/service quality are expressed as actual number rather than percentages of defect-free products/services.
   ___ ⑤ Strongly agree ④ Agree ③ Somewhat ② Disagree ① Strongly disagree

Safety/environmental/public responsibility measures

36. The organization collects data on safety and environmental performance at least once a month, using several different metrics.
   ___ ⑤ Strongly agree ④ Agree ③ Somewhat ② Disagree ① Strongly disagree

37. Measures of safety are more behavioral and preventative in nature rather than the typical lost time accidents.
   ___ ⑤ Strongly agree ④ Agree ③ Somewhat ② Disagree ① Strongly disagree

38. Environmental measures go beyond those mandated by the EPA and other regulatory agencies.
   ___ ⑤ Strongly agree ④ Agree ③ Somewhat ② Disagree ① Strongly disagree

39. The organization collects data on measures of public responsibility such as hours of community service or awards received from community/civic groups.
   ___ ⑤ Strongly agree ④ Agree ③ Somewhat ② Disagree ① Strongly disagree

40. The organization has developed a public responsibility index that is an aggregation of safety, environmental, and community service measures.
   ___ ⑤ Strongly agree ④ Agree ③ Somewhat ② Disagree ① Strongly disagree

Part III: Reporting and analyzing data

41. The organization reports data from all sections of its scorecard in a single report to all key managers.
   ___ ⑤ Strongly agree ④ Agree ③ Somewhat ② Disagree ① Strongly disagree

42. Data are presented graphically in an easy to read format that requires minimal analysis to identify trends and levels of performance.
   ___ ⑤ Strongly agree ④ Agree ③ Somewhat ② Disagree ① Strongly disagree

43. Data on customer satisfaction, employee satisfaction, and public responsibility are reviewed as often and by the same executives as data of financial, operational, product/service, and supplier performance.
   ___ ⑤ Strongly agree ④ Agree ③ Somewhat ② Disagree ① Strongly disagree

44. The organization has done research to identify correlations between customer satisfaction levels and financial performance.
   ___ ⑤ Strongly agree ④ Agree ③ Somewhat ② Disagree ① Strongly disagree

45. The organization understands the relationship between all the key measures in its overall scorecard.
   ___ ⑤ Strongly agree ④ Agree ③ Somewhat ② Disagree ① Strongly disagree

46. Performance data are analyzed and used to make key decisions about the organization's business.
   ___ ⑤ Strongly agree ④ Agree ③ Somewhat ② Disagree ① Strongly disagree

47. The key measures are consistent with the organization's missions, values, and long-term goals and strategies.
   ___ ⑤ Strongly agree ④ Agree ③ Somewhat ② Disagree ① Strongly disagree

48. The organization continuously evaluates and improves its measures and the methods used to collect and report performance data.
   ___ ⑤ Strongly agree ④ Agree ③ Somewhat ② Disagree ① Strongly disagree

49. Automated and human (e.g. surveys/checklists) measurement devices are calibrated on a regular basis to assure accuracy and reliability.
   ___ ⑤ Strongly agree ④ Agree ③ Somewhat ② Disagree ① Strongly disagree

50. The measures in the organization's scorecard are the same ones on which annual and longer-term goals are set during the planning process.
   ___ ⑤ Strongly agree ④ Agree ③ Somewhat ② Disagree ① Strongly disagree

Calculating your score — Questions 1-5 relate to your entire measurement system, so they are worth more than the rest of the questions. Add up the total for questions 1-5. A perfect score would be 25, if you answered Strongly Agree for all five questions. Write the total for questions 1-5 in the space below.

Proceed by adding up the total for questions 6-40. Next add up the total points for questions 41-50, and multiply this number by 2.

Add the three sub-totals to give yourself a grand total score. A perfect score on this assessment is 330, so if you ended up with more than that, go back and check your math.

Total questions 1-5 _____ X2 = _____
Total questions 6-40 _____ = _____
Total questions 41-50 _____ X2 = _____
Grand total = _____

Interpreting your score

Scores of 276 -330 — If your score on this survey ended up in this top band, you truly have a worldclass approach to measuring your organization's performance. You have narrowed down your database to a few key metrics and must have a well-balanced set of metrics. It also is evident that you actually use the data you collect to make decisions about improving organizational performance. Yours should be an organization that others benchmark for measurement.

Scores of 226-275 — If your score ended up in this second band you have a systematic approach to measurement that approaches being well-balanced. Chances are you are weak in measure of customer satisfaction and employee satisfaction, and may not do a good job of aggregating individual metrics into summary statistics, and analyzing the data to improve organizational performance. You have made a great deal of progress in improving your organization's approach to measurement. However, additional refinement is needed over time, and more research needs to be done to identify correlations between long-term measures such as customer satisfaction/ employee satisfaction and shorter-term measures such as financial performance. Being in this band probably means that your measurement system is better than 75-80 percent of organizations in North America.

Scores of 176-225 — A score in this range puts you in about the middle, which says that you are off to a good start in re-engineering your approach to measurement. You probably have a good set of measures for some of the seven boxes on an organization's score card. You also probably have some major weaknesses in some types of measures. You are probably strong in financial, operational, and product/service quality data, and weak in the other four areas. Chances are you still have too many measures, and

have inconsistencies across the different units/locations in your organization. A score in this range says that you are making some refinements in your approach to measurement, but still need to do quite a bit of work to put together a good solid measurement approach.

Scores of 175 or less — This puts you at the 50 percent or below level, which means that you are a long way from having a balanced score card. You're in good company at this level, however. In my experience, this is where most businesses are, and where almost all government and healthcare organizations are. Most business organizations are only just starting to measure customer satisfaction and employee satisfaction. Government and healthcare organizations are weak in these two areas, and also tend to be weak in product/service quality data and measures of supplier performance. Organizations that score at less than 50 percent on this survey probably still have not convinced upper management that strategic longer-term measures are just as important as the traditional financial and operational metrics.

A New Perspective for Statistics

Statistical theory is helpful for understanding differences between people and interactions between people; interactions between people and the system that they work in, or learn in.
—W. Edwards Deming[5]

Since all work is a process that exhibits variation, and quality aims for consistently excellent results, **quality improvement** can be defined as using the context of process-oriented thinking to:

• understand observed variation

• reduce unintended and inappropriate existing variation

• control the influence of detrimental outside variation, including uncontrolled variation in human behavior.

Statistics is the only sound theoretical basis for interpreting variation and coming to objective conclusions. However, it could be terribly misleading to use statistics on any data set unless one can answer the questions:

• What is the objective of these data?

• How were these data collected?

Analyses must be appropriate for the way the data were collected.

Also implicit in proper QI statistical applications is a proactive data strategy that considers *data to be the basis for action*. Unless the objective of data is clear, data collection can merely add cost without adding value, and statistical analysis can be inappropriate and misleading.

So, within the context of QI:

Statistics is the *art* and science of *collecting* and analyzing data.

Whether or not people understand statistics, they are already using statistics to interpret observed variation.

Every day, many decisions are made based on data, whether planned or unplanned, real or anecdotal, statistically analyzed or not. When people use data, they perceive, interpret, and react to observed variation in order to make a prediction. As will be

discussed shortly, the variation in a given situation is generally one of two types. It is a common error to mistake one for the other, and action based on this error actually *makes things worse*.

These concepts are summarized in the Data Inventory Considerations of Figure 4.4. Look at the data you work with every day. Can you answer the five questions? They can be the basis for discussion about your current measurement set.

Figure 4.4: Data Inventory Considerations

1. What is the **objective** of these data?

2. Is there an unambiguous **operational definition** to obtain a consistent numerical value for the process being measured?

   Is it **appropriate** for the objective?

3. How are these data **accumulated/collected**?

   Is the collection **appropriate** for the objective?

4. How are the data being **analyzed/displayed**?

   Is the analysis/display **appropriate**, given the way the data were collected?

5. What **action**, if any, is currently being taken with these data?

   Given the objective and action, is anything "wrong" with the current number?

Unfortunately, the framework within which statistics often is taught in academia incorrectly treats statistics as sets of techniques to perform on existing data sets. An (unaffectionate) acronym for this type of analysis is PARC. The letters in the acronym have a variety of meanings. Some examples are Practical Accumulated Records Compilation, Passive Analysis by Regression and Correlation, Profound Analysis by Relying on Computers, and Planning After Research Completed.

Of course, such acronyms exist for a reason. Service industries and medicine are flooded with data. The availability of databases and computers with "user-friendly" statistical packages generating literally thousands of reports gives people the illusion of knowledge and control of their processes. Analysis in this context generally gives a PARC analysis in reverse. Appropriate phrases might be Continuous

Recording of Administrative Procedures or Constant Repetition of Anecdotal Perceptions. The acronym and interpretation are left as an exercise for the reader.

One need not be a statistician to use statistics effectively in QI. The statistical thinking mindset involves four skills:

- Choosing and defining a problem/opportunity in a process/systems context

- Designing and managing *a series of* simple, efficient data collection processes to expose and assess variation

- Using graphical display methods which are understandable to persons at all levels: colleagues, management, and other staff

- Assessing interventions and maintaining gains.

Significant improvement can occur only when statistics are utilized in a framework of both appreciating a system and understanding its variation. Only such understanding can result in effective decisions based on planned data collection. Neither a focus solely on results nor arbitrarily imposed numerical goals or standards will improve a process.

Enumerative vs. Analytic Statistics

The statistics encountered by most people are known as **enumerative** methods. These include descriptive statistics (e.g., averages, standard deviations), hypothesis tests, using the normal distribution, and regression. This has created an incorrect impression that one can draw accurate conclusions by passive application of statistical techniques to huge, randomly accumulated data sets collected without objectives. It has also resulted in a tendency to display and use data through highly aggregated tables and descriptive statistical summaries. The objective of enumerative analyses is estimation, not predictive action. It is only through an **analytic** framework that the latter objective can be tested.

Enumerative studies are designed to freeze a process. They represent a snapshot in time. The objective is usually an estimate of the current state: no more, no less. Variation is seen as a "nuisance," clouding the "true" number. Any stated confidence level refers to the accuracy of the estimate. The United States census is a perfect example.

However, the processes we are trying to improve function continuously. The factor of time becomes a major consideration in the data planning and collection. Therefore, we use analytic statistics to assess the ongoing, continuous processes that produce these snapshots. The analytic process asks:

- Since these data reflect the process frozen at one moment in time, is it a typical snapshot?

- How does this snapshot relate to previous summaries? Is the process that produced the current data set the same as the process that produced previous data sets?

- What are the significant sources of variation?

- Do people agree on how these numbers should be measured?

- What can be predicted from these data?

The primary objective of analytic statistics is assessment of the stability of the process producing the data. Variation is a nuisance clouding whether an intervention is necessary or not. The obsessive accuracy of the number is not an issue. If the process is statistically stable (to be discussed in the next example), one can assess its current performance and take action either to predict future performance or to measure the effects of an improvement intervention.

Enumerative studies simply assume a stable process. Testing of stability is, in fact, *not even an objective.* The data are assumed "frozen" and have no time identity (a concept of great importance that will be discussed in the cardiac mortality example). The order in which the data are collected is typically ignored, and usually isn't even a consideration—a disastrous paradigm if data are collected for the predictive purposes of an analytic study.

Summary techniques for enumerative studies may not be appropriate for analytic studies. The difference between enumerative and analytic analyses is illustrated in Figures 4.5 and 4.6. Artificial data on cardiac mortality from three different clinics are plotted.

Figure 4.5 contains histograms (graphs showing the spread of the data) for each clinic. Each bar indicates the number of months with mortality in the range associated with that bar. For example, Clinic 1 had two months with 2 percent plus or minus 0.25 percent.

Figure 4.5: Histogram Comparison of Three Clinics - No Apparent Difference

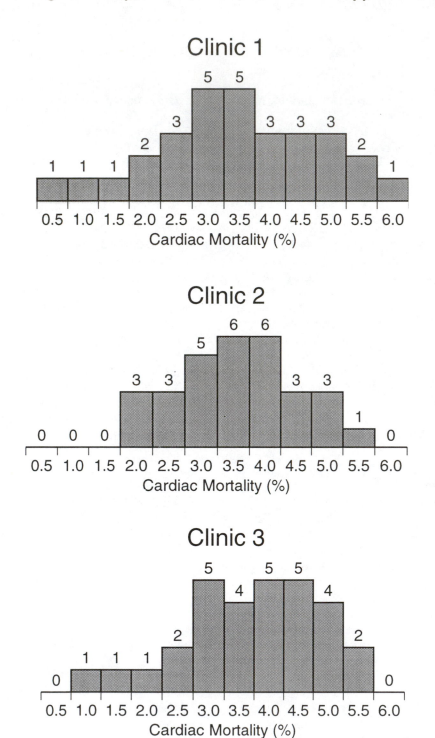

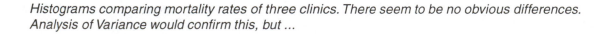

Histograms comparing mortality rates of three clinics. There seem to be no obvious differences.
Analysis of Variance would confirm this, but ...

Figure 4.6: Time Plot Comparison of Three Clinics - No Difference ?!

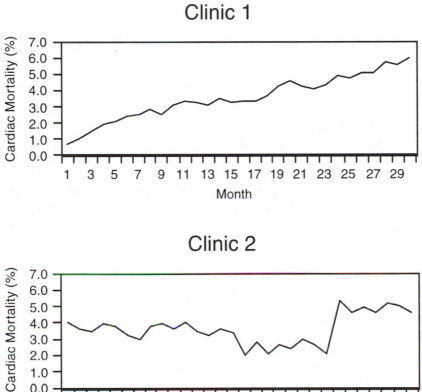

Clinic 1

Clinic 2

Clinic 3

Time plots of the same mortality rates from the three clinics. Now they can be seen to differ significantly.

The plots appear fairly similar. All have the familiar bell-shaped curve and seem to cover about the same range. A typical enumerative analysis such as analysis of variance or t-test would conclude no statistically significant differences among the three clinics. The analysis assumes that each data set comes from a stable process, which leads to the incorrect conclusion that the clinics exhibit no difference.

If "prediction of future mortality" were the objective presented to prospective buyers, the time order of the data becomes important. Looking at plots of the data in time sequence for each process (Figure 4.6), would you reach the same conclusion? No difference?! Clinic 1 increases during the entire time period and Clinic 2 is subject to abrupt shifts. Clinic 3, while highly variable, appears to be stable over time.

After looking at the time order plots, do "averages" for Clinics 1 and 2 have any meaning at all? In fact, the appropriate answer to the question, What is the average of Clinic 2? is When?! Over the time period of the data collection, Clinic 2 had three distinct averages. What can you predict about future performance?

Typical enumerative "stats," e.g., average, standard deviation, etc., are inappropriate for the processes from Clinics 1 and 2. The process from Clinic 3 is stable and can be summarized in its current form. That does not mean it is necessarily the most desirable process, only that its current performance can be accurately assessed. Suppose these were presented as three "one-point summaries," i.e., the past averages of three different health systems and their cardiac mortality, or other key results? Would you prefer to make a decision with the one-point summaries or the plots of monthly results? Which summary allows you to ask more meaningful follow-up questions?

It is a much higher yield strategy, after observing the time plots, to ask questions about Clinics 1 and 2. What changes were made during this time? The nature of the plots would result in different questions. Have any gains been held? Is Clinic 3 even capable of achieving desired, consistent results? What is different about their individual processes and practice environments? What is different about their results? Additional data will be needed to answer these questions.

Rather than relying on single-number summaries of huge, aggregated, random samples, the analytic framework ensures predictive stability by using smaller samples taken more frequently over time. Ignoring the time element implicit in every data set can lead to incorrect statistical conclusions. Applications of descriptive and enumerative statistics (e.g., averages, standard deviations) to an unstable process are invalid.

In a healthcare context, contrast the questions each type of statistical analysis would ask:

Descriptive: "What can be said about this **patient**?"

Enumerative: "What can be said about this **group** of patients?"

Analytic: "What can be said about the **process** that produced this group of patients?"

Whenever presented with a data summary, one should ask, What was the objective of these data? How were these data defined and collected? What action is being contemplated? A good rule of thumb is to make no decision that you would also not make by looking at a time plot of the data.

Common and Special Causes

The different patterns in the time plots from Figure 4.6 demonstrate the key concepts of common and special causes of variation.

All processes vary. Some of the variation is inherent in the system. Numbers differ for whatever reason, but there is no discernible pattern in the data—the variation appears to be random. This inherent variation is called **common cause** and is present to some degree in all processes.

The process of flipping coins and counting the number of "heads" is a simple example. Suppose 50 people in a room each have a coin, and at a signal, they simultaneously flip them. Some sample data are plotted in Figure 4.7. The average number should be 25. However, when the process is repeated, successive flips don't yield exactly 25 every time. It can be shown statistically that the number of heads would usually be between 18 and 32, and occasionally could extend as far as 14 or 36.

Suppose we didn't know the probability of heads. The enumerative framework would try to estimate the "true" value, i.e., 25. The analytic frame would evaluate the sequence of heads to see whether it represents a consistent process and to make predictions.

Figure 4.7: Plot of Coin Flip Data

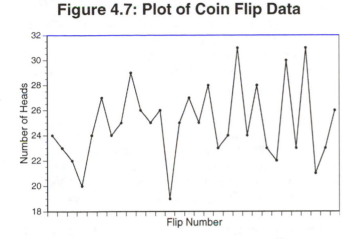

Figure 4.8: Plot of Coin Flip Data Before and After Process Change

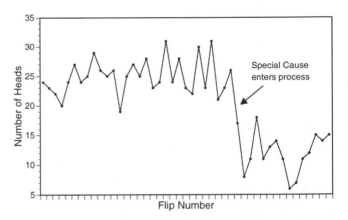

Another type of variation comes from outside the system and causes noticeable shifts or trends in the data. This type of variation is called **special cause**. For example, a special cause is acting on Clinic 1 and causing its output to steadily increase. Special causes entered Clinic 2's process after observations 15 and 23, causing the output to shift. Special causes are not necessarily present in all processes —Clinic 3 shows no signs of special causes. A simple technique for statistically assessing stability will be discussed in Chapter 7.

Returning to the coin flipping example, suppose a special cause enters and the process changes. People are told to flip their coin twice, and only those obtaining heads on both flips will be tallied. These data are plotted in Figure 4.8. With this process, the numbers will fall in the range of 4 to 21. How long would it take for an observer of the data to detect the change? Note that this range (4-21) overlaps the range of the previous process (14-36), so it may not be immediately obvious.

Enumerative analyses would not detect this difference, and instead may focus on determining the number of flips necessary to get a good estimate. Unbeknownst to the study designers, the estimate would be contaminated and invalid due to the special cause. What if the U.S. census was half-complete and an incident comparable to the famous flu epidemic suddenly broke out? The census is reported as if the final data were collected in one day. In reality, it makes the assumption that each day is "typical."

The analytic perspective is less concerned with the actual value, and more interested in the process stability. Once the process has achieved stability, enumerative statistics are appropriate.

Chapters 6, 7, and 8 will discuss common and special cause variation in the context of several examples. Through the application of simple statistical theory, identification, interpretation, and appropriate strategies for handling each variation type will be demonstrated. There will also be discussion of the consequences of inappropriate action. For now, suffice it to say that a process with only common cause is predictable within limits, although it is impossible to predict where any individual result will lie within those limits. The limits may or may not be acceptable to one's pre-conceived desires.

Special causes may occur randomly and make a process virtually unpredictable at any future time period. How can one determine whether this has happened?

Understanding the difference between common and special causes is crucial to statistical thinking. The strategy for improvement is very different for processes with special causes than it is for processes with only common causes of variation.

Think of the three clinics. The strategy for Clinics 1 and 2 is to identify the specific events or special causes that created the patterns in the data. Those which had a negative impact should be eliminated, and those with a positive impact should be incorporated. Finally, a strategy should be in place to hold and maintain the gains at a desirable level. Subsequent graphing of data would assess intervention efforts.

The strategy for Clinic 3 is not a matter of finding specific events, but rather understanding and discovering hidden opportunities for improvement. Studying and comparing the individual data points would be a no-yield strategy. Inappropriate action due to the failure to distinguish between common and special causes will generally make things worse.

Enumerative statistics do not make sense on processes with special causes because they assume a predictable process. Analytic statistics, by looking at the process, attempt to identify special causes and suggest strategies to make the process more predictable.

QI vs. Clinical Trial Research: Unstable and Stable Environments

Most physicians' experiences with statistics are through clinical trials, which use enumerative methods to analyze results. Enumerative methods are appropriate for clinical trials where all six of the process inputs are heavily controlled to minimize variation. The difference in "methods" between control and treatment groups is deliberately varied. This variation is created with the assumption that any observed variation in outputs is due to that factor only. *Creation of a stable process is inherent in the methodology.* Clinical studies take place over time, but great lengths are taken to "freeze" the lurking presence of outside influences. It is assumed that nothing will change over time. The data collection and "measurements" are well-planned, and the analyses are appropriate to the processes. Variation due to the remaining process inputs: people, machines, materials, and environment, is minimized through the choice of patients, trial protocol and clinical centers. This deliberate (and necessary) minimization is quite expensive.

After the clinical trial, however, the results are applied in an environment in which the investigators' control over the situation is lost. Variations in both practice and individual environments can compromise the quality of the trial's results. Unintended human variation in interpretation of the protocol and in patients chosen for the treatment add variation through Deming's Funnel Rule 4, which paraphrased is, "Treat each patient with what worked for the previous one."[4] Scientifically, the result is random movement continuing further away from the original result, also known as a "random walk" or in physics, "Brownian motion."

While clinical trials generate useful innovative medical treatments, attempts to impose their enumerative form of statistical analysis in a real world practice environment can have dangerously misleading results. In our dynamic work situations, QA's enumerative framework is not necessarily valid to summarize and compare the relative performance of events in several environments. This is especially true if the environments themselves have contributed unintended variation, typically a positive "spin," to the measurement. One-number summaries are not accurate when unstable processes tend to be the rule and not the exception.

In the real world, variation is a fact of life and must be taken into consideration when planning. To make better predictions and decisions, analytic statistics must be used to assess deviations from expected process results and pinpoint sources of variation. The objective of each analysis is to answer the questions, Have we created a stable process where the proposed gains are uniformly achieved and held? and Are there further opportunities for improvement? The six sources of problems with a process (Figure 3.5) should be used as a guide. If serious variation is observed, one must investigate the process producing it to see whether the variation could possibly be appropriate given the inputs to the process.

When Is Variation Appropriate?

There are times when variation from special causes is inevitable and quite appropriate for the situation. Suppose data show mortality rates to be unusually high for one cardiologist. A typical assumption is that her treatment "methods" are different (and by implication, worse) than the other cardiologists. Remember though, methods are only one input to a process. If she is a highly-regarded specialist who gets the "toughest" and "nearly hopeless" cases, her mortality rate is likely to be higher than other physicians because the "people" inputs to her process are different.

Special causes in data show only that things (processes) are different. They allow people to ask the right questions. Not all variation is bad or undesirable, but we are better off at least being aware of it, and possibly making a conscious decision to take no action.

Summary

Statistical thinking through process focus is the key to continuous improvement. A summary appears in Figure 4.9. The role of statistics is to enhance prediction by:

- understanding existing variation

- reducing inappropriate and unintended variation in a context of systems thinking

- controlling the detrimental influence of outside variation.

The traditional educational emphasis on enumerative methods has been well-meaning but misguided.

Enumerative methods focus solely on process outputs and implicitly assume that the data come from a stable process. Their objective is assessment, and they are often not appropriate for prediction. Unless there is awareness and evaluation of the stability of the process inputs, improper inferences about causation can result. Unstable processes tend to be the rule, not the exception. Even analytic methods will tend to be marginally effective when used without appreciation for the fact that a process is producing the observed data.

Whether or not people understand statistics, they are already using statistics. It is not necessary for everyone to become a statistician to participate in a QI effort. However, everyone must become aware of the continuous presence of variation and how to deal with it.

4

Figure 4.9: Summary of Process-Oriented Thinking

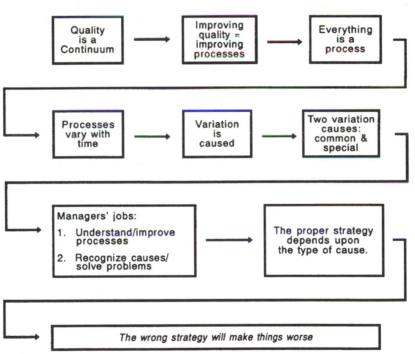

Notes to Chapter Four

1.   Hacquebord H. "Health care from the perspective of a patient: Theories for improvement".

2.   Brown, MG. "Is Your Measurement System Well-Balanced?"

3.   Rummler GA and Brache AP. "Improving Performance".

4.   Brown, MG. "Is Your Measurement System Well-Balanced?"

5.   Neave HR. *The Deming Dimension*.

Chapter Five
Some Human Factors—Overcoming Resistance to Change

Key Ideas

- Work exists as a cultural pattern.

- Any change has implicit social consequences which can create problems in the culture.

- The reasons initially given for resistance may not be the root reasons.

- Change has a deliberate pace. Allow sufficient time for it to happen.

- Use Juran's "Rules of the Road" to help overcome resistance.

Introduction

Up to now we've aimed our focus mostly toward Juran's diagnostic journey discussed in chapter 2. It is now time to turn our attention to the remedial journey, and in particular, resistance to change.

Figure 5.1 gives more detail about the steps in the remedial journey as shown previously in Figure 2.3. This chapter addresses the issue of resistance to change. Chapter 7 goes into more detail about holding the improvement gains.

Figure 5.1: Remedial Journey—A Breakthrough in Behavior

Standardization
- Overcome cultural resistance to change
- Use Juran's "Rules of the Road"
- Ongoing training
- Formal documentation

Hold gains
- Data collection to assess ongoing current state of process

Change Would Be Easy If It Weren't for All The People

Many QI projects come to excellent solutions only to mysteriously return to the same problems six months later. An obvious beneficial remedy to a situation should create no problems. However, an unexpected backlash of delaying tactics or outright rejection of the remedy often occurs. These come from various sources: a manager, the workforce, an external customer, or a union. The reasons given for resistance may seem quite puzzling, senseless, or even illogical to the advocates of the change. Many times resistance comes from the very people who will benefit from the change!

Because improvement means change, resistance to change must be considered in each improvement plan in order to bring about effective, lasting improvement.

Juran[1] has done extensive study of the resistance phenomenon and named it "cultural resistance to change." He has identified two elements common to all change:

1) The change itself (usually technological)

2) A social consequence of the change.

The social consequence of change is usually the source of resistance because it is an "uninvited guest" in the culture. Figure 5.2 contains key factors in resistance to change. It is critical to understand and plan for the nature of the social consequence of any change.

5

Figure 5.2: Why People Resist Change[2]

Loss of Control	Change requires people to go from being on top of things to being unsure and out of control. Change is exciting when done by us, threatening when done to us.
Too Much Uncertainty	The future is not obvious and every day it feels like you are about to walk off a cliff. Simply not knowing enough makes comfort impossible.
Surprise, Surprise!	We like novelty, but hate surprises. People are easily shocked by decisions sprung on them without groundwork or preparation.
The "Difference" Effect	Habits are efficient, effective, and mindless. Changing abruptly to new habits and ways of doing things is uncomfortable, because we notice the differences from our previous pattern.
Loss of Face	If accepting a change means admitting that things were done incorrectly in the past, people are certain to resist.
Concern for Competence	People always question their ability to master the new. "Can I do it or will I get fired?" Sometimes new ways require new skills that people don't have.
Ripple Effects	Change sometimes disrupts plans, projects, or family activities that have nothing to do with the job. Anticipation of these disruptions causes resistance.
More Work	Change involves more energy, more time and greater stress. People may not want to put forth the effort.
Past Resentments	Unresolved grievances from the past can hamper the change effort. The cobwebs of the past get in the way of the future.
The Threat is Real	Sometimes a change creates winners and losers. People may lose status, power, and comfort because of a change.

Work as a Cultural Pattern

As an organization grows and matures, its culture develops patterns. Change is difficult when these patterns are disrupted. Society is defined as a continuing body of human beings engaged in common purposes. Without exception, all human societies exhibit cultural patterns—habits, status, beliefs, traditions, practices. These patterns stem from real needs of law and order: to defend the society against danger, to explain mysterious phenomena, and to continue the perpetuation of the society itself. Once a pattern is established, all members are "taught" the accepted pattern of behavior, and new members must conform to this pattern or face unpleasant consequences.

The cultural pattern is a stabilizer and reinforces existing emotional boundaries. We count on the pattern's predictability for comfort. Any change is perceived as a threat to this predictability and must be examined in light of what threat it poses to the culture.

All proposed improvement solutions must be evaluated in the context of the question, What threats will this change pose to our organization's cultural pattern? It is certain that the organization's members will make precisely such an evaluation! Because proposed change comes from the change advocate's cultural perspective, it seems perfectly logical *to the advocate*, but not necessarily to another context or culture.

Simple awareness of the existence of cultural resistance is necessary but not sufficient to overcome it. One must discover precisely what—which habits, whose status, and what beliefs—are threatened by proposed changes.

The "Stated" Reasons vs. the "Real" Reasons

One must listen carefully to those whose work lives will be affected by a change. Their reasons for resistance tend to be a mixture of stated reasons and unstated real reasons hidden in the psychology of the culture. While some of the stated reasons are true concerns, they can also contain distracting baggage that masks deeper issues.

Stated reasons for resistance may include:
- specific points of a change
- concern for another person
- issues about safety or quality.

These are all legitimate considerations. However, the *real* reasons may be concerns about the individual's status, security, respect, and stress level. A complicating factor is that the mixture of stated and real reasons applies to *both* the advocates of change as well as the members of the work culture that change will affect.

Any team proposing a solution should consider whom the solution will affect, how they will be affected, and how they are likely to react. To understand, ask:

- Are people being asked to perform new, unfamiliar tasks?

- Are they being asked to work harder, do someone else's job, or take on additional (or fewer) levels of responsibility?

- Are they losing autonomy?

- Will employees lose contact with long-time associates and/or need to interact with new people?

- Will daily work schedules and activities, including lunch and break times, need to change?

Depending on the proposed solution, the reactions can include fear, hostility, overt resistance, passive resistance, and stress.

The "Rules of the Road"

Faith Ralston developed a useful model (Figure 5.3) for implementing cultural change. It places strong emphasis on identifying and acknowledging personal feelings and business needs. While individuals may perceive a conflict between the two, if business needs are separated from personal needs, and facts are separated from feelings, the chance of success is significantly greater.

Figure 5.3: A Model for Implementing Cultural Change[3]

> 1. Acknowledge the presence of strong feelings.
>
> 2. Clarify individual feelings and needs.
>
> 3. Identify and respect the needs of the business.
>
> 4. Create a win-win solution for individuals and the organization.
>
> 5. Be truthful and compassionate in the process.

Juran provides clarity on these points. He has studied the recommendations of several anthropologists and developed guidelines for implementation of a solution. The rules are quite simple, relevant to any improvement effort, and can have a profound impact on improvement planning, piloting, and implementation.

1) Provide participation.

We have all been, at one time or another, a victim of NIH (Not Invented Here). Resistance often results when key participants in a process are not meaningfully involved in both the planning and implementation of the change. Soliciting ideas from participants throughout the improvement process helps them develop ownership in the change and facilitate its eventual acceptance. Providing participation during data collections and sharing results make the project goings-on less of a surprise. If the solution can be kept at a general enough level, the participants (the culture) should help design its details, since they know the actual situation the best. This ensures a smoother and more successful pilot.

This is especially important with clinical leaders, who are often mistakenly left out of "administrative" improvements. One coding project site found that when physician leadership was actively involved, the team was able to successfully implement change, while a very similar team working on the same process without physician leadership was not.

2) Provide sufficient time.

Change cannot be rushed. People need time to change. They must evaluate the merits of the change in relation to their habits, status, and beliefs. There is always the additional need to develop or negotiate an accommodation with the proposed change.

Start small. Always pilot a proposed change on a small scale. This reduces risk and facilitates acceptance by proponents of *both* the new and old ways. Pilots have the additional benefit of containing unforeseen "bugs" in the process that would cause untold damage to the project if rolled out and experienced on a larger scale. They also provide another opportunity for the culture to evaluate and accept the change.

Avoid surprises. Cultures thrive on predictability and continuity. Sudden surprises are shocking and disturb the peace. Maintain constant communication at all levels and allow appropriate time for adequate planning.

Choose the appropriate time for change. Are too many other changes going on? Is there negative "fall out" from previous QI efforts? Will current relations with management sabotage this effort before it is begun?

3) Keep solutions free of excess baggage.

Solutions should address deep, root causes. Only so much change can be absorbed at one time. A typical resistance strategy is to distract from the major issue by focusing on the "baggage," not the basic merits of the proposal. Acknowledge that many issues will be addressed during the improvement process, but continually redirect attention and energy toward the root cause.

4) Work with the recognized informal leadership of the culture. Which front-line workers have earned the respect of their colleagues?

5) Treat people with dignity and understand their position.

Listen actively, ask for input, respond seriously and directly to input provided.

6) Name the resistance for what it is and deal directly with it.

Demonstrate flexibility and change specific objectives that can either benefit or have a neutral effect on the solution.

7) Offer a quid pro quo: in exchange for their support, offer those affected something in trade that they value. The trade does not have to be related to the change!

Mountain States Employers Council, Inc. has developed a similar set of strategies which are listed in Figure 5.4.

Figure 5.4: Strategies For Making Change Happen[4]

- Involve as many people as you can in the change-planning process. Participation leads to ownership and enthusiasm.

- Communicate clearly—and often—the vision of what you are trying to achieve, and give people as much detail as you can.

- Divide the implementation of change into manageable, digestible steps. Make the steps as familiar as possible. Keep the first steps small and easy to insure success.

- Give people advance notice and a chance to readjust their thinking.

- Let commitment grow—don't ask for a pledge of allegiance to new, untried ways.

- Going forward may mean going back. Let people air past resentments and reach closure.

- Make clear what is expected of people after the change. Carefully and fully communicate standards and requirements.

- Reward achievement and effort. When people try the new ways, reward them. When people succeed at the new ways, reward them. Reward progress, don't expect perfection.

- Seek out those who learn and succeed early in the change. Use these people as positive examples. Acknowledge their successes publicly. Use them as role models.

- Provide the extra resources and training people need to adapt to something new. Change takes extra time, extra energy, extra support. Make it available.

- Anticipate the fact that some people will be losers. Be honest and compensate that loss. Keep the losses from being so obvious to people.

- Celebrate the past. Don't bad-mouth what was. Allow time for expressions of grief, nostalgia, loss. Bury the past with honor...then build a sense of excitement and anticipation about the future.

- Minimize or reduce the number of differences introduced by the change, leaving as many habits and routines as possible in place. Make people comfortable.

- Introduce change with flexibility so people can make transitions without major disruptions in other areas of their lives. Give people choices.

Beyond a Project Context

When undertaking a quality improvement effort, meeting customers' expectations (both internal and external) for service and product performance becomes an organization's central focus. John Grinnell[5] argues that beneath the measurable quality targets of the product or service lie six sublevels of quality that must first be considered. These sublevels get progressively more fundamental, with the first three considered the "engine" of the organization and the remaining three considered the "fuel" for that engine.

Most efforts are spent on the first three, yet note how levels four through six are set up to tap hidden human energy: energy lost to poor self-esteem and poor interpersonal and interdepartmental relationships. The six levels address the problem of resistance in a more macro context, which will ultimately benefit project implementations. (Emotional issues are also implicit in the third level because people are not necessarily trained to manage their ego reactions to feedback in healthy ways.)

1. Quality of doing — the processes employees use to do their jobs.

    Focusing on processes, not outcomes. "Results orientation" typically makes employees work harder to do what they've always done, which is fruitless. Working smarter implies learning. "Doing" is the result of many human-system factors.

2. Quality of thinking and decision-making that supports the "doing."

    Refining thinking skills will sharpen decision-making capability. Many of the traditional quality tools do just that. Focusing just on tools, however, as has been the experience in many quality efforts, ignores the other five sublevels.

3. Quality of information that influences employees' thinking.

    The generation and successful flow of information affect employees' thinking and decision-making. This should include statistical feedback from technical and administrative processes. Again, this is the tendency, but it is not enough.

    Accurate, timely, and useful interpersonal feedback from employees who work in the processes daily is also needed. However, people usually are not trained to manage their ego reactions in healthy ways, and dysfunctional processes of communication develop and perpetuate. "Canned" approaches tend to minimize conflict, but conflict must be seen as a basis for learning.

    It is imperative to deal directly with the interpersonal barriers that clog the information flow between people and between organizations. By deftly bringing to the surface and addressing people problems, fear and defensiveness within the organization will be reduced.

4. Quality of relationships through which the information flows.

    Within the human system, relationships are the conduits through which information flows. The degree to which the human system is emotionally blocked by a bad relationship will determine the amount, quality, and timeliness of information flow between people. The human system approach is to bring interpersonal problems to the surface and deal with them in a way that does not put blame on those involved. New, mature skills are needed to overcome long-standing cultural patterns.

5. Quality of perceptions and feelings that influence employees' relationships with others.

    The quality of relationships rests on how people perceive others. It takes great efforts to defuse negative situations by getting feedback, becoming aware, choosing to change behavior, and acting differently. It takes time and great discipline to alter perceptions and behavior patterns.

6. Quality of mind-sets — the operating beliefs and values that employees bring to service processes.

    Beneath perceptions lie deeper psychological structures of beliefs and values *that are learned early in life* as a child or adolescent. They virtually determine perceptions and business decisions made as an adult and also affect relationships. When these unexamined beliefs are threatened by information contrary to conscious or unconscious beliefs, defensive behavior results, which keeps one close to the familiar and safe status quo. This will sabotage needed learning, change, and improvement.

A needed catalyst in a quality effort is for everyone to have awareness of his or her beliefs and values and be prepared to alter them to accomplish a task or human interaction. Awareness can be defined as the ability to stand outside (or be intellectually and emotionally detached from) a system to view, and thereby understand, it. This is extremely difficult to master and requires time as well as listening to and assimilating feedback. An excellent practical framework and skill set for dealing with this issue, "Gaining Control, the Franklin Reality Model," is available through Franklin International Institute, Inc. It features Hyrum Smith, a dynamic speaker who deals with human behavior in a way that puts the emphasis on people's <u>behavior</u>, not the people themselves. It depersonalizes issues and minimizes the risk of defensive responses. As Smith makes clear, *it is what's going on anyway*, so let's "name" it and get on with it for the good of everyone involved. If allowed to continue, the company's long-term needs will not be met.

Summary

"People don't resist change, they just resist being changed." The psychology of cultural change is not trivial. In any QI effort, there are two aspects to change:

1) the overall cultural philosophical change required by a QI approach

2) changes caused by implementation of specific project solutions.

The concept of a work culture that thrives on predictability can help to explain the many reasons for resistance to change and improvement. You will get many stated reasons, but real reasons often have to do with perceived value and status in the current culture. The "rules of the road" are useful and clear for managing resistance.

Management must both demonstrate the expected change and reward those behaviors in their staff.

Although beyond the scope of this book, societal change is exploding at an unprecedented pace. This is no doubt causing cultural "angst" in every organization. An extremely valuable book, *Thinking in the Future Tense*, has been written by Jennifer James, a cultural anthropologist. It is witty, intellectually exciting, and highly practical. She also has a video series.

Another valuable resource is the video "Just GET It!" by Morris Massey. Whereas Jennifer James takes an anthropological approach, Massey takes a sociological approach that rests on the coexistence of several layers of society. Each has been shaped by different events, which has implications for both workplace relationships and customer relationships.

Both videos cited in the previous two paragraphs are listed in the Bibliography.

5

Notes to Chapter Five

1. Juran JM. *Managerial Breakthrough: A New Concept of the Manager's Job.*

2. Sandberg J. "Why People Resist Change."

3. Ralston F. *Hidden Dynamics.*

4. Sandberg J. "Strategies for Making Things Happen."

5. Grinnell JR. "Optimize the Human System."

Chapter Six
Data Skills I: Understanding Current Processes Using the QI Process

Key Ideas

- Data currently collected are often not the data necessary for improvement.

- Data necessary for improvement are frequently available, but not currently collected.

- Any improvement situation should use data collection to isolate and focus the effort on a major opportunity.

- Improvement opportunities break down into the "vital few" and the "useful many." Formal projects should result from the "vital few;" the "useful many" need to be integrated into normal work or less formal projects.

- Stratification helps identify special causes and localize future data collection. Further data collection may identify special causes within the common cause system.

- Data collection for improvement is a disturbance of the work culture and therefore must be simple and efficient. To minimize the disturbances, there is a sequential strategy of data aggressiveness.

- The set of six sources of problems with a process (from Chapter 3) is the underlying foundation of most effective improvement sequences. This foundation drives all data collection and use of statistical tools.

Introduction

Processes are repetitive procedures with potentially measurable data as outputs. The process flowcharting work that begins a QI project generates key questions which further define data collection needs.

There is no such thing as a one-time "broad-brush" special data collection that gives all the answers. (This type of temporary data collection sometimes becomes "permanently temporary.") Knowledge about a process or situation increases through a *sequential* process of successive, small, simple, well-defined data collections designed to address variation exposed by preceding sets of data.

People often are unaware of the wealth of data they could easily capture in their daily work. Consequently, they do not generate the data they really need for improvement. Reconsider the five questions posed by Berwick, initially presented in Chapter 2, and reprinted here. After each question, some follow-up questions suggest data that, if collected, may clarify the situation.

1) "Do you ever waste time waiting, when you should not have to?"

   Exactly how long, how often, and under what circumstances? What accounts for the bulk of it? What about time wasted in meetings? Does it happen to anyone else?

2) "Do you ever redo your work because something failed the first time?"

   Which things? What accounts for the bulk of it? How often? What percent of your total work time does it take? Does it happen to anyone else?

3) "Do the procedures you use waste steps, duplicate efforts, or frustrate you through their unpredictability?"

   Which procedures? Are there a few procedures that cause the bulk of this rework? What caused the need for such procedures? What have you noticed as a result of these procedures? Does it happen to anyone else?

4) "Is information that you need ever lost?"

   Which information? What accounts for the bulk of it? How often? What happens as a result? Does it happen to anyone else?

5) "Does communication ever fail?"

   Exactly what does this mean? What observable events does this cause? Does it happen to anyone else?

6

The data suggested by the follow-up questions are not the type of data normally collected in an organization. The data needed to run a business are often quite different from the data needed to improve its processes. However, when operating in a pre-QI environment, the business data are the only data that exist.

The medication error example discussed in this chapter demonstrates the **Pareto principle**. The principle described in detail in the sidebar is critical to improvement efforts. The example shows how the Pareto principle can be used in conjunction with the concepts of special and common causes of variation to identify major improvement opportunities. These simple concepts are the primary guide for designing many data collections. The example incorporates these concepts into a process that uses existing data or simple data collection strategies. From an initially vague project definition, this process isolates and localizes major improvement opportunities.

A series of data collections and the questions they generate demonstrate a powerful statistical technique: exposing major sources of process variation by stratifying data along their process inputs. A significant source of variation is identified by isolating special causes. This allows specific action to focus on solving the problem. The example illustrates how simple analysis of an existing work situation can yield significant improvement through focused, simple, efficient data collection.

The Pareto Principle

In the 1920s, Juran noticed that when faced with an improvement opportunity, 80 percent of the observed variation was generally caused by only 20 percent of the process inputs. For example:

- 20 percent of the customers usually account for 80 percent of the sales.

- 20 percent of one's expenses probably account for 80 percent of one's monthly checking statement, either individually or by class.

- 20 percent of the types of food bought make up 80 percent of one's food bill.

- 20 percent of a company's products produce 80 percent of its sales.

- 80 percent of an organization's "quality problems" are due to 20 percent of the potential improvement opportunities.

- 20 percent of the diagnoses classes represented or 20 percent of the physician's panel of patients account for 80 percent of a physician's practice activity.

Juran called this phenomenon the **Pareto principle**, after a renaissance Italian economist who studied the distribution of wealth.

QI uses this principle to its fullest advantage. When studying an improvement opportunity, doesn't it make sense to isolate and attack the 20 percent of the variation causing 80 percent of the problem? This gives the greatest return on investment of precious time.

Juran calls the 20 percent the "vital few" and the others the "trivial many" or more recently, the "useful many." It should be emphasized that these problems are most assuredly not trivial to the people who must work in those situations. They are trivial only in terms of their current impact on the entire organization. As the more significant opportunities for improvement are solved, some of these "trivial" opportunities will either be addressed in the context of a larger problem or eventually become "vital."

The "vital few" are generally long-standing, perennial opportunities that have never been solved despite repeated efforts. Their root causes are deeply entrenched in the culture of interconnected processes of many departments, and they will require more formal and higher level guidance and participation to be addressed, including that of top management. Their solution processes will be lengthy and require patience and persistence. However, the solutions should have a significant impact on organizational culture.

The "useful many" are important to individuals. However, because of their sheer number, there is a common tendency for them to distract teams from their primary tasks. This is particularly true if the team's mission is not clear. The useful many take just as much time to solve as the more significant problems, but with less value to the organization. The best reminder is that "There is no such thing as improvement in general." The goal must be to expose and focus, and then further focus on a major opportunity.

What About the Useful Many?

If all of the organization is educated in statistical thinking and awareness of processes and customers, the existing work teams can form *informal* "task teams" (generally intradepartmental) of two to three months', duration to work on these problems. In other words, "working on their work" should become a routine part of people's daily jobs. These projects are very important for educational purposes. They empower people by giving them proof that they are making a difference in the organization as well as solving a frustrating work problem, thus providing people with more joy in their current job.

These task teams should be ad hoc. Forcing them to become part of an organization's "quality machinery" drains their inherent energy by bogging down a seemingly spontaneous effort in dreadful formality. Ideally, QI becomes the organization's work culture, existing in parallel with the necessarily more formal higher level improvement efforts. Managers and supervisors are part of this culture, communicating with each other through an informal network to share results with other similar groups in the organization.

The Medication Error Problem

Part 1

A hospital pharmacy instituted a quality program. A Pareto analysis of "cost of poor quality" data gathered over a year showed that medication errors represented a significant improvement opportunity. The six pharmacists were informed of this, told of the potential impact on the organization, and instructed to be extra careful in their jobs. They were given a goal: reduce errors by half over the next year with a target of at least a 10-15 percent reduction per quarter. Data collected during the next month produced a baseline of 70 errors. To help the pharmacists, a "challenge" was issued—their first month with less than 50 errors would be rewarded with a free pizza lunch. The next three months yielded 63, 60, and 75 errors, respectively.

Questions about Part 1

1) How are they doing relative to their goal?

2) What are your comments regarding this program?

3) Do you have any questions or further suggestions?

Commentary on Part 1

1) How does one correctly interpret the sequence of numbers 70, 63, 60, 75 when the goal is "at least 10-15 percent reduction per quarter?" Statistically there is only one interpretation (to be explained in Chapter 7), but there easily could be as many general interpretations as there are people reading this.

While the goal intuitively seems to make sense, the lack of an operational definition makes it difficult to really interpret and enforce. Does the 10-15 percent reduction per quarter mean that the year-to-date quarterly average should be 10-15 percent below the baseline? Does it mean that every future quarter should be 10-15 percent below the baseline? Does it mean that all future quarters should be 10-15 percent below their preceding quarters? Everyone at one time has been a participant in a well-meaning management program like this, issued as a relatively friendly albeit serious challenge. When it comes time to report results, it's easy to mold one's figures to fit such a "squishy" goal.

2) Undesirable variation (errors) was observed consistently, so management decided to do something about it. They apparently felt that telling people to "do their best" and reporting their performance by measuring the process outputs would eventually improve the process. As explained in Chapter 3, people are not the only type of input to a process. There are five others to consider as well (methods, machines, materials, measurements and environment).

3) By telling all the pharmacists to do their best, management is making the implicit assumption that everyone is contributing more or less equally to the problem. In other words, they are assuming all the variation is due to common causes.

How could this assumption be tested? Should errors be traced to individual pharmacists? While this approach could generate useful information, it must be taken with the objective of further questioning the work processes, and not a search to "shoot the offenders."

If this information were to identify special causes among the pharmacists, what should those pharmacists do differently? Think about how a program for improvement based on special causes could affect daily interactions among the pharmacists.

Part 2

Some of the pharmacists complained that they were already doing "above average" work–it wasn't their fault the goal wasn't achieved. Management was also concerned about the disturbing "upturn" to 75 at the end of the quarter. During the next month they established traceability of the errors to individual pharmacists. This is an example of **stratification** of a process output by the input of "people." During the month, 85 (!) errors occurred and were detailed as follows:

Pharmacist A:	8 errors
Pharmacist B:	27 errors
Pharmacist C:	2 errors
Pharmacist D:	4 errors
Pharmacist E:	40 errors
Pharmacist F:	4 errors

These data were presented to the pharmacists. Some of those with above average performance felt vindicated. However, despite the exposure of two special causes, management still was not pleased by the total of 85 and stated that this trend must stop. They added the "incentive" that if the trend continued in the next month, the pharmacists' upcoming raises would be delayed and Pharmacists B and E's raises even further delayed until they could exhibit "above average" performance for two months in a row. Management asked the pharmacists to help each other by working as a team.

Questions about Part 2

1) How do things look relative to the goal?

2) What are your comments on this data process?

3) What about the action taken?

4) Further questions or suggestions?

Commentary on Part 2

1) Management is concerned about the increase in errors over the past two months. Things don't look good relative to the goal. Again, management is making an implicit assumption. In this case they assume that the increases to 75 and 85 errors are due to special causes. In other words, this interpretation represents the belief that the process has truly changed each month.

   A common cause perspective would hold that the work process did not change. The varying numbers over the months were due to variation inherent in the process itself, e.g., the coin flipping example from Chapter 4.

   Is the variation over time due to common causes or are there special causes present as well? Chapter 7 will discuss run charts and control charts that can help make this distinction.

2) The data collection method seems to have been useful. If the errors were equally distributed, i.e., common cause, one would have expected approximately 15 errors per pharmacist. However, intuition (in this case correct) says that Pharmacist B's 27 errors and Pharmacist E's 40 errors are not even close to 15. Thus, their error rates differ from the other pharmacists' due to special causes. They seem to have different work processes, *for whatever reason*. Their work processes exhibit excessive, undesirable variation from the rest of the department. These numbers are consistent with the Pareto Principle. Two pharmacists (33 percent) account for 79 percent of the errors.

Note that if all pharmacists made approximately 15 errors, the variation among pharmacists would be due only to common causes and would range from 3 to 26. It then would be a mistake to say that the one with the fewest mistakes performed better than the one with the most, since it would essentially be random luck that generated the numbers. The next month could see a complete turnaround with no changes in the process. (Think of people flipping coins 50 times each and ranking them by the number of "heads." With numbers ranging from 14 to 36, this could be done easily, but would be ludicrous.)

3) While management's action seems logical, it is based purely on motivation. Since everyone's raise is partially determined by the entire group's performance, management hoped that the other pharmacists would help B and E. What do you think? How do you think Pharmacists B and E feel?

   Management believes that since Pharmacists A, C, D and F seem to have no trouble doing the job, there should be no reason Pharmacists B and E shouldn't be able to achieve the same results by trying just a little harder. Management now expects results instead of alibis. The troubles with Pharmacists B and E are being attributed only to the "methods" input to their processes.

4) While exposure of a special cause allows a person to zero in and take an action, was management's action appropriate? The question, "Well, what should I (a pharmacist) do differently from what I'm doing now?" has not really been answered. By encouraging them to "Do better work," management is treating variation within each pharmacist's work as common cause. Could there be special causes in the individual pharmacist inputs? If special causes are present, will they be the same for each pharmacist?

   When talking about Pharmacist B and E's raises, what does management mean by "above average" performance? If the six pharmacists are compared only to each other, someone will always be below average. (Think of the coin flips–half of the people will be below 25, but is it necessarily anything special they've done?)

Part 3

Secretly, management was puzzled. Pharmacist B was perceived to be one of the up-and-coming workers, yet the data clearly showed otherwise. Their quality consultant said to make decisions with data, not perceptions, so the action was considered fair.

Pharmacist B's supervisor was very troubled. While reading a book on quality tools, the chapter on Pareto analysis inspired her to collect data in a way that would recognize the presence of different error types. This is an example of stratification by the "measurements" input to the process since errors are measurements of the process output.

After discussion with the quality assurance audit inspectors, B's supervisor discovered that there were 29 different error types. The next month while keeping the errors separated by pharmacist, she also tracked the occurrences of the 29 individual error types. There were 80 errors, which stratified as follows:

Table 6.1 Breakdown of Medication Errors by Worker and by Error Type

By Worker	By Error Type	
Pharmacist A: 6 errors	Error Type 1:	4
Pharmacist B: 20 errors	Error Type 2:	2
Pharmacist C: 8 errors	Error Type 3:	19
Pharmacist D: 3 errors	Error Type 4:	1
Pharmacist E: 36 errors	Error Type 5:	13
Pharmacist F: 7 errors	Error Type 6:	7
	Error Types 7-29: All less than 6 each	
Total: 80 errors	Total:	80

Questions about Part 3

1)   What about the performance of Pharmacists B and E? The other workers?

2)   Has another source of problems been found?

3)   What action should be taken to improve?

Commentary on Part 3

1)   There seems to be some "marginal" improvement overall (6 percent) from the previous to current month. Pharmacist B reduced his errors by about

25 percent and Pharmacist E reduced his by 10 percent. However, Pharmacist C had four times as many errors and Pharmacist F had almost twice as many errors as in the previous month. Are these differences (i.e., variations) real (special cause) or not (common cause)? What should be done?

2)   Stratification by the process measurement was helpful. Six percent of the Error Types (3 and 5) accounted for 40 percent of the total errors! Once again, both intuitively and statistically, these two types indicate special causes. Note once again how stratification allows us to localize a problem.

3)   A typical, logical reaction would be to hold a half-day in-service for everyone to talk about Error Types 3 and 5 and how to prevent them. But this would again assume common cause (all pharmacists equally responsible for these error types) when special causes could be present.

Suppose there were special causes. Suppose some pharmacists are more prone to make certain error types than others. How would that make the pharmacists who didn't need to be at such an in-service feel? This *presentation* of the data does not address it. Is there a better way to present the data?

Part 4

The analyst who prepared the report discovered another page that had been lost behind the printer. This page stratified by pharmacist and error type simultaneously. Table 6.2 shows the last data collection exhibited this way.

Table 6.2 Stratification Grid of Pharmacist and Error Type

Error Type	Pharmacist						Total
	A	B	C	D	E	F	
1	0	0	1	0	2	1	4
2	1	0	0	0	1	0	2
3	0	16	1	0	2	0	19
4	0	0	0	0	1	0	1
5	2	1	3	1	4	3	13
6	0	0	0	0	3	0	3
.	.	.	.	.	.	.	.
.	.	.	.	.	.	.	.
27	.	.	.	.	.	.	.
28	.	.	.	.	.	.	.
29	.	.	.	.	.	.	.
Totals	6	20	8	3	36	7	80

Questions about Part 4

1) Has this presentation of the data clarified the situation?

2) What should happen next?

3) What about the goal?

Commentary on Part 4

1) Revisit Pharmacist B's current month of 20 errors. Do any further special causes exist within his performance? Yes: Error Type 3! Other than this error type, how is the rest of his work? Excellent! Does any other pharmacist have a problem with Error Type 3? No. What are the odds for rectifying this situation? Virtually guaranteed!

On the other hand, look at Pharmacist E. There are no further special causes in his error pattern. For some reason, he is "nickel and diming" the organization. Did he receive proper orientation and training? Does he handle more complicated medications? Is he right out of school? Is the stress of the job affecting him? Is he even up to the job?

Error Type 5 also shows common cause behavior. It would be incorrect to say that Pharmacists B and D have something to teach the others because they had the fewest errors of this type.

That would be treating common cause as if it were special. Things could be completely reversed the next month. Statistically, Type 5 errors would typically range from 0 to 6 (although over time, Pharmacist E would probably have the highest number).

2) Think back to the action taken when Pharmacist B was first exposed as a special cause. The action, threatening his salary increase and telling him to do better, treated his entire performance as common cause variability. It did nothing to understand why his performance was different. The natural reaction of Pharmacist B was frustration. He was already doing his best and, for the most part, doing excellent work. It was not until his special cause was localized and identified as Error Type 3 that clear action could be taken. It answered the question, What should I be doing differently than what I'm doing now? because the rest of the data showed that this process was capable of keeping Type 3 errors to a minimum. In general, reacting to special causes as though they are common causes will make things worse.

What if management had held an in-service seminar for Error Type 3? That, too, would be treating variation containing a special cause as if it were common cause, and it would have angered four people by wasting their time.

The appropriate action is different in the case of Pharmacist E. It would be a mistake to observe from Table 6.2 that Pharmacist E made more errors of Type 5 than any other error, and give him special training in Error Type 5. This would be an example of treating common cause variation as though it were due to a special cause. It would be ineffective, because the problem with Pharmacist E is not Error Type 5, it is with how he does his job, i.e., his work process. Treating common cause variability as though it is special cause is known as **tampering**, and generally makes things worse.

In such a common cause situation, clear, localized action is not possible. Pharmacist E does not seem to be capable of giving the required results. Further study of Pharmacist E's work process and its inputs is necessary to understand his problem.

The process for improving Error Type 5 is similar to that for Pharmacist E. The prescription filling process does not seem to be capable of avoiding that error because *all* the pharmacists make it

6

consistently at the same level. The data only yield questions that require further data collection to answer and rectify the situation.

The fact that all pharmacists exhibit this error indicates something inherent in the process of prescription filling (the inputs of which include the prescription writing process) is affecting the error rate. It could also represent a misinterpretation between the pharmacists and the QA inspectors as to what constitutes an error, i.e., the lack of an operational definition understood by everyone.

Once again, the final localized solution is not clear, but at least the process has been localized from 29 possibilities down to one. Many questions and possible theories can be generated and tested. Ultimately the process will need to be modified. This could include redesign of a form, relocation of materials, additional training of pharmacists and/or QA inspectors, or any number of other solutions.

3) What about the goal? The goal can now be seen as *irrelevant* to improvement of the situation. By focusing on the output of the process (total number of errors), common cause variation was being treated as special cause variation, resulting in inappropriate action (and lots of it!). The theory management implicitly used stated that the cause of variation (errors) was, "You are not working carefully enough." Percent ups and downs that compare successive monthly outputs from a process generally treat common cause in a process as if it were special cause. This will be thoroughly discussed in Chapter 7.

It was only by *focused study of the process producing the output* that opportunities for improvement became clear. During the six months that the process was studied, Pharmacist B *continued* to make Error Type 3, Pharmacist E *continued* not to be up to the job, and all pharmacists *continued* to make Error Type 5.

The pharmacists were never given the answer to the logical question, Well, what should I be doing differently than what I'm doing now? Only through data collection on the process can that important question be answered.

A one-month stratification as shown in Table 6.2 would have had an *immediate* impact of reducing total errors by approximately 70 percent! A typical reaction to the thought of such data collection would be, "But that's so much work!" However, it

would only have to be done *once*. By taking the easy way out and not doing it, nothing would change, and overreaction to common cause would actually further complicate the situation. Like many initiatives, well-meaning people take the path of least resistance: simple, obvious, and wrong.

Data Aggressiveness: What Level of Study Is Needed?—Four Strategies

While data collection is very important, there is a tendency to overuse it in the early stages of understanding an improvement opportunity. If the data collection is not carefully defined, it is easy to accumulate too much data with vague objectives, leaving people scratching their heads about what they should do with it. Sometimes any resemblance between what the team intended and what actually gets collected seems purely coincidental!

When data collection objectives and methods are unclear, the project team unduly inconveniences the work culture involved in the collection. Those providing data understandably become peeved when told, "We're sorry. We forgot to think about _____ [Fill in the blank]. Would you mind doing it again?" Credibility for the project is lost as well as credibility and cooperation for future collections and projects. In addition, this error feeds into some of the natural initial cultural cynicism about "this QI stuff."

Do not lose sight of the fact that *data collection itself is a process*. People collecting the data must be educated in the objectives of the data, the forms used to collect it, and operational definitions of what they collect. Forms also must be "user-friendly," i.e., allow the data to virtually collect themselves because, once again, people's jobs already take up at least 100 percent of their time.

In the course of designing a data collection, project teams should also ask the questions: "What is our plan for using these data? Suppose we had the data in hand right now. What is the potential action? What specifically would we do with them? What analysis is inherent in our collection process? What tools would appropriately analyze them? Would we know the right processes for interpreting the analysis and taking action?"

Recall the six sources of problems from Figure 3.5:

- inadequate knowledge of how a process works

- inadequate knowledge of how a process should work

- errors and mistakes in executing the procedures

- current practices that fail to recognize the need for preventive measures

- unnecessary steps, rework, wasteful data collection

- input and output variation.

Apply them to the data collection process as well as the process under study. Can you think of examples where a data collection was not as effective as it could have been? Was this due to the effects of the first five types as well as failing to consider input variation? Did the data collectors understand how the data were to be collected? Did data have to be retaken? Remember the envelope data? The pharmacy data?

Each source of process problem requires its own unique data collection based on understanding its contribution to the variation in the work process. Without awareness of variation and what can cause it, people tend to overcomplicate a situation and perceive it to be full of special causes. Reacting to each observed variation as if it were a special cause slowly adds unnecessary complexity to a situation.

This discussion demonstrates one of the many "non-mathematical" aspects of statistics and statistical thinking. To paraphrase Yogi Berra, who once said about baseball, "Ninety percent of this game is half mental," "Ninety percent of statistics is half planning."

The key is to have extremely focused objectives on major opportunities. This encourages an inherent strategy of a series of simple, efficient data collection processes that progressively zero-in on the significant root causes of variation. When they exist, exposing special causes of variation allows localization of both problem and solution. The medication error data followed this pattern.

Four basic data collection strategies exist to accurately understand a situation and test potential improvements. They will be discussed in ascending order of "aggressiveness," i.e., disturbance to the daily work habits of people involved. Careful consideration

of the impact of a data collection on a department or other group will go a long way in obtaining that group's cooperation. This can extend into further buy-in by actually involving key department personnel in the design of the data collection.

Strategies of low aggressiveness should be used to expose major potential sources of variation and opportunity. Low aggressiveness strategies can sometimes help screen out initial theories regarding causes of the problem.

Exhaust Existing Data

The first strategy is to **exhaust already existing in-house and routine data**. It can be dangerous to use data that originally were collected with no objective in mind. However, at a project's early stage, simple stratifications, scatterplots, and time plots of existing data may shed light on possible significant sources of variation and their causes, *which can then be tested by subsequent, properly designed data collection.*

In-house and routine data frequently consist only of process outputs. Because they normally cannot be traced directly to their inputs, outputs themselves are not necessarily helpful for improving processes. However, output collection can establish a *baseline* for evaluating the *progress* of improvement strategies. As shown in the medication error example, the number of errors in and of itself was useless for improving the process. However, once the process was improved, detailed stratification was no longer necessary. Through techniques to be demonstrated in Chapter 7, continuous plotting of the total errors would indeed show whether any gains have been maintained.

It is a common error to have only an anecdote as a pre-existing measure of a quality improvement opportunity. Do not underestimate the value of in-house data to provide a crude insight into an anecdote or at least a baseline on a macro measure of it. Beware of projects with no sources of baseline data. These tend to be thinly disguised opportunities for implementing an anecdotally "known" solution. Remember, "In God we trust...".

It is wrong to institute a change or solution based strictly on in-house data. However, they can be a rich source for suggesting significant theories to be tested. Since someone went through the trouble to collect the data, they may as well be used for what they're worth. This also creates an opportunity to assess the value of continuing to collect these data.

Study the Current Process

The second strategy is **study the current process**. This allows work processes to proceed normally while recording data that are virtually there for the asking. It's almost like taking a "data movie" of the work as it occurs. Usually this involves stratification of an important output to *trace* the sources of its inputs. The medication error data demonstrated this simply and beautifully. Through minimal additional documentation of normal work, stratification and Pareto analysis can expose potentially significant sources of variation. This is particularly useful in finding the third source of problem with a process, "errors and mistakes in executing the procedures."

The first two levels of aggressiveness, looking at routine data and studying the current process, expose many sources of special causes and allow localized efforts to fix these obvious but previously hidden problems. They may also bring to the surface the fourth source of problem with a process, "current practices that fail to recognize the need for preventive measures." Solutions to these problems frequently involve redesigning the process to include an "error-proofing" element.

When data show a problem to be common cause, it means that, given the current process, occurrences of the problem are inevitable. They are not under the control of people working in the system. The cause could even be due to the limitations of human attention, sometimes called MSR – Multiple Simultaneous Responsibilities. A robust process redesign that inherently forces use of the desired behavior or technique is often a good strategy.

Error Type 5 was a common cause among the pharmacists. The root cause may have been "inadequate knowledge of how a process should work," or "current practices that fail to recognize the need for preventive measures." Some examples of preventive measures and error-proofing include a written script for receptionists or a computerized billing system that does not accept incomplete forms.

Identifying deep causes of variation can also expose some elements of the fifth type of problem in a process, "unnecessary steps, rework, wasteful data collection." Examples include extra paperwork (especially inspections and pseudo-inspections) and time buffers which merely condone an inefficient process.

An analogy could be made to a restaurant which scrapes and documents every piece of burnt toast. Should it become excessive, they may feel the need to hire more toast scrapers. Shouldn't the issue be, "Why is the toast burnt?" Couldn't data collection help identify areas in processes with significant "burnt toast" and resulting no-value processes (i.e., scraping) which were created to cope with it?

Many times additional steps are unnecessarily added to the process due to one-time events that created chaos for workers in the past. They were added as a "knee jerk" reaction to a special cause (happened only once) that was treated as a common cause (perceived potential to happen often in the future). Think of some legislation. Sound familiar?

There is a tendency for processes to grow over the years with many steps losing whatever value they once had. Elimination of this slack strengthens and improves the process by addressing root causes of variation and reducing opportunities to add further variation to a process.

Now that many of the special causes of variation have been addressed and eliminated, one can assess the *value* of each step of the process by review and revision of the original flowchart. Has process redesign eliminated the need for some of the non-value work?

Cut New Windows

The third strategy is **cut new windows**. This takes study of the current process one step further by gathering data that are not routinely collected. More disturbance in the daily work flow is required to get at these data. In essence, a possible improvement opportunity has been identified, but the process has to be *dissected* beyond routine requirements or easily obtainable data to find the major source of variation.

For example, if "lab turnaround time" is identified as a major problem, strategy 1 or 2 could employ stratification to zero-in on the lab procedures accounting for the majority of complaints. Initial studies of the current process could be based on a global definition of "lab turnaround time" such as the elapsed time from the test being ordered to the time the result is available to the patient. (It would be interesting to stratify these results by words on the order such as "STAT", "STAT!!", "RUSH", "Priority", etc. Do they really make any difference?)

If the times are still unacceptable, "lab turnaround time" would have to be broken or "disaggregated" into its major component times to study their contribution to the total. Such component times would include transportation to the lab, waiting in the work queue, performing the test, communicating the result to the physician or hall nurse, etc.

Breaking apart the total time is, in effect, cutting new windows into the process—looking at it from different perspectives and in smaller pieces. A detailed flowchart would expose these leverage points and allow creation of an effective checksheet (see "Summary of Data Collection" later in this chapter) to determine the major bottleneck. If future data collection is focused primarily on the bottleneck, then gathering the required information will involve no more people than necessary. Data collection in other areas would add little value for the effort expended. This study of the process for lab procedures with the most complaints could also provide some benefit for *all* procedures.

Designed Experimentation

The final strategy is **designed experimentation**. This involves making a *major fundamental change* in the way a process is performed and measuring whether the it is indeed an improvement. It also involves major disturbance to the daily work culture and should be used only sparingly. The first three strategies should initially be used to expose all existing special causes of variation. They also provide necessary insight into how the current process came to be and allow construction of a baseline for assessing the effects of a designed experiment. This allows optimization of the current process to its fullest capable extent. If the process remains incapable of meeting customer needs and some root causes still have not been addressed, a designed experiment is appropriate to evaluate a fundamental redesign of the process.

Again, it is common for teams to implement "known" solutions based on anecdote; lack of problem definition compounds this error. This approach jumps right to the most aggressive strategy, i.e., making a fundamental change in the process, and will cause much disturbance to a work culture that thrives on predictability. The lack of good baseline data, the presence of unexposed special causes, and reliance on poorly planned data collection can make evaluation and prediction from the experiment no better than looking into a "crystal ball." They also inhibit cooperation and understanding from the department involved in the experiment.

To summarize, flowcharts and data collections allow people to focus on the significant improvement opportunities, ensuring that the right solution is applied to the right process. The team will gain substantial political credibility if it considers the work culture's feelings and time during the project, demonstrates its competency in the improvement process, and involves members of the work culture at the appropriate times.

Candidates for solutions should be generated, prioritized and initially tested on a small scale. *One always should pilot any proposed solution on a focused, small scale first.* It is not desirable to put a large work environment through a major disturbance. It will create unintended variation and cloud the results. A pilot will expose the lurking *unexpected* problems that compromise the experimentation process itself.

It is crucial to have baseline data describing the problem. A plot comparing the pilot and the baseline will determine whether the change was indeed effective. The question, How will we know if things are better? must be answered in the planning of the experiment and answered with appropriate data collection.

Data aggressiveness is summarized in Figure 6.1. Each level of aggressiveness is listed along with its purpose, common approaches, and the amount of "jerkaround" or disruption to the work processes.

6

Figure 6.1: Data "Aggressiveness"

1. Exhaust In-house Data
    (Minimal disturbance)

    *   Establish baselines to assess current process.
    *   Isolate process problems.
    *   Expose variations in perceptions of data definitions.
    *   Suggest theories needing further consideration for possible testing.

    — Pareto analysis to localize problems

2. Study Current Process
    (Tolerable disturbance)

    *   Establish extent of problem(s).
    *   Establish baseline for measuring improvement efforts.
    *   Develop operational definitions suited to data collection objectives.
    *   Reduce data contamination due to "human" variation.
    *   Further localize problems.

    — Use current data collection methods to establish traceability to process inputs.
    — Capture and record available data that, while currently uncollected, are virtually there for the taking.
    — Pareto analyses and stratified histograms to localize problems

3. "Cut New Windows" — Process Dissection or Disaggregation
    (Uncomfortable disturbance)

    *   Intense focus on a major isolated source of localized variation.
    *   Split process into sub-processes for further study.

    — Collect data not needed for routine process operation – the data collection process may be awkward and disruptive to routine operation.

4. Designed Experimentation
    (MAJOR disturbance)

    *   Test a process redesign suggested by one of the previous three levels.

    — Use run/control chart to assess success.

A Word On Surveys

One of the authors is of the opinion that there should be a temporary ban, perhaps ten years, on the use of written, mailed surveys. Of course, this is overly dogmatic and silly, but experience has shown...

When a survey is planned to address a problem, many questions are typically brainstormed about "how the customer might feel" (Please rank from 1 to 5) and "Oh, yes that would be nice to know, too" (age, sex, day of the week born, favorite color, shoe size, etc.). The result is an amorphous 5-10 page survey which generally gets a return rate of 5-30 percent, usually from Mr. Grumpy and Ms. Ecstatic. What about Mr. and Ms. Average? *Imagine you have the data in hand. What are you going to do with them?* Remember, data are a basis for action. To paraphrase Joiner, "Vague data with vague objectives yield vague results." Are you committed to use what you learn? How?

Generally, one's knowledge after a survey isn't really very useful and doesn't present any particular surprises (except perhaps: We were rated 4.56 on this last time, but only 4.42 this time.) It is a waste of time to ask what you already know. This is not an especially useful customer focus, and it tends to bring out the "What happened? Who's to blame?" mentality, or sometimes, "Let's send it out again and see if the results are better next time."

Again, these comments refer primarily to mailed, written surveys answered independently, not those asked orally by an interviewer in person or over the phone. The assumptions of survey designers tend to be different from the answerer's understanding of what is being asked. It is very hard to tell what those assumptions are and equally difficult to come up with an unbiased, unambiguous question. People's responses to mailed surveys tend to reflect their current, transient reactions. One does not know how they may have felt in the past and is unable to probe for such important information. Generally the customers' comments after answering the survey are far more interesting.

"Before and after" surveys merely represent two points in time. How does one explain the difference? Do the differences mean anything? Are they due to common causes or special causes?

The people who designed the survey sometimes put their own (generally positive) "spin" on survey results to confirm their entrenched perceptions. Or, if they don't like the results, they may send out another survey, or blame the customer since "the customers don't know what they want anyway!"

In fact, customers do know what they want. However, it may not be what they need. Customers often need education to learn their real needs. Hacquebord[1] lists as his first principle for improvement of quality in healthcare: "Improving quality includes customer education, because the customer does not always know what he or she needs. The customer does, however, judge what he has received, and can only specify what he wants based on his past experiences, or what he has heard others experience."

What should be done instead? Generally, open-ended comments are more useful, especially when kept in the customer's language, and give insight into what the customer is actually thinking. Transforming organizations increasingly conduct *face-to-face focus groups* with both internal and external customers. *Customer Focused Quality* provides some excellent guidelines for focus groups. They also have a nice summary of many methods for understanding customer needs, which is reproduced in Figure 6.2. Can you think of any better way to find out how your processes should work?

6

Figure 6.2: Tools to Aid in Understanding Customer Needs[2]

Methods	Advantages +	Disadvantages -
Internal Brainstorming	Multiple ideas from internal sources. Lots of ideas quickly.	Can be misled by the internal paradigms of your organization.
Casual Comment Cards	Collects large amounts of information from many customers in an unobtrusive way.	Can be somewhat difficult to administer. Workers may simply fail to listen or record casual comments if they do not see the effect they are having.
Interviews and Focus Groups	Allows for specific dialogue with customers. Facilitates completion of thoughts and clarification of meaning.	Requires a considerable amount of the customer's time. Also, several interviews may be required to understand the attitude of "many" customers. Surveys may be required to verify what is learned.
Friends Comments	Excellent source of honest opinions and ideas.	Only provides one point of view. Must be supplemented with other information.
Observing other businesses with the same customer base	Allows you to pick up on ideas that may have been missed by others in your industry. Good source of innovation by understanding the need that is being addressed.	Not totally reliable. Needs to be supplemented by other methods.
Surveys	Collects comments and opinions from large numbers of people. Good for validation of ideas from other methods.	Responses are often superficial and polarized. Somewhat intrusive. No chance for dialogue and explanation.
Pilot Studies	Provides a method to stop bad ideas before the customer is affected. Also provides a means to observe customer/product interaction.	May prevent rapid deployment of new ideas. Requires ideas be fundamentally complete before study is done.
Mystery customer	Allows management to experience and evaluate service experiences from a customer perspective.	Risks being used as a tool of fear. May also be very subjective.

The gap of customer preference can be assessed vis-à-vis the current process. The process observation sheets from Joiner Associates (Figures 3.10, 3.11, and 3.12) are a means for accomplishing this.

One must ask questions, *listen*, and have the wisdom to probe deeper to understand the customers' *real needs* as opposed to what they may be superficially and literally asking for. Record comments in the customers' language.

Once again use the Pareto principle to determine the major opportunities for the organization. *Focus resulting surveys and action there.* After summarizing a focus group session, surveys can be used *to test the conclusions drawn from the data gathered face to face.*

A Summary of Summaries

The material presented thus far may make improvement appear to be an overwhelming challenge. The rest of this chapter summarizes the information needed to guide you through the process. Refer to it as you work on improvement. The summary is divided into three parts:

- data collection as a process

- the improvement process itself, and

- "tools" that are useful for improvement.

They are intended as guides for you to continually refer to as you work on improvement. We've presented them with the recognition that different people have different learning styles. For example, we show several different views of the improvement process. Our recommendation is that you look them over and try what you think will be useful.

Data Collection as a Process

Good data collection is crucial to process improvement, yet it is rarely taught as a skill. The teaching of passive analysis through traditional tools is no substitute. Untold precious time can be saved by knowing the skills of simple, efficient data collection. In addition to simply collecting the data, the skills include awareness of human factors which may add unintended, contaminating variation. Figure 6.3 should be referenced frequently.

Figure 6.3: Summary of Data Collection

Data collection is a process in and of itself. As a process, it can always be improved. The following is a list of considerations for any good data collection plan:

1)   Questions should relate to *specific* information needs of the project. For the best, simplest, most efficient collection, objectives should be as narrow and focused as possible and relate to a potential major source of observed variation.

     People involved in the actual data collection should have confidence that the team knows *exactly* what it is asking and looking for *and* that it is going to do something with the information.

     The level of data "aggressiveness" should be appropriate for the stage of the project.

2)   Imagine you have the data already in hand: Have the necessary data been collected to truly answer your question? What data tools will be used? Is the proposed analysis *appropriate* for the way the data will be collected?

3)   Where is the best leverage point in the process to collect the data? Where will the job flow suffer minimum interruption?

4)   Who should be the collector? Is this person unbiased with easy and immediate access to the relevant facts?

5)   *Understand the data collectors and their environment.*

     What effect will their normal jobs have on the proposed data collection? Will data be complete? Do the forms allow efficient recording of data with minimum interruption to their normal jobs?

6)   Design of a data collection form (checksheet) is not trivial. Whenever possible, involve some of the collectors in the design.

     Reduce opportunities for error; design traceability to collector and environment; make the form virtually self-explanatory; make its appearance professional. *Keep it simple!*

7)   Prepare simple instructions and possibly a flow chart for using the data collection forms.

8)   Train the people who will be involved. Have a properly completed form available.

     Answer the following natural questions of the collectors: What is the purpose of the study? How will the data be used? Will the results be communicated to them?

     Reduce fear by discussing the importance of complete and unbiased information.

9)   *Pilot the forms and instructions on a small scale.* Revise them if necessary using input from the collectors. Do they work as expected? Are they filled out properly? Do people have differing perceptions of operational definitions? Are they as easy to use as originally perceived? When possible, sit with and observe the people collecting the data.

10) Audit the collection process and validate the results. Randomly check completed forms and occasionally observe data collection during the process.

     Are data missing? Any unusual values? Is bias being reflected in the data collection process?

A Process for Improvement

Several figures from *The TEAM Handbook* are useful to summarize what, at this point, may seem like a forbidding task. However, if one can bring a process-oriented framework to a situation and utilize it within the "six sources of problems with a process" from Figure 3.5, a startlingly logical, intuitive plan emerges.

Figure 6.4, "The Project Selection Checklist," contains excellent business, human and practical issues to consider when choosing a project/ situation to study. Note that we say project/ situation. As will be explained in Chapter 9, projects are necessary but not sufficient for improvement. The goal is to transform daily work life so that QI is imbedded in all aspects of the culture. In terms of the concepts discussed in this chapter, items 9 and 10 are especially relevant.

If people are not careful, the concept of a mission statement can become dreadfully formal and misunderstood in early QI efforts. It cannot be summarized in a few paragraphs. While extensive discussion is beyond the scope of this book, *The TEAM Handbook* is an outstanding resource.

Figure 6.5, "Project-Oriented Model of Progress," is a visual guide to the thought process used for organizational transformation. It is presented in a top-down flowchart form. Our book is mainly concerned with the "Improvement Loop" portion of this model, yet you should be aware of the non-trivial elements which sometimes get lost by bogging down in tools. Figure 6.6, "Transformational Model of Progress," gives the same guide as Figure 6.5, but is oriented toward organizational change.

Figure 6.7, "Project Progress Checklist," is the information from Figure 6.5 presented in a checklist format for a project context. It expands the generalities of the top-down flow chart into specific actions.

6

Figure 6.4 The Project Selection Checklist[3]

Instructions: If you have selected and defined an appropriate project, you should be able to check most, if not all, items listed below. If you can't check all of these items, you may want to re-evaluate your choice.

___ 1. The process or project is related to key business issues.

___ 2. The process targeted for improvement has direct impact on the company.

___ 3. The process or work area has a lot of visibility in the company.

___ 4. All managers concerned with this process—at all levels of the organization—agree it is important to study and improve this process.

___ 5. Enough managers, supervisors, and front-line personnel in this area will cooperate to make this project a success.

___ 6. This process is not currently being changed in any way, nor is it scheduled to be overhauled in the near future. (This criterion does not apply if the project team is being commissioned to study how the change might occur.)

___ 7. The project is defined as one clearly defined process that has easily identified starting and ending points.

___ 8. This process is not being studied by any other group.

___ 9. One cycle of the process is completed each day or two. (That is, there is quick turnaround time. Again, this is most important when selecting initial projects. Once a team has some experience, it can tackle longer, more complex processes.)

___ 10. The mission statement for this team describes a problem to be studied, or an improvement opportunity, not a solution to be tried.

Figure 6.5: "Project-Oriented" Model of Progress[4]

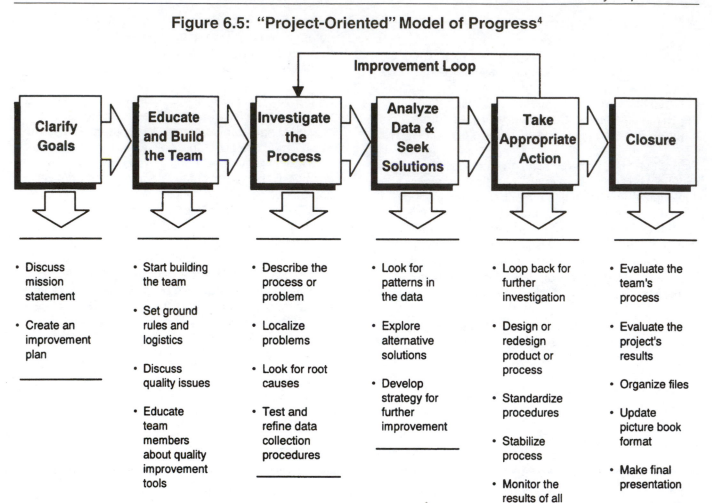

Clarify Goals	Educate and Build the Team	Investigate the Process	Analyze Data & Seek Solutions	Take Appropriate Action	Closure
• Discuss mission statement	• Start building the team	• Describe the process or problem	• Look for patterns in the data	• Loop back for further investigation	• Evaluate the team's process
• Create an improvement plan	• Set ground rules and logistics	• Localize problems	• Explore alternative solutions	• Design or redesign product or process	• Evaluate the project's results
	• Discuss quality issues	• Look for root causes	• Develop strategy for further improvement	• Standardize procedures	• Organize files
	• Educate team members about quality improvement tools	• Test and refine data collection procedures		• Stabilize process	• Update picture book format
				• Monitor the results of all changes – evaluate and refine as needed	• Make final presentation
				• Document progress	• Recommend follow-up activities

Figure 6.6: Transformational Model of Progress[5]

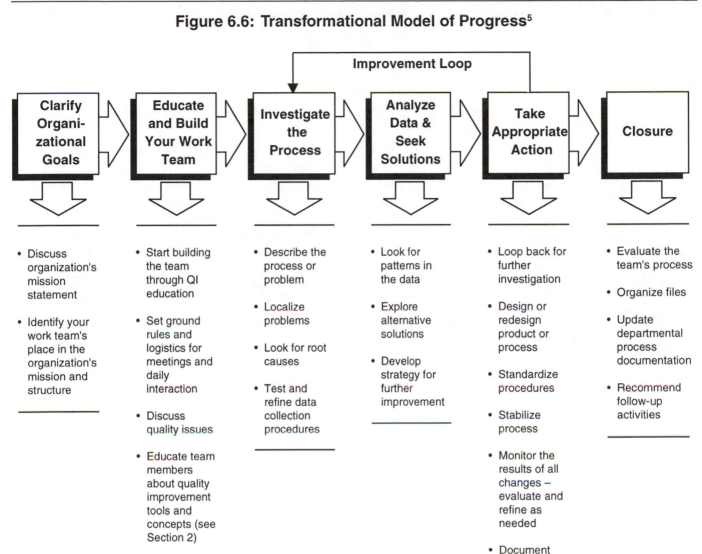

Improvement Loop

Clarify Organizational Goals	Educate and Build Your Work Team	Investigate the Process	Analyze Data & Seek Solutions	Take Appropriate Action	Closure

- Discuss organization's mission statement

- Identify your work team's place in the organization's mission and structure

---

- Start building the team through QI education

- Set ground rules and logistics for meetings and daily interaction

- Discuss quality issues

- Educate team members about quality improvement tools and concepts (see Section 2)

- Describe the process or problem

- Localize problems

- Look for root causes

- Test and refine data collection procedures

- Look for patterns in the data

- Explore alternative solutions

- Develop strategy for further improvement

- Loop back for further investigation

- Design or redesign product or process

- Standardize procedures

- Stabilize process

- Monitor the results of all changes – evaluate and refine as needed

- Document progress

- Evaluate the team's process

- Organize files

- Update departmental process documentation

- Recommend follow-up activities

6

Figure 6.7: Project Progress Checklist[6]

Instructions: Refer to this list occasionally to monitor the team's progress. This list can also give you clues of what to do if your team gets stuck between phases of the project. Some of these items may not pertain to your team—or you may be able to identify other milestones that are not listed here that you want to add.

Mission statement
- Receive from management
- Clarify; modify if necessary
- Get management approval for mission revisions
- Define goals and objectives related to mission

Planning
- Select team members
- Develop logistical system for team meetings
- Create an improvement plan
- Develop a top-down flowchart of project stages

Education/team-building activities
- Introduce team members
- Explain roles and expectations
- Orient to group's process
- Introduce basics of new approach: 14 points, Joiner triangle, key quality improvement concepts
- Provide training in needed scientific tools
- Develop ownership in project

Study the process
- Construct top-down flowchart of process
- Interview customers to identify needs
- Design data gathering procedures
- Gather data on process
- Analyze data to see if process is stable
- Identify problems with process

Localize problems
- Identify possible causes of problems
- Select likely causes
- Gather data to establish root causes
- Analyze data
- Rank causes
- Develop appropriate, permanent solutions

Make changes/document improvement
- Develop a strategic plan to test changes
- Implement test
- Gather data on new process
- Analyze data, critique changes in light of data
- Redesign improvements in process and repeat this step if necessary
- Implement further changes, or refer matter to appropriate person or group
- Monitor results or changes
- Establish a system to monitor in the future

Closure
- Prepare presentation on project
- Deliver presentation
- Evaluate team's progress
- Evaluate team's product
- Document

Figure 6.8 shows the improvement process from the perspective of actual improvement activities and a service or administrative perspective. It does not contain the project-administration detail of Figure 6.5 which, albeit necessary, can sometimes obscure people's perspective. Figure 6.8 is just a different "cut," if you will, of Figure 6.5. It was developed by Joiner Associates as "The Seven Step Method." While the authors do not necessarily advocate this method exclusively, we note that it is virtually identical to FOCUS-PDCA and the 10-step method in the project summaries. *Any good process comes from the same theory.*

Figure 6.8: **The Joiner Seven Step Method** (with emphasis on administrative processes)[7]

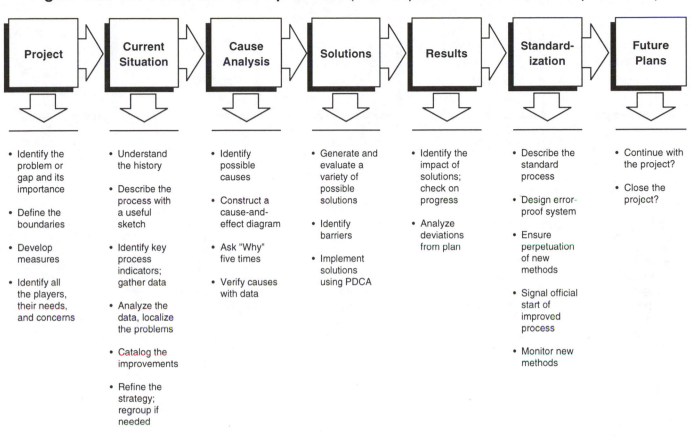

Project	Current Situation	Cause Analysis	Solutions	Results	Standard-ization	Future Plans
• Identify the problem or gap and its importance • Define the boundaries • Develop measures • Identify all the players, their needs, and concerns	• Understand the history • Describe the process with a useful sketch • Identify key process indicators; gather data • Analyze the data, localize the problems • Catalog the improvements • Refine the strategy; regroup if needed	• Identify possible causes • Construct a cause-and-effect diagram • Ask "Why" five times • Verify causes with data	• Generate and evaluate a variety of possible solutions • Identify barriers • Implement solutions using PDCA	• Identify the impact of solutions; check on progress • Analyze deviations from plan	• Describe the standard process • Design error-proof system • Ensure perpetuation of new methods • Signal official start of improved process • Monitor new methods	• Continue with the project? • Close the project?

6

Figure 6.9, "A General 5-Stage Plan for Improvement," expands the "Improvement Loop" of Figure 6.5 into a top-down flowchart, ties in the "six sources of problems with a process," and incorporates the four levels of data aggressiveness.

Figure 6.9: A General 5-Stage Plan for Improvement[8]

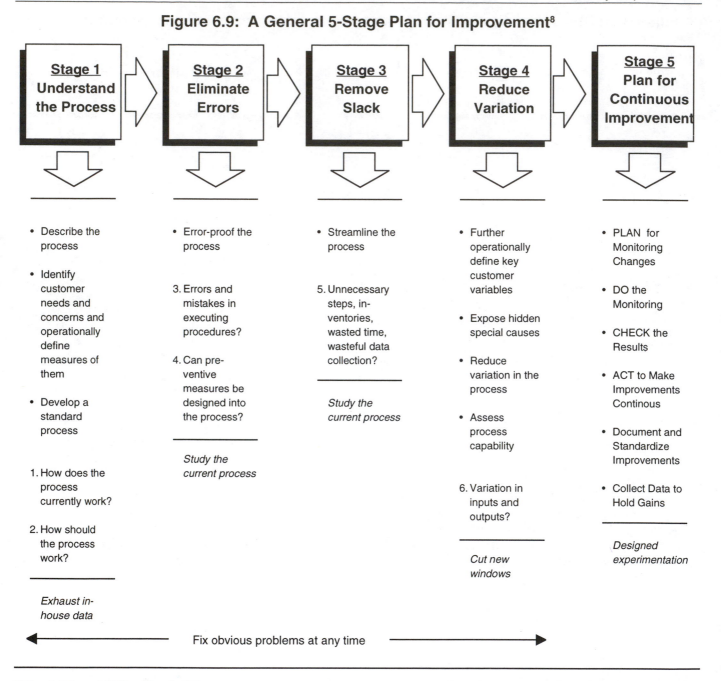

* Describe the process

* Identify customer needs and concerns and operationally define measures of them

* Develop a standard process

1. How does the process currently work?

2. How should the process work?

_____

Exhaust in-house data

* Error-proof the process

3. Errors and mistakes in executing procedures?

4. Can preventive measures be designed into the process?

_____

Study the current process

* Streamline the process

5. Unnecessary steps, inventories, wasted time, wasteful data collection?

_____

Study the current process

* Further operationally define key customer variables

* Expose hidden special causes

* Reduce variation in the process

* Assess process capability

6. Variation in inputs and outputs?

_____

Cut new windows

* PLAN for Monitoring Changes

* DO the Monitoring

* CHECK the Results

* ACT to Make Improvements Continous

* Document and Standardize Improvements

* Collect Data to Hold Gains

_____

Designed experimentation

← —————————— Fix obvious problems at any time —————————— →

_____

What About "The Tools"?

Tools and their mechanics are secondary to the statistical thinking behind their use. The overall motivation in quality improvement is to understand variation. When teaching a process for improvement, i.e., the "Improvement Loops" of Figures 6.5 and 6.6, the emphasis should be on:

* process-oriented thinking through **flowcharts** (as discussed in Chapter 3)

* proper planning of data collection through

appropriate **data aggressiveness** and design of a **checksheet/data sheet**

* identification of possible sources of variation and special causes in inputs to a process through an **Ishikawa (Fishbone) diagram**, stratification **(Pareto analysis, stratified histogram),** and **scatterplots**

* assessment of stability of processes in time and their capability (desired vs. actual performance) through **run charts/control charts**, which will be covered in detail in Chapter 7.

Good **checksheets** will result from using the Summary of Data Collection (Figure 6.3). The project case studies provide further examples and critique of some data collection tools.

The **Pareto principle** was demonstrated in the medication error example. To turn a stratified data collection into a Pareto diagram bar graph, plot the bars in descending order and show the individual percent contribution of each. Figure 6.10 contains a Pareto diagram of the medication error Part 2 data stratified by pharmacist. It is initially useful to brainstorm possible categories of stratification when "studying the current process."

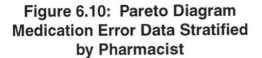

Figure 6.10: Pareto Diagram Medication Error Data Stratified by Pharmacist

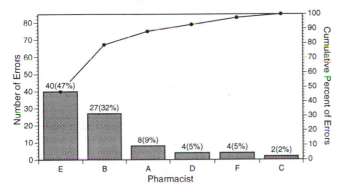

Ishikawa (Fishbone) diagrams help organize brainstormed ideas about causes of undesirable variation. They are developed by the project team working on the process and represent the relationship of a problem to its major inputs: people, methods, machines, materials, measurements, and environment. *They should be used sparingly*, usually after proper flowcharting and stratification/Pareto analysis have localized a major opportunity. Otherwise, they quickly become unwieldy! Figure 6.11 illustrates a fishbone diagram that has become overly complicated.

Figure 6.11: Ishikawa Cause and Effect Diagram: Vague vs. Localized

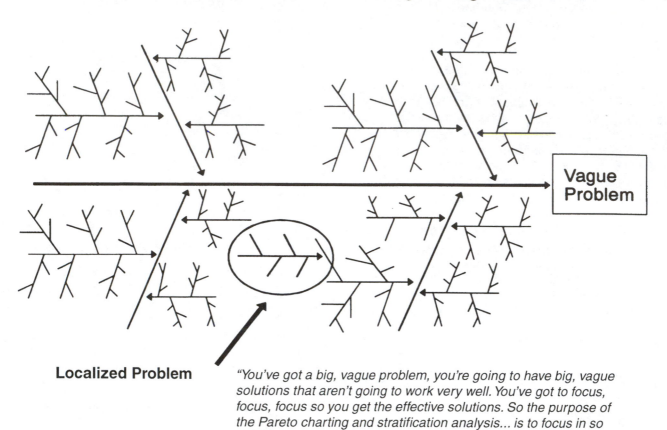

Vague Problem

Localized Problem

"You've got a big, vague problem, you're going to have big, vague solutions that aren't going to work very well. You've got to focus, focus, focus so you get the effective solutions. So the purpose of the Pareto charting and stratification analysis... is to focus in so you get right to the solution..."

—*Brian L. Joiner*

A **scatterplot** graphically tests a simple theory about whether an input affects a process output. By plotting the output on the vertical axis and the theorized input on the horizontal axis, one of three patterns can be observed: A positive relationship (output increases as the input increases), a negative relationship (output decreases as the input increases), or no relationship (the data appear as a "shotgun" pattern). Figure 6.12 contains a scatterplot of charges vs. length of stay. The plot shows that as the length of stay increases, the charges rise as well.

Scatterplots can be useful when exhausting in-house data and studying the current process. Linear regression is a statistical analysis typically performed on these type of data. The graph provides much more information than a linear regression analysis, even a statistically significant one, because again, such an analysis may not be appropriate. "A picture is worth a thousand numbers."

Regression without plots may also fail even when a relationship exists if the relationship is not linear. Linear regression analysis of a non-linear relationship could be misleading. Additional danger lurks when a tenuous linear relationship is extrapolated for future prediction beyond the range of the current data.

It is also important to remember that just because an input and an output show a pattern on a scatterplot, it does not guarantee a cause-and-effect relationship. For example, ice cream sales and the murder rate show a positive relationship on a scatterplot. Does this mean that ice cream causes murder? A more likely explanation is a third variable—temperature—whose increase causes both ice cream sales and the murder rate to rise.

Figure 6.12: Scatterplot of Charges vs. Length of Stay

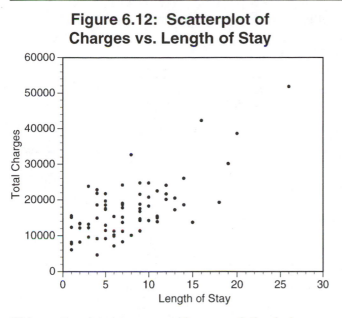

This scatterplot shows a positive association between length of stay vs. total charges.

A **stratified histogram** is another method of stratifying data. Unlike a Pareto chart, which is used when the data represent the number of times an event has occurred, a stratified histogram uses "continuous" data - numbers based on measurements. An example appears in Figure 6.13.

Figure 6.13: Stratified Histogram of Emergency Room Admissions by Time and Day

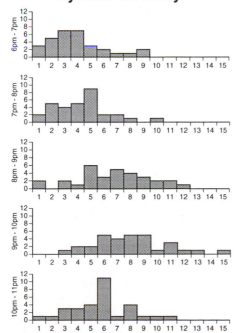

The stratified histogram shows that admissions do not occur randomly throughout the evening.

The TEAM Handbook contains more extended explanations of these tools and gives good capsule summaries and examples. *Our message is: Do not get bogged down in the mechanics and minutiae of the tools.* **Their purpose is to understand variation!**

Figures 6.14 and 6.15 relate various tools to the improvement process. Figure 6.14 lists the steps of Joiner's Seven Step method (Figure 6.8) and some questions and activities that are part of each step. Figure 6.15 is a chart showing which tools go with which steps. Following the data thought process as outlined will help you decide when it is appropriate to use a particular tool.

6

Figure 6.14: Process Improvement Tools: Questions and Activities

1) Situation selection

2) Assess current situation
   a) How does the process work?
   b) How should it work?
   c) What data are already available?
   d) Is there a historical baseline?

3) Cause analysis
   a) Are there errors and mistakes? Do they contain special causes or are they common cause?
   b) Can we localize a major opportunity?
      1. Should we "study the current process?"
      2. Should we "cut new windows?" (Disaggregation)
   c) Is the current process capable vis-à-vis desired performance?
   d) Does the process need to be redesigned?

4) Solutions
   a) Technically, what will solve the problem?
   b) How will this solution affect the work culture?
   c) Where should we pilot the solution on a small scale?
   d) How will we know if the solution works?

5) Results
   a) Is the problem basically solved?
   b) Can additional waste be eliminated from the process?
   c) Were there any unexpected side effects?
   d) Have we sufficiently addressed cultural resistance?

6) Standardization
   a) Has everyone been properly trained?
   b) Are there any cultural side effects?
   c) Is the proper data collection in place to hold gains?

7) Future plans

Figure 6.15: Grid of Process Improvement Steps and Process Improvement Tools

Process Improvement Tool

Improvement Step	Flowchart	Cause-and-Effect Diagram (Ishikawa)	Pareto Chart / Stratification Analysis	Scatter Plot	Stratified Histogram	Run Chart/ Control Chart	Operational Definitions	Checksheet
1. Situation Selection	x		x			x		
2. Current Situation	x	x	x		x	x	x	x
3. Cause Analysis	x	x	x	x	x	x		
4. Solutions	x	x						
5. Results			x		x	x		
6. Standardization	x					x		
7. Future Plans	x	x	x		x			

Notes to Chapter Six

1. Hacquebord H. "Health care from the perspective of a patient: Theories for improvement."

2. Mowery N et al. *Customer Focused Quality.*

3. Scholtes PR. *The TEAM Handbook.*

4. *Ibid.*

5. *Ibid.*

6. *Ibid.*

7. *Ibid.*

8. *Ibid.*

Chapter Seven
Data Skills II: Studying a Process in Time

Key Ideas

- The element of time is a key process input. Time affects process data collection, use of statistical tools, and analysis.

- Traditional report formats using "two-point trends" and aggregation usually do not accurately represent true variation. One commonly used managerial summary technique renders statistical analysis invalid. Decisions based upon these formats can lead to wasted resources because the solutions do not meet real needs.

- Knowing how the data were collected is crucial to performing a good analysis.

- The key question when looking for special causes is, "Is the process which produced this observation the same as the process which produced other observations?"

- Run charts and control charts must become routine analysis tools.

- A true statistically-defined trend is a relatively rare occurrence.

- Some common cause patterns can easily be misinterpreted to be the results of special causes.

- Preconceived notions of special causes can result in biased, inappropriate displays of data.

- Tampering—reacting to common cause variation as though it is special cause—results in incalculable losses for the organization.

- The capability of any process being improved must be assessed, i.e., its actual inherent performance vs. its desired performance. Any goals must be evaluated in the context of this capability, and an appropriate strategy must be developed to deal with gaps.

- QA analyses that use rankings must be re-evaluated in a common cause context.

- Routine use of ongoing run and control charts for common clinical conditions has tremendous potential.

- Whether they realize it or not, people are already using variations of the ideas presented in this chapter.

Studying a Process in Time

In addition to the six types of inputs (people, machines, methods, materials, measurements and environment), there is one other major consideration when characterizing a process. This final element is time. Its presence affects process analysis, data collection, and the use of statistical methods. *Every* process occurs over time.

Some Unfortunate Common Practices

It is a common practice and seemingly part of human nature to treat the difference between two consecutive numbers as a "two point trend," i.e., a special cause, with the implication that two different processes produced the different numbers.

A partial list of two-point trend examples includes:

- monthly sales
- unit costs
- quarterly reports
- weekly production reports
- annual financial reports
- monthly absenteeism.

This practice is evident in questions like:

- Days per 1000 are up eight percent from last month, what are you doing about it?

- Enrollment is down four percent from last year, what are you doing about it?

Managers demand explanations as to why current results differ from previous results. "Bad" results are punished. Workers are motivated by reward for good results. Sometimes goals are stretched even further after good results are received.

When results are graphically displayed, it is often in the form of a bar graph over time (see Figure 7.1). As will be seen later, the bar graph is difficult to interpret and can hide important information. Reports in "rows and columns" format are also quite common, comparing the current result to the previous one, and also to the result during the same time period of the previous year. Aggregated year-to-date summaries are typically presented along with the "variance" from previous reports and corporate goals. Are there other, more useful alternatives?

Figure 7.1: Bar Graph of Patient Counts

Patient Counts

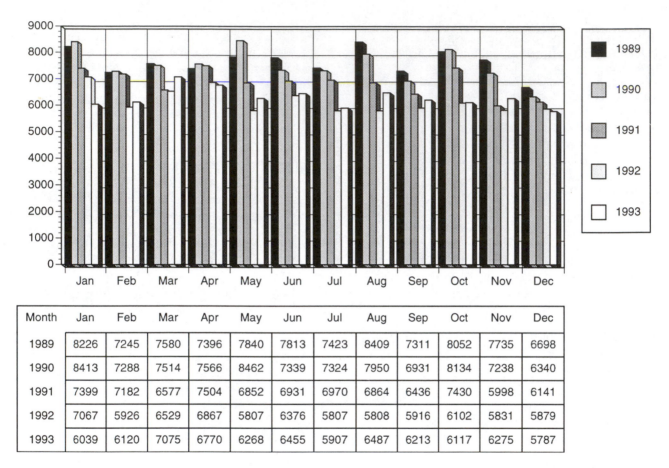

Month	Jan	Feb	Mar	Apr	May	Jun	Jul	Aug	Sep	Oct	Nov	Dec
1989	8226	7245	7580	7396	7840	7813	7423	8409	7311	8052	7735	6698
1990	8413	7288	7514	7566	8462	7339	7324	7950	6931	8134	7238	6340
1991	7399	7182	6577	7504	6852	6931	6970	6864	6436	7430	5998	6141
1992	7067	5926	6529	6867	5807	6376	5807	5808	5916	6102	5831	5879
1993	6039	6120	7075	6770	6268	6455	5907	6487	6213	6117	6275	5787

Bar graphs are a poor way to plot data over time.

Think about data reported monthly. Instead of looking at a single point, consider a graphical display. As shown in Figure 7.2, one option is to include the result from the previous month. Is this plot useful?

Figure 7.2: Time Plot of Data From Two Consecutive Months

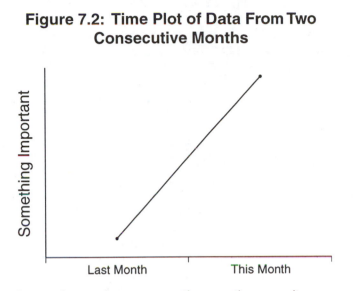

Comparisons of two consecutive months are quite common. When viewed graphically, this comparison is not very enlightening.

Graphs such as this are rare because a plot of two points really doesn't give much information. Would it be better to look at these numbers in a broader context?

How about adding the same period from the previous year? This allows one to keep a finger on two important trends, or does it? As it turns out, a plot of these data (Figure 7.3) is not very useful, either. As in Figure 7.2, the data are not presented in the context of the process that produced them. No information is provided about the variation inherent to that process.

Figure 7.3: Time Plot of Two Consecutive Months and the Month One Year Prior to the Current Month

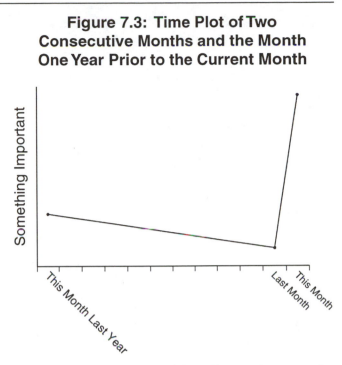

Even when the same month from the previous year is included, the comparison of the months is not very enlightening.

Consider three time periods of a process. The results from each period are different. How should the data be interpreted? Figure 7.4 shows the six possible sequences of these numbers, each followed by a word that could be used to "explain" the variation. This is similar to the three months that make up a typical business quarter.

7

Figure 7.4 Six Possible Sequences of Three Different Points

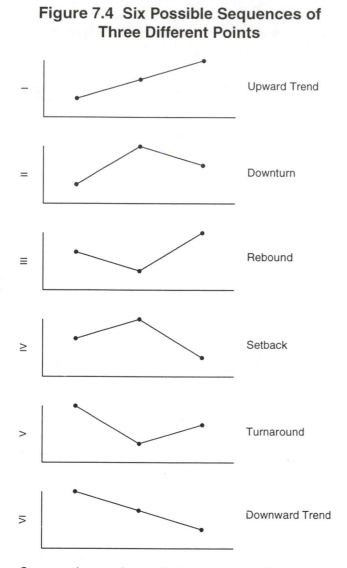

Consecutive numbers will almost always differ from each other. The terms ascribed to the above sequences imply a special cause interpretation, i.e., concluding something changed between each point. If the variation is due to common causes, it is of little value to attempt to explain the individual differences from point to point.

Aren't the terms in Figure 7.4 making a special cause interpretation of the observed variation? They imply that the numbers are different because the process has somehow changed.

What if the numbers differ merely by common cause, e.g., three bowling or golf scores, or a room of people on three separate occasions flipping coins and counting the number of heads obtained? Yes, the numbers are different, but they were all produced by the same process. What are the consequences of

attributing a special cause to the observed variation? How would the action differ? Are the terms in Figure 7.4 appropriate for this variation? Is the variation really due to common causes? Special causes? With only three data points it's difficult to tell.

Three questions one could ask about these presentations of data are:

- Why are the ten months between the first two data points in Figure 7.3 ignored? A common explanation is "seasonality."

- Why is January used as an essentially arbitrary cut-off point for data? This approach makes the previous year virtually cease to exist except for the current month. The bar graph in Figure 7.1 implies no continuity between December of one year and January of the next year.

- It is a common practice to display only the last twelve months, at most, of data. Why?

On what *theory* are these analyses based? Right or wrong, any display and analysis of data has an inherent theory. The theory usually reflects the displayer's bias toward a particular special cause interpretation or "mental model" about a situation. Unfortunately, many are arbitrary and based on intuition.

A Perspective of Statistical Theory

Variation in time is unique and different from aggregated variation. The difference results from both the lack of recognition of the time factor and the implicit mixture of process inputs. Further confusion results when one realizes that each input stream also occurs (and varies) in time!

Variation in time is like taking a series of photos of a process. Small details will vary depending on the time at which it is taken, but the overall large details do not. The small details are analogous to common cause variation, while changes in the large details would be due to special causes.

All processes have common cause variation, but only some are affected by special causes. Those processes without special causes can be considered statistically stable. Stability in time of process inputs and outputs is essential if you want to predict the process outputs. Returning to the photo analogy, if no special causes affect the large details of the picture, we can predict how the picture will look day after day.

Studying any process in time is crucial to:

- assess current process performance

- establish a baseline for improvement efforts

- assess improvement efforts

- predict future performance

- ensure that improvement gains are held.

Any data set has an implicit time element (recall the cardiac mortality data from Figure 4.3). It cannot be overemphasized: ignoring the time element can lead to incorrect statistical conclusions.

Suppose the envelope exercise presented in Chapter 4 were repeated. Would the numbers be different from the previous ones? Of course they would! Would it depend on whether objectives and a measurement process were discussed? Not necessarily! What could be said about the process which produced these measurements? Is it the same? Has it improved? How would you know?

Statistical analysis of a process should begin with a plot of the data in the time order in which it was produced. By analyzing patterns in the plot, two important questions about the process can be answered:

- Did these data come from a stable process?

- If the process is stable, how much variation is naturally inherent in it?

Figure 7.5 contains two scenarios. The last two points in each plot are the "two point trend" data from Figure 7.2, but now they are put in the perspectives of their previous history. How do these graphs help interpret the difference between these points? The first plot (Figure 7.5a) shows this last difference to be quite atypical when compared to its previous history: it is a special cause, i.e., truly different. It seems that a different process was at work during this time period. The second plot (Figure 7.5b) shows the same increase in the last two points, but when placed in the context of its previous history, it is no different than other increases and decreases experienced by the process. One would not immediately see it as different, and the difference could be attributed merely to common cause. The underlying process itself hasn't really changed. Inherent random variation is acting within a predictable range.

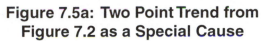

Figure 7.5a: Two Point Trend from Figure 7.2 as a Special Cause

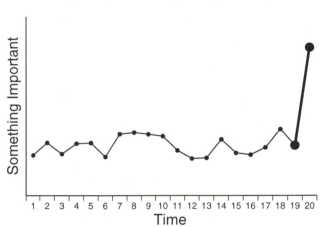

The difference between the last two points (the two points from Figure 7.2) is clearly different than the normal variation in the process. This means the difference is due to a special cause.

Figure 7.5b: Two Point Trend from Figure 7.2 as a Common Cause

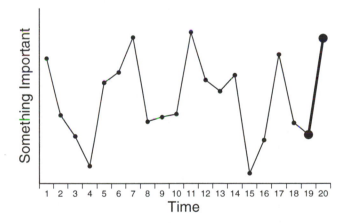

The difference between the last two points (the two points from Figure 7.2) is no different than the normal variation in the process and can be attributed to common causes.

Again, the cornerstone concept in quality improvement—understanding the distinction between **common** and **special** causes of variation in a process—aids in formulating an appropriate response to a given situation.

Instead of asking the obvious, "Is the current data point different than the previous data point?" the key question to ask when comparing two points in time is:

*Is the **process** which produced this current data point the same as the **process** which produced the previous data point?*

This is a deeper, more fundamental question that radically affects one's approach toward process improvement. Using statistical theory to correctly interpret a situation and answer this question minimizes the probability of inappropriate action.

Common vs. Special Cause in a Time Perspective

The output over time from a common cause process represents the aggregated effect of a consistently present set of forces. These forces are inherent in the process and act on it in a seemingly random manner. Think of the individual differences of one's consecutive bowling scores, golf scores, car gas mileage, amounts spent at the supermarket, times to get to work. They're not exactly the same. One's natural obvious reply is, "Of course, they're not!".

People sometimes feel that because they can explain the specific reasons for individual ups and downs of common cause processes (like Figure 7.5b) that these are indeed special causes. **However, the ability to explain a change after the fact does not make it a special cause**. There are many sources of common cause variation. We can't predict in advance which particular sources will affect the process at any given time – we only know that some will. To paraphrase Gilda Radner's Roseann Roseannadanna character from *Saturday Night Live*, "It's always something¡!...You know? If it isn't one thing, it's another."

Since common causes are consistently present it is reasonable to ask, "What range of variation do they normally exhibit?" The aggregated effect of the specific forces acting on a common cause process at any one time cannot be predicted in advance. Each force contributes a random, small amount of variation. Thus the individual data points are not, *and never will be*, predictable. However, when studied over time the *range* of the resulting process outputs can be predicted, i.e., we can determine maximum and minimum values that the outputs will almost never exceed. As long as the output stays within this range, the effects of inherent, common cause forces on the process have not changed. In fact, this inherent common cause is the "yardstick" that determines when the observed variation is excessive. *When variation is excessive and attributable to forces that are not typically part of the process, it is special cause variation.*

A common misconception holds that a process with only common cause variation, i.e., no special causes, cannot be improved. This is inaccurate and will be discussed subsequently at great length. Common cause just means that the points cannot be treated and reacted to *individually*. They must be considered in their *aggregate* because they were all produced by the same process. The power of aggregation can expose the hidden, underlying, consistent pattern that characterizes the process in a seemingly random manner.

In considering Figure 7.5a, the last increase can truly be considered a special cause. Its behavior is different from the previous history. It obviously represents the action of a force not usually present in this process. Treating this point as unique would be a high yield strategy. There is something to be found.

If this result is beneficial, discovery of the cause could have true improvement potential. Or it could signal the effect of a known intervention: perhaps the special cause was intentionally created for testing a possible improvement or problem solution.

If the result is not beneficial, a process may need to be established to prevent future occurrence. Or, it could just turn out that this represented a strictly one-time occurrence and no further action is needed.

Special causes represent the effects of forces not typically inherent in the process. Neither their specific occurrences nor their effects on the process can be predicted except in the case of a known intervention. In any event, special causes require unique investigation and action.

There Is No Choice: You're Already Using Statistics

As previously stated, whether or not people understand statistics they are already using statistics. Without statistical theory, however, there is human variation in interpretation of organization performance tables and reports as everyone filters them through their own unique "statistical ouija board".

It is not necessary to wait to form a project team before using statistics for effective problem-solving. All routine data reports must be evaluated using a common, agreed-upon theory: statistical theory. Statistical theory allows the reports to be placed into contexts that reduce the human variation in perceptions. It cannot be emphasized enough:

All decisions are predictions based on interpreting patterns of variation in data (real, anecdotal, or "one point" comparisons to a goal). All variation is caused and can be classified into one of two categories: common cause or special cause. Treating one as the other will usually make things worse.

The term coined by Deming to characterize the specific case in which a common cause is treated as special cause is **tampering**. This is by far the most prevalent error made in work cultures. Deming has said that the losses caused by tampering are incalculable.

Work cultures tend to treat each situation requiring action as a special cause. Problems march into one's office, people are told to "do something about it," and action is taken immediately.

Let's think about if from another perspective. Can't undesirable situations be considered variation? Something has happened to indicate a process did not produce the desired result. Isn't action, in essence, a prediction that the problem will be solved? It might be a higher yield strategy to consider whether this observed variation is a common or special cause. Is it unique (special) or could it happen under similar circumstances to different people in the future (common, or randomly inherent in the process)? Is the action going to solve a specific problem (special cause) or has this same problem been repeatedly solved in various guises (common cause)? A better action would be to ask questions to understand the variation so it can be properly evaluated and acted upon.

Everyone in an organization needs knowledge of variation. As individuals learn to appropriately respond to variation the whole improvement process itself improves.

An Example: Daily Incoming Medical Information Calls

This example describes one practice's experience with data intended to monitor incoming Medical Information (MI) calls. Many medical centers have purchased expensive telephone and software systems to try to manage phone usage and staffing. It is not unusual for data from these systems to be presented in a table format with averages, summaries and other "stats" aggregated in a typical "rows and columns" format. When common and special causes are not understood, management frequently circles high and low numbers, and demands explanations about apparent changes in productivity. These numbers frequently are used to change staffing levels. Incorrect data collection or analysis could result in overstaffing, understaffing, or an inappropriate staffing mix.

For our example, five months of phone data were aggregated and statistically analyzed (Figure 7.6). The objective was to gain insights into the number of MI calls received. Since the data were collected daily, one obvious theory was that phone calls varied by day of the week. Thus, "day of the week" was a possible special cause. A stratification, shown in Figure 7.7, revealed this to be true: Mondays averaged 254 calls; Tuesdays, 194 calls; and Wednesdays through Fridays, 207 calls. Three distinct "processes" are present in this phone system. What can be expected on a typical day?

Figure 7.6: Medical Information (MI) Telephone Data

Hourly Calculations Box for ABC Shift 9:00 - 19:00									
HOUR	AGENTS WORKING	TOTAL RECEIVED	TOTAL ANSWERED	TOTAL ABANDONED	PERCENT ANSWERED	AVG TIME BEFORE ANSWER	PERCENT ANSWERED IN 60 SECS	# OF CALLS ANSWERED IN 60 SECS	ADJUSTED % ANSWERED IN 60 SECS
9:00-10.00	5	68	60	8	88%	20	95%	57	83%
Month Ave	6.3	85.9	80.1	5.9	93.1%	20.7	93.3%	74.7	86.9%
10:00-11:00	4	65	60	5	92%	30	90%	54	83%
Month Ave	6.3	82.9	75.5	7.4	91.1%	26.1	88.2%	66.6	80.3%
11:00-12:00	4	57	56	1	98%	14	98%	54	94%
Month Ave	5.4	68.7	64.7	4.09	4.2%	18.6	94.7%	61.3	89.2%
12:00-13:00	2	38	33	5	86%	16	97%	32	84%
Month Ave	3.8	61.9	55.9	6.0	90.3%	19.9	93.6%	52.3	84.5%
13:00-14:00	4	55	52	3	94%	25	90%	46	83%
Month Ave	4.9	62.6	55.7	6.9	89.0%	25.6	90.6%	50.5	80.6%
14:00-15:00	4	40	39	1	97%	10	100%	39	97%
Month Ave	5.2	58.4	51.7	6.7	88.5%	24.8	88.2%	45.6	78.1%
15:00-16:00	3	39	34	5	87%	27	82%	27	69%
Month Ave	3.7	42.5	37.2	5.3	87.5%	22.3	88.8%	33.0	77.7%
16:00-17:00	3	15	11	4	73%	15	91%	10	66%
Month Ave	3.3	24.8	19.6	5.2	79.2	20.7	90.3%	17.7	71.5%
17:00-18:00	1	8	8	0	100%	28	88%	7	87%
Month Ave	0.8	10.4	7.1	3.3	68.3%	30.0	80.3%	5.7	54.8%
18:00-19:00	1	3	3	0	100%	25	67%	2	66%
Month Ave	0.8	5.3	3.9	1.4	74.3%	24.1	85.9%	3.4	63.8%
DAY TOTAL	31	388	356	32				328	
HOUR AVG	3.1	38.8	35.6	3.2	91.8%	20.7	92.1%	32.8	84.5%
FM DAY AVG	40	503	451	51				410	
FM HOUR AVG	4.0	50.3	45.1	5.2	89.7%	22.6	91.9%	41.1	81.6%

When presented in a tabular format, the data and "stats" provide little insight into the process. Even labels can be confusing!

Figure 7.7: Stratification of MI Data by Day of the Week

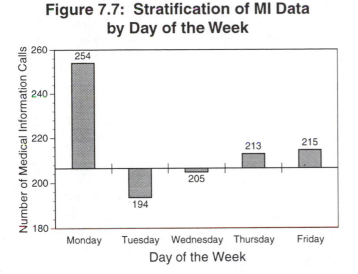

Three systems exist in the MI phone call process. A stratification and further statistical analysis (discussed in Chapter 8) shows that: 1) Wednesdays - Fridays represent one system; 2) due to its higher average, Mondays are in another system; and 3) due to its lower average, Tuesdays are in yet a third system.

Figure 7.8 shows a special kind of time plot known as a **control chart** for Tuesday's call pattern. A control chart shows data plotted in their natural time order. Three horizontal lines appear on the plot to show the average and the limits of the natural, inherent range, i.e., common cause variation, of what can be expected in the process. *It is crucial to note that these limits are calculated from the data. They have nothing to do either with a desired range of values or arbitrary numerical goals needed for business survival.* Calculation and interpretation of the limits will be discussed in more detail later in this chapter.

Figure 7.8 Control Chart for Tuesday Medical Information Phone Data

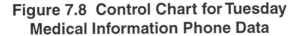

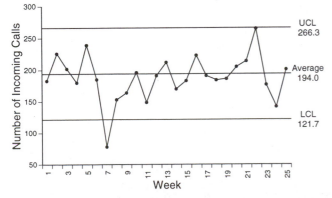

Note that the seventh point in Figure 7.8 lies below the lower horizontal limit. This signifies a special cause unique to that point only. Given the normal course of

events, a value this low would not be expected. Investigation showed this to be December 24, Christmas Eve day. Is this a reasonable explanation? One would think so. Then does it also seem reasonable that this date should be *excluded* from the calculation of the average for Tuesdays?

Yet, *overall* daily averages for months are routinely reported. With all the special causes in this process (day of the week, Christmas Eve day), what does that average mean? Can that average help people determine staffing requirements? If the average is taken at face value, it is similar to someone saying, "If I stick my right foot in a bucket of boiling water and my left foot in a bucket of ice water, on the average, I'm pretty comfortable." Also, note the common cause variation of plus or minus 72 calls for *any one day*. This was a much wider range than anyone expected. Without this simple, statistical, graphical summary, is it any wonder that the temptation to tamper cannot be avoided by merely reacting to a table of numbers? **Without knowledge of the range of common cause variation, it is easy to mistake routine day-to-day variation for special causes.**

Note that data point 22 lies extremely close to, but does not exceed, the upper horizontal limit. Subsequent investigations revealed nothing unusual about that particular Tuesday. It was just an extremely busy day. A day this busy will happen *occasionally*.

Notice how during the subsequent week, calls returned to well within range of the average. Suppose staffing had been adjusted as a result of that demand? The result would have been tampering. Extra costs would have been caused for no reason. Natural variation (common cause) would have been treated as if action were needed (special cause).

This process is stable and predictable. It is the inherent result of the aggregation of all the inputs of the process. Assessment of its current performance can be used to ask questions as to whether that level of performance is acceptable and what implications there are for staffing. The common cause of plus or minus 72 calls is also inherent in the process as reflected in this data collection.

What is the objective of these data? Suppose they are used for staffing. Does one staff for the average, or does one staff for slightly higher than the average? Staffing for slightly above the average will result in better customer service, even though the phone system will be overstaffed on some days.

7

Could these data be stratified further? Should there be a breakdown by time of day to see whether there are special causes at certain times of the day? This could result in better predictability because variability from any "time of day" special cause is currently included in the common cause range. When this special cause is removed from the data, the common cause range will be smaller than plus or minus 72 calls. Follow-up action could involve staffing higher only at certain times of the day, and perhaps decreasing the phone staff at other times.

Note how the questions needed to answer a common cause situation aren't as simple as taking action based on a single data point. In understanding common cause, fundamental questions which require further data collection must be asked about the underlying process. The hope is to eventually expose a hidden special cause thus allowing a focus on both a significant source of variation and appropriate solution.

The key issue is not whether one data point is different from another data point. Variation virtually guarantees that. The more fundamental question again is, "Is the **process** that produced this particular data point the same as the **process** that produced the other data point?".

The concept of a process, especially an administrative one, as having a center (or average) with observed, inherent, predictable, common cause variation can be extremely difficult to grasp. The center for the Tuesday MI process is 194 calls with common cause variation of plus or minus 72 calls. This means that while the Tuesday average is 194 calls, on any given Tuesday, the clinic could expect between 122 and 266 calls.

This concept is especially hard to understand when a corporate goal lies between the common cause limits. (This would occur if, as an example, the medical center had a goal of receiving a minimum of 225 calls per day.) The result is that the goal will be "achieved" in some, but not all of the time periods. As stated in the previous paragraph, numbers as high as 266 could randomly be produced by common cause variation from this process, even though it is centered at 194. ***Processes do not understand goals***. A process can only perform at the level that its inputs will allow. If this level does not allow the goal to be consistently achieved, fundamental changes will have to be made to the process.

In addition, each process input also occurs in time and special causes contained within a particular input stream will aggregate. As a result, variation caused by both the process input and the special causes

contained in it aggregate in and affect the output. Recall the Medication Error example from Chapter 6. The "people" input was one source of variation in that process. Pharmacists B and E were special causes inside the "people" input, and there was a further special cause (Error Type 3), with Pharmacist B. All these special causes were combined and aggregated with normal day-to-day variation. This produced the predictable outputs seen by the management. Understanding variation and prediction is rarely as easy as the numbers seen in a summary table.

The following examples demonstrate two simple yet very important techniques, the **Run Chart** and the **Control Chart**. These tools are essential to assess and quantify variation inherent in any data set collected over time.

Assessing Data in Time Through Trend Analysis and Run Charts: The Accident Data Problem

The following example is based on actual experience. It is typical of many routinely collected data sets that focus on numbers important to an organization. If an organization does no more than to apply run charts to its routine data, untold amounts of tampering will be avoided. Thus, in theory, better decisions can be made from better data display.

Safety is extremely important in an industrial environment. A manufacturing facility kept monthly data on the number of accidents in their factory (Table 7.1) and found 45 such accidents in 1989. The company set a safety goal: reduce accidents by at least 25 percent in 1990. The resulting 32 accidents in 1990 showed a 29 percent decrease. Time to celebrate...or is it?

TABLE 7.1: Industrial Accident Data

1989		1990	
Month	Accidents	Month	Accidents
January	5	January	2
February	4	February	1
March	5	March	3
April	7	April	2
May	1	May	3
June	3	June	7
July	2	July	0
August	6	August	3
September	2	September	1
October	3	October	5
November	7	November	5
December	0	December	0
Total 1989	45	Total 1990	32

Every month, a safety report similar to Figure 7.9 was posted. One can see that it is a thinly disguised variation of the two-point trend. Does this information help people improve, especially if the variation is common cause? Think of an accident as variation—an undesired result. One definition of accident is: a hazardous situation which was unsuccessfully avoided.

As discussed earlier in this chapter, we are not asking whether the numbers are different from month to month or year to year; we are asking whether the process that produced those numbers has changed. Thus the key question when determining if safety has improved is whether the underlying situations have changed or whether people were just luckier in avoiding them in 1990.

Figure 7.9: Accident Data Safety Recap

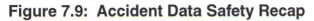

Figure 7.10 shows a typical display of such data: the "Year-Over-Year" plot. One could conclude that 1990 was better because eight of its months were lower when compared to the same months in 1989. Intuitively, this seems to makes sense, but what does statistical theory say? Believe it or not, purely random data could generate this result 23 percent of the time!

Why 23 percent? It's the odds of flipping a coin 11 times and getting eight heads or tails—the law of probability. Here, we compare 11 months (December had the same number of accidents both years and doesn't count in the comparison) and find eight of them to be lower.

Thus, if one were to conclude that 1990 was truly better, i.e., the result of a special cause, there is a 23

percent chance of treating common cause variation as if it were special. When considering the risk of tampering (taking the wrong action, or action when you shouldn't), a rule of thumb is to make this risk **5 percent or less**.

Figure 7.10: "Year-Over-Year" Plot of Accident Data

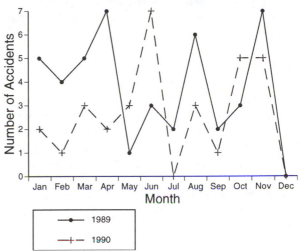

When data are plotted in this format it implies that special causes may be associated with the same months in each year.

Figure 7.11 shows another common data display. The individual data points are plotted as a scatter plot in their naturally occurring time order with a "trend line" superimposed. Literal interpretation of the line could cause one to conclude that accidents were cut almost in half! However, the probability of this being due to a linear trend special cause is only 21 percent. Once again, are these odds worth betting on?

Figure 7.11: "Trend Analysis" of Accident Data

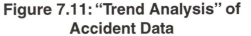
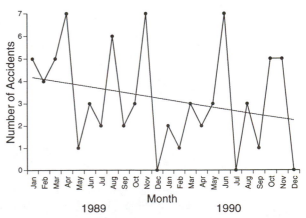

When data are plotted in this format it implies that a special cause has created a linear trend.

There is a common fallacy that "you can prove anything with statistics" as well as Mark Twain's famous "lies, damn lies, and statistics." These ideas result when statistical techniques are inappropriately (and usually unintentionally) used until the desired special cause is found (sometimes known as "data torturing"[1]). The two presentations of the accident data are typical. Similar analyses occur every day. Even though the conclusions seem intuitively correct, they are just random, common cause patterns of variation incorrectly interpreted as special cause.

Before drawing conclusions from other analyses, it is necessary to first assess the stability of the process that produced the data. The first assessment of process stability comes from a **trend analysis**. Since everything is a process, the accident data should initially be considered as just 24 measurements of a process output. Let the data themselves determine whether they should be plotted year-over-year or whatever. The concepts of year and January are human inventions of convenience. The process doesn't know when a new year begins. *What do the data say?*

Trend Analysis

Figure 7.12 is a plot of the data over time. The first question to ask is whether any "trends" exist. **A true**

trend as defined by statistical theory is: **seven consecutive points all in either ascending or descending order** (Figure 7.13).

Figure 7.12: Time Order Plot of Accident Data

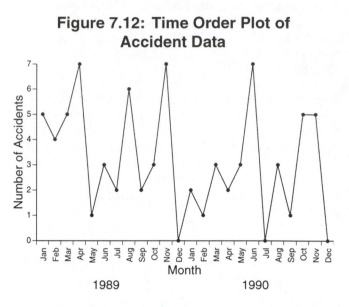

Plotting the data in time order removes the biases created by assuming the presence of special causes.

Figure 7.13: Statistical Definition of Trend

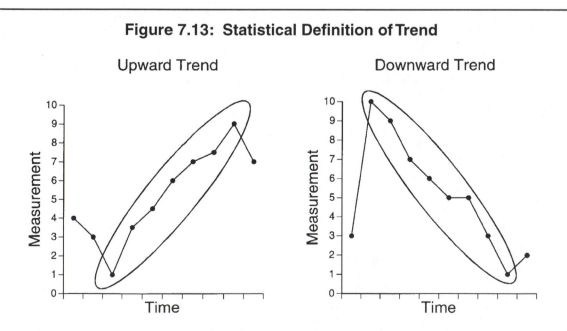

Special Cause - A sequence of SEVEN or more points continuously increasing or continuously decreasing - Indicates a trend in the process average.

Note: Omit entirely any points that repeat the preceding value. Such points do not add to the length of the run nor do they break it.

A trend is statistically defined as a sequence of seven consecutive points, all decreasing or all increasing.

There are two exceptions to this rule. First, if the number of data points plotted is *20 or less, six* consecutive points all in ascending or descending order would define a trend. Second, if two consecutive points have the same value, they only count as one point in the trend. Thus if there were seven points all in ascending order in a plot of 30 data points, it would be considered a trend. However, if two of those points had the same value, an eighth point in the same ascending or descending order would be required to declare it a trend.

Refer back to Figure 7.4 where the six different possibilities for three data points are displayed. It can be seen that with three points, two out of the six possible combinations exhibit "trend" behavior. Do three successively ascending or descending data points really represent trends? If one chose to interpret them as such, there would be a 33 percent chance that random (common cause) behavior is being interpreted as a special cause. Statistically, it takes a trend of seven to minimize this risk to an acceptable level.

To summarize, it takes at least six (or five, with 20 data points or less) *consecutive* increases (or decreases) to define a true trend and to have a low risk of treating common cause as a special cause. (Note that seven consecutive points in ascending order represent six increases.) However, if a data point *exactly* repeats its preceding value, it neither breaks the trend nor adds to it: ignore that data point for trend analysis purposes. Quite frankly, true trend behavior as defined by this test is observed quite rarely.

The accident data exhibit no such trend behavior. The plot in Figure 7.12 shows the longest sequence of increases or decreases to be three months. Sequences of three occurred three times during the time period, once from February - April of 1989, again from September - November of 1989, and finally from April - June of 1990.

Run Chart Analysis - Determining the Median

A **run chart** is a time plot with a horizontal line drawn at the median value. The **median** of the data set divides the data into two equal portions: Half of the data values are larger than the median, and the other half have values smaller than the median. The box shows two examples of the median calculation.

Calculating the Median

The median divides the data so that half the numbers are larger than the median and the other half are smaller than the median. Two examples will demonstrate the following step-by-step sequence.

A) Sort the data from the smallest value to the largest.

B) Count the number of data points. We'll refer to this number as "N."

C) If N is odd, calculate $\frac{N+1}{2}$. Begin counting at the smallest value from Step A. When your count reaches $\frac{N+1}{2}$, stop. The associated data point is the median.

D) If N is even, calculate $\frac{N}{2}$. Begin counting at the smallest value from Step A. When your count reaches $\frac{N}{2}$, stop. Calculate the average of this data point and the next number in the list from Step A. This average is the median.

A good check of the calculation is that the result should be the same regardless of whether the counting goes up from the smallest or down from the largest value in steps C and D.

Example 1

Suppose we have the numbers 18, 12, 29, 19, 16. The median calculation is as follows:

A) Sort the data from the smallest value to the largest.
When sorted, the numbers are 12, 16, 18, 19, 29.

B) Count the number of data points. We'll refer to this number as "N."
In this case, N = 5.

C) If N is odd, calculate $\frac{N+1}{2}$. Begin counting at the smallest value from Step A. When your count reaches $\frac{N+1}{2}$, stop. The associated data point is the median.
Since N is odd, $\frac{N+1}{2} = \frac{5+1}{2} = \frac{6}{2} = 3$. We start counting at the smallest value from Step A. The median is the third number, which is 18. Thus the median is 18. Note that two numbers are larger than 18 and two numbers are smaller than 18.

Note that we could also have started at the largest value from step A (29), and counted down three numbers. We still would end at 18.

Example 2

Suppose we have the numbers 18, 12, 29, 19, 16, 23. The median calculation is as follows:

A) Sort the data from the smallest value to the largest.
When sorted, the numbers are 12, 16, 18, 19, 23, 29.

B) Count the number of data points. We'll refer to this number as "N."
In this case, N = 6.

C) This step is skipped because N is even.

D) If N is even, calculate $\frac{N}{2}$. Begin counting at the smallest value from Step A. When your count reaches $\frac{N}{2}$, stop. Calculate the average of this data point and the next largest. This average is the median.
Since N is even, $\frac{N}{2} = \frac{6}{2} = 3$. We start counting at the smallest value from Step A. The third number is 18.
We must take the average of 18 and the next number in the list from Step A, which is 19. The median is the average of 18 and 19, which is 18.5. Thus the median is 18.5. Note that three numbers are larger than 18.5 and three are smaller than 18.5.

Note that we could also have started at the largest value from step A (29), and counted down to the third and fourth largest numbers. These would still be 18 and 19, and the median would remain 18.5.

Table 7.2: Sorted Accident Data

Month	Accidents	
December 1989	0	1st (Smallest)
July 1990	0	2nd
December 1990	0	3rd
May 1989	1	4th
February 1990	1	5th
September 1990	1	6th
July 1989	2	7th
September 1989	2	8th
January 1990	2	9th
April 1990	2	10th
June 1989	3	11th
October 1989	3	Median is 12th
March 1990	3	average of 13th
		12th & 13th
May 1990	3	14th
August1990	3	15th
February 1989	4	16th
January 1989	5	17th
March 1989	5	18th
October 1990	5	19th
November 1990	5	20th
August 1989	6	21st
April 1989	7	22nd
November 1989	7	23rd
June 1990	7	24th (Largest)

Figure 7.14: Run Chart of Accident Data

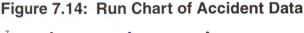

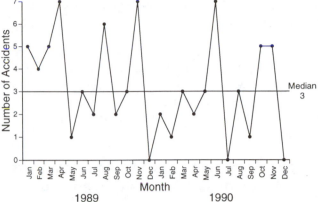

A run chart is a time plot with a line drawn at the median

Table 7.2 shows the accident data sorted in ascending order. The total number of data points, "N" is 24. Since N is even, we calculate $\frac{N}{2}$, which is 12, and start counting the numbers in Table 7.2. The 12th value is 3. The actual median is the average of the 12th and 13th values. Since the 13th value is also 3, their average, and thus the median, is 3.

To create the run chart then, we simply take the time order plot from Figure 7.12, and draw a horizontal line at the median, in this case 3, as shown in Figure 7.14.

Now what? In this or any time plot, what does "special cause" actually mean? Look again at the fundamental question to be asked: Was the process that produced the 1990 data the same process that produced the 1989 data? If a special cause were present, it would mean that at least two different processes were at work during this time sequence. For an improvement in safety, we would hope to see evidence of a different process with a lower level of accident occurrences in 1990. So far, the trend test gives no indication of such a special cause, since there is no sequence of seven consecutive decreasing points. What additional tests based in statistical theory can be used?

Run Chart Analysis - Counting the Length of Runs

A **run** is defined as a consecutive sequence of data points all on the same side of the median. If the data points are connected with a line, a run ends when the line *crosses* the median. A new run starts with the next point. Points on the median are ignored in runs analysis. They neither add to nor break any run.

Figure 7.15 shows the run chart of Figure 7.14 with each run circled and numbered. The runs can be interpreted as follows. The first four data points, January – April of 1989 represent a *run of length 4* above the median. The run is broken when the line going from April to May crosses the median.

As the line continues from May it reaches the median in June, but does not cross it, and stays below the median in July. The data point from August, though, brings the line across the median, thus the second run goes from May to July. While three months are included in this run, one of them (June) is on the median. *For the purpose of determining the length of the run*, the June data point should be ignored. Thus, the second run is of length 2.

This analysis continues until all the plotted points are assigned to a run. Figure 7.16 shows the lengths of each run, as well as the run number. Note that runs 2, 4, 6 and 8 all include points on the median, which makes their run lengths less than their actual number of months.

Figure 7.15: Run Chart of Accident Data With Individual Runs Circled and Numbered

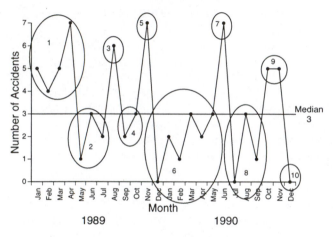

A run ends when the line connecting the data points crosses the median. If the line touches the median without crossing it, the run continues.

Figure 7.16: Run Chart of Accident Data Showing the Length of Each Run

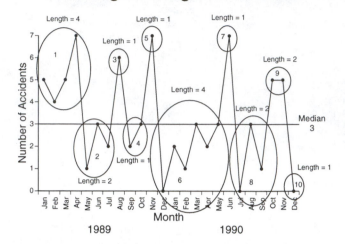

Note that points on the median are not counted when determining the length of a run.

How long must a run be to indicate a special cause? We can make an analogy to flipping coins. When flipping a (fair) coin, there is a 50 percent chance of getting heads and a 50 percent chance of the coin landing tails. Similarly, if all variation in the accident data were due to common causes, each point would have a 50 percent chance of falling above the median, and a 50 percent chance of falling below the median. Special cause patterns can be determined quite easily from statistical theory.

To minimize the risk of tampering, we use a run length of eight to signal a special cause. In other words, *a special cause has occurred if eight or more points fall on the same side of the median.* There is only a 0.8 percent chance of this happening due to common causes alone. If eight points in a row are on the same side of the median, there is almost surely a special cause present in the process. Figure 7.17 contains an example of a run of eight points.

Figure 7.17: Special Cause as Defined by a Run

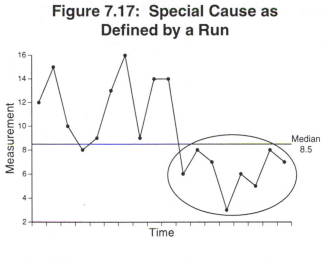
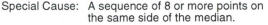

Special Cause: A sequence of 8 or more points on the same side of the median.

Note: Exclude any point that falls exactly on the median. It does not break the run, nor does it add to its length.

A special cause is indicated if eight or more consecutive points are on the same side of the median.

Returning to the accident data, if 1990 were truly lower in accidents, there might be a run of length eight below the median to signify it and/or a similar run of length eight above the median in 1989. As Figure 7.16 shows, this did not happen. So far, no special cause has been found.

Run Chart Analysis - Counting the Number of Runs

Figure 7.18 shows a set of data with two runs of length 7 followed by two runs of length 1. Suppose an improvement team had made some recommendations which were implemented after the fifth data point. This intervention is equivalent to *creating* a special cause for a desired effect. Did it make a difference? Obviously, there is no statistical trend (despite the trend of length 5 from observations 5-9). Neither is there a run of length 8. So, would one want to conclude that the intervention had no effect? What if the Joint Commission were coming next week? This plot certainly looks as though something has happened.

Figure 7.18:   Run Chart of 16 Points Showing Two Runs of Length 7

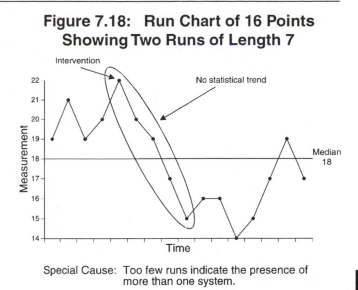

Special Cause: Too few runs indicate the presence of more than one system.

This chart fails none of the tests discussed so far, but it does not look like random, common cause variation. The test for number of runs will show a special cause.

There is a third test used in conjunction with the trends and runs tests. It is based on the number of runs observed in a data collection. Figure 7.18 shows that the 16 data points yielded only four runs (of lengths 7, 7, 1, and 1). Returning to the coin-flipping analogy, even though it might be possible to obtain seven consecutive heads (i.e., points above the median), it would be extremely unlikely to immediately follow it by flipping seven consecutive tails (i.e., points below the median). One might expect to see shorter runs, e.g., two - four heads, followed by one or two tails, etc., but not the type of clustering displayed in Figure 7.18.

Table 7.3 is based on the total number of runs observed above and below the median. Across from each value in the left column, "number of data points," are the minimum and maximum number of runs one would *expect* from a common cause process. With 16 data points from a common cause system, 5 to 12 runs are expected. Figure 7.18 contains only four runs. Since this is below what would be expected from common cause variation, *a special cause exists*. It would seem the intervention had the desired effect.

Table 7.3: Tests for Number of Runs Above and Below the Median

Number of Data Points	Lower Limit for Number of Runs	Upper Limit for Number of Runs
10	3	8
11	3	9
12	3	10
13	4	10
14	4	11
15	4	12
16	5	12
17	5	13
18	6	13
19	6	14
20	6	15
21	7	15
22	7	16
23	8	16
24	8	17
25	9	17
26	9	18
27	9	19
28	10	19
29	10	20
30	11	20
31	11	21
32	11	22
33	11	22
34	12	23
35	13	23
36	13	24
37	13	25
38	14	25
39	14	26
40	15	26
41	16	26
42	16	27
43	17	27
44	17	28
45	17	29
46	17	30
47	18	30
48	18	31
49	19	31
50	19	32
60	24	37
70	28	43
80	33	48
90	37	54
100	42	59
110	46	65
120	51	70

Revisiting the accident data, Figure 7.15 shows 10 runs. Recall that in runs analysis, points on the median are ignored, so the number of data points for Table 7.3 is not 24 because five points fell on the median. Instead we must look at the entry for (24 - 5) = 19 data points. Six to 14 runs would be expected if this were a common cause system. We obtained 10—no surprises.

According to these data, there is no evidence of a special cause. In spite of the fact that 1990 saw fewer accidents than 1989, we have no evidence that it was necessarily a safer place to work in 1990. As far as we can tell, the process which produced 32 accidents in 1990 was the same process that produced 45 accidents in 1989. The variation in the numbers was most likely due to common causes. The fact that 1990 met the goal is probably purely coincidental, confirming a fundamental statistical theorem:

> Given two numbers, one will probably be smaller (or bigger) than the other one.

Since evidence points to a common cause system, we can make predictions. If these data were plotted on a control chart we would learn that, if nothing in the work process fundamentally changes in the next year, there will be a total of 20 to 57 accidents in 1991, with any individual month having zero to nine accidents!

This does not mean that one must passively accept the current situation. It does mean, however, that the current process of reducing accidents has been ineffective. What to do instead will be discussed shortly.

Run Chart Analysis - Sequence of Alternating Points

Figure 7.19 shows a fourth test, indicated by 14 consecutive data points alternating up-and-down. This behavior occurs occasionally and indicates a special cause in the data collection process. It may indicate that two different process inputs are being reflected by being sampled alternately, i.e., measurements alternating between two people. It can also stem from accounting: were the figures from the last day of the month entered into the data base on the last day of the month or the first day of the succeeding month? The fact that months contain differing numbers of working days can also affect this.

Figure 7.19: Run Chart Showing 14 Points in a Row Alternating Up and Down

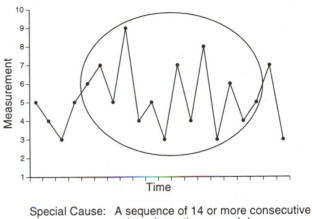

Special Cause: A sequence of 14 or more consecutive points alternating up and down – suggests a bias or systematic sampling from different sources

This type of special cause can result from alternating between two process inputs when collecting the data.

Another unfortunate possible cause of this variation is made-up data. In an atmosphere of fear where certain goals must be met, people can be very clever in creative reporting of results – slightly above average one month, slightly below the next, not wanting to call attention to themselves. In many cases these people are simply victims of their processes, which are incapable of meeting the goals. (Do these data add value to the organization?)

Figure 7.20 summarizes construction and analysis of a run chart. In a runs analysis, the occurrence of *any one* of the tests is sufficient to infer the presence of a special cause.

7

Figure 7.20: How to Construct a Run Chart

1) Obtain a sequence of data in their naturally occurring time order.

2) Plot the data from left to right in this time order.

3) Look for **trends**: Is there a sequence of seven or more consecutive points which go up (or down), i.e., do you observe a sequence of points where there were six or more consecutive increases (or decreases)?

   Note: Any value in the sequence which is an *exact* repeat of its preceding data point should be ignored in this test. It neither adds to nor breaks the sequence you are testing.

4) Look for a sequence where at least 14 points consecutively alternate "up-down-up-down-etc." or "down-up-down-up-etc."

   If this occurs, it indicates that there could be a special cause in the way the data have been sampled. For example, data could have been collected from two or more sources, or it can mean that data are not precise and have been "guesstimated."

5) Determine the **median** of the data, the number which divides the data so that half the data are smaller than the median and the other half are larger:

   A) Sort the data from the smallest value to the largest
   B) Count the number of data points. We'll refer to this number as "N"
   C) If N is odd, calculate $\frac{N+1}{2}$. Begin counting at the smallest value from Step A. When your count reaches $\frac{N+1}{2}$, stop.

      The associated data point is the median.

   D) If N is even, calculate $\frac{N}{2}$. Begin counting at the smallest value from Step A. When your count reaches $\frac{N}{2}$, stop.

      Calculate the average of this data point and the next number in the list from Step A. This average is the median.

   E) Check your calculation by starting at the other end of the data.

6) Draw the median line on the time plot of the data.

7) Draw circles around each run. A run is a series of points that do not cross the median. A run is complete when a subsequent point in the current sequence *crosses* the median. It is not unusual to have a run of length one.

   Note: A point exactly on the median should be *ignored* in the runs analysis—it neither adds to nor breaks the sequence of the current run.

8) An individual run *of length eight or greater* (eight or more *consecutive* points either all above or all below the median) indicates the presence of at least one special cause. Over the time period covered by the data, the process exhibited at least two different averages or centers. The special cause may not necessarily have occurred at the beginning of the run.

9) Count the number of runs obtained and compare it to the "Test for the Number of Runs Above and Below the Median" (Table 7.3).

   To obtain the "Number of Data Points" to use in this table, count the total number of data points and subtract the number of points exactly on the median. The total number of data points = N.

   If the number of runs is less than the lower limit from the table, the interpretation is the same as in 8) above. The process exhibited more than one average. It could also indicate the presence of a cycling effect in the process. Looking at the pattern of the graph would be useful in distinguishing between these two.

   If the number of runs is greater than the upper limit from the table (which rarely happens), this indicates either a problem with the way the data was collected (see 4, above) or else an extremely unstable process. It could also be evidence of tampering with the data.

The presence of any one of (3), (8), or (9) is enough to signal a special cause. Subsequent analysis and interpretation depend on one's "master knowledge" of the situation. Situations (4) or the "Too many runs" case of (9) indicate more fundamental issues in data process design or sampling.

A Very Common Misconception: Strategies for Common Cause

When people are first exposed to the concepts of common and special cause, they often are left with the impression that special causes mean one can immediately do something about a situation, whereas, with common causes, one is powerless and "stuck" with the current conditions. True, the key objective in quality improvement is to expose and reduce inappropriate significant sources of variation, and exposing special causes allows one to do that. Exposing special causes localizes the opportunity for improvement, and swift action can be taken to utilize the information for improvement.

However, it is not generally understood that special causes can exist in common cause systems, and a different, additional strategy is needed for exposing them. For example, one worker in a system may be producing a result that is 95 percent correct while another worker produces 85 percent. The combined or aggregate output would exhibit consistent, common cause behavior predictable at 90 percent. The process appears stable over time, but special causes are operating within the time periods.

Exhortation and goals would accomplish little, and an obvious, immediate opportunity for improvement would continue unrecognized. The two people are probably unaware of the variation. Yet it would seem there is a good possibility to improve the process to at least 95 percent, especially if the 85 percent worker is willing to learn. Again, one must focus beyond the process outputs. Plots of highly aggregated outputs have a tendency to exhibit stable behavior. This only means that the process is predictable over time. If nothing more is done about it, the process will continue to be predictable at its current level. After studying the process inputs and dealing with the special causes within the time periods, the process will continue to be predictable, but at a new, improved level.

This is analogous to the performance of the pharmacists in the Medication Error example from Chapter 6. The medication errors were consistent over time (as far as we know), but there were special causes within the system, namely Pharmacists B and E, and Error Types 3 and 5.

Reconsider the accident data, a common cause system. It is tempting to search for reasons that zero accidents occurred in some months as well as the reasons that some months had more accidents than average. Unfortunately, this strategy would yield

results: reasons *would be found,* but they would likely not be the correct reasons. When we look at a common cause system and pick out certain individual points to investigate, we are treating them as special causes. This is a natural tendency, perhaps because it results in immediate action and a feeling of "having done something." However, it generally results in well-meaning tampering that does not get to the root causes and actually adds complexity with no value.

Once again, consider the exercise where a roomful of people flip coins. The goal is to have as many people as possible obtain "heads" on each flip. One of the authors collected hard data "proving" that if everyone in the room took off their shoes and flipped coins with their left hands, it would maximize the number of heads. That was the method used by the person who had gotten the most heads when a coin flipping "evaluation audit" was completed. When this theory was "tested" on the next flip, the room got its highest total ever. Hence, that became the new work policy.

Of course, proper statistical analysis of the data would have shown a common cause system. It just so happened that this person had the highest number, but it was not due to anything special about her method. If the exercise had been repeated, *someone else* would most likely have had the highest number. It was a lottery. The high number of heads obtained in the subsequent test could have been shown to be merely common cause also.

It is virtually guaranteed that if one looks for reasons for pseudo-special causes, one will find them. What should be done to really differentiate common from special causes?

Because the accident process exhibits common cause, all the points are equally important. The data must be looked at as an aggregate from a process, i.e., there are 77 accidents to explain (45 from 1989 plus 32 from 1990). Questions must now be asked about the process and its inputs. Theories must be generated to drive *further data collection*.

Examples of questions to be asked might include:

- How were these data collected?

- What exactly is meant by "accident?"

- Do they include accidents by office staff? (Yes, mostly paper cuts!)

- How many different kinds of accidents are there and how many of each occurred?

- Which day of the week did they occur?

- What specific times of day did they occur?

- On which shifts did they occur?

- In which departments did they occur?

- Do they occur more often on certain equipment?

- When normalized by hours worked, are rates different for each department?, etc.

These questions are the motivation for tools to organize theories about the variation. An Ishikawa (Fishbone) diagram discussed in Chapter 6 could be helpful in this case.

Team members may have theories. But without further data collection to locate and isolate major opportunities (usually stratification of the process inputs), solid answers will not emerge. Note how all the questions address process inputs. Through Pareto analysis of the stratified data, major improvement opportunities can be found (the 20 percent of the reasons causing 80 percent of the accidents). This was the approach taken with the medication errors. Solving a common cause situation requires a more patient, long-term strategy than the approach for special cause problems. Common cause variation is reduced by working on fundamental issues of the process and its design.

Think about your organization's current data collections. How many of them consist of aggregated summaries such as the accident and medication error data with no traceability to the process inputs? Do people react as though every undesirable event is a special cause requiring an explanation? Are month-to-month comparisons made? Do people make comparisons to goals and treat the differences as special causes? We've shown how a run chart allows assessment of the process. This assessment helps to guide people toward the proper improvement actions. We will shortly do the same with control charts.

A Word About Goals

Improvement comes from *not focusing solely on the output but on the process*. Are the dangers of arbitrary numerical goals becoming more apparent? They cause distraction by comparing *individual* results to a goal and treating the difference as a special cause. This ignores the fact that this output is generated by a *process* which exhibits an inherent range of results.

Goals themselves are not bad. It's all in how they are used. By what method is an organization going to try

to achieve a given goal? Numerical goals have a tendency to be arbitrary. Have you noticed such goals tend to end in "0" or "5" with the exception of, specifically, "3". What's the theory behind this? What specific processes need to be improved? Exhortation to achieve goals treats a culture with special causes (obvious opportunities for improvement) as common cause ("Come on everyone, do it!")? What effect does this have on morale? What exactly are they supposed to do differently? Remember, there is no such thing as "improvement in general."

As an example, consider a prominent Fortune 500 company that created a financial index in 1977 and concluded that, for reasons of "business survival," this index needed to be at least 27 percent. The history of this index was studied via yearly annual reports from 1977 through 1994. It is presented in Table 7.4. A run chart analysis determined that years 1980-1994 represented a stable process. The first three years of the index seem to come from a different process.

A control chart, based on the stable years and calculated in a manner similar to the Medical Information phone example, is presented in Figure 7.21. The index's average is 23.0 percent. It has a common cause band of variation of plus or minus 6.3 percent *for any one year*. This results in a range of 17 percent to 29 percent! The goal of 27 percent is contained within the common cause! While the index could be met in an occasional year, it will not be met consistently given the current system. Achieving it once could be due merely to a fortunate aggregation of circumstances outside the company's control.

Table 7.4: Financial Index Data

Year	Index	Year	Index
1977	27.4%	1986	23.2%
1978	31.4	1987	24.4
1979	31.0	1988	26.8
1980	27.6	1989	26.9
1981	25.2	1990	24.5
1982	21.0	1991	20.2
1983	22.4	1992	19.7
1984	23.7	1993	19.1
1985	20.0	1994	20.7

Figure 7.21: Control Chart of Financial Index

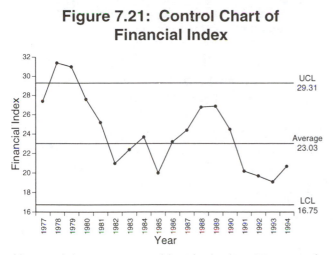

No special causes are evident in the last 15 years of this plot. The common cause range of variation is 17 percent to 29 percent.

The company's current process of operation has yielded a consistent result *over the last 15 years*! The numbers from 1989 through 1993 show a steady decline, but none of the runs rules have been violated. The reason given by management for the low (19.1 percent) 1992 number was "pricing pressures and negative currency effects," essentially, the economy, implying a special cause.

Of course it was the economy! "It's always something…, you know?!" But who could have *predicted* these conditions? They occurred randomly! The *specific result*, i.e., the index in any particular year, is unpredictable.

Going to work, there are days when all the traffic lights are red (or all green). How did we know it was going to happen? We didn't! How can we prevent the all red case from happening or get all greens all the time? We can't! It's out of our control despite our desire for the best possible situation (all green). We know the reason for the variation, but we could not have predicted it in advance, nor, with the current process design, have much control over it.

If extreme variation was a problem , how should we try to improve the situation?   Should we change our route (process), or should we do nothing? Would changing our route be a high yield strategy or would it be over-reacting to one bad day?

Continuing with the example of traffic, speed limits could also be considered arbitrary goals. Given a speed limit, traffic tends toward some average, usually higher than the limit. This is the result of the

enforcement process. If one exceeds the limit by the same amount as everyone else on a heavily traveled road (common cause), chances of getting a ticket are slim; they are pretty much a lottery. But if only one or two drivers distinguish themselves from the pack by excessive speed (special cause), they incur a much higher probability of a ticket. For speed limits to be more effective, the *process* of enforcement must be changed. The speed limit could also be lowered (creating a special cause in the process) theorizing that the result will still be higher than the limit but lower than the current average. However, data will be needed to know *exactly* how much higher than the speed limit people typically drive on the average.

How does this apply to the financial index?   When trying to improve the performance of this financial index, runs analysis would help determine whether the goal is ever truly achieved or at least heading in the right direction. As an interesting side note, should the company ultimately achieve the goal, i.e., move the average to 27 percent, half of the years would *still* be below 27 percent due to the random nature of variation! A key consideration should be *how the goal is operationally defined*: Is it a number that should *always* be attained or is it a goal for the *process average*?

Once the goal is defined, the fundamental question becomes, "Is the current process *capable* of meeting this goal?" The time plot of the data will answer that question. However, the individual data points will not. The plot and analysis of the process variation will then drive questions that need to be asked and the strategy for improvement.

Since we agree that most (85-97 percent) problems are based in systems, the data needed for improvement must be routinely collected from that perspective. It is a natural tendency to collect and react to individual results and outputs. The good news is that plotting the current output data can give *baselines* from which a process's capability and the improvement attempts can be assessed.

Solution implementations can be thought of as attempts to deliberately create beneficial special causes. These causes would be detectable on run charts and control charts. The other good news is that as questions are asked for stratification purposes (or any of the six sources of problems with a process in Figure 3.5), the answers will require small, focused, simple, efficient, one-time data collections on the work while it is performed by the people (as opposed to a retrospective view).

7

Additional Common Cause Strategies

Aside from stratification, another technique for understanding variation in a common cause system is called **disaggregation**. This is a form of "cutting new windows," previously discussed in Chapter 6. It involves separation of a measured output into its smaller components to identify the component causing the major source of variation. For example, take "x-ray turnaround time". A doctor could operationally define this as the time from when an x-ray is ordered to when the dictation is in the chart. Suppose a run chart of these turnaround times shows a common cause system at an unacceptable level?

It would be tempting to brainstorm reasons for "unacceptable turnaround time," but this almost seems like another "world hunger" problem, i.e., trying to bite off too much at once. (Recall the big, vague problems of Figure 6.10.) Wouldn't it make sense to separate or disaggregate turnaround time into its various components first to isolate the major bottleneck? Might it also be a good idea to do this on the 20% of the departments accounting for 80% of the problem? This could easily be established via stratified histograms of complaints or volume by department.

Design of a good data sheet and, perhaps, a week's worth of data collection in the departments involved would be well-worth the effort. The Pareto principle virtually guarantees that 80 percent of the variation is caused by 20 percent of the process. Disaggregation would help focus the improvement effort on the right process step and the right people, making the problem seem less overwhelming. Once again, to quote Joiner, "Vague solutions to vague problems yield vague results." Localize wherever possible.

A final way to address common cause, as discussed in the "Data Aggressiveness" portion of Chapter 6, is to *create* a special cause through designed experimentation. This would be "positive" variation which is theorized to be beneficial to the process. If the less aggressive strategies have shown no obvious special causes and the level of performance is still unacceptable, the experiment will involve a major process redesign. To get the current process to its best possible performance level before attempting major experimentation, it is always best to stratify and disaggregate. Redesign is so upsetting to a culture that one should exhaust the current potential opportunities by exposing and exploiting heretofore hidden special causes. By using current performance as a baseline, the effect of the intervention can be

measured by application of the run rules as will be demonstrated in the next example.

Using Run Charts to Assess an Intervention and Hold Gains: The Menopause QI Team Example

Figure 7.22 shows a run chart of the frequency of Follicle Stimulating Hormone (FSH) test ordering for women ages 40 to 44. A special cause is signaled by the run of the last eight data points below the median, beginning with November 1991. Thus, during this time period, the process has exhibited more than one "center," i.e., average. What special cause happened in November?

Figure 7.22: Run Chart of FSH Ordering Frequency

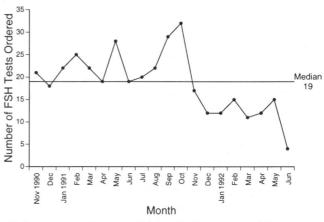

Eight consecutive months are below the median at the end, signaling a special cause.

November 1991 is when a team distributed their recommendations regarding the diagnosis of menopause. Guidelines were presented regarding the appropriate use of FSH testing. Their intervention lowered the use of the test, creating the desired effect. Now, how do they hold their gains?

Figure 7.23 shows a more appropriate picture of the data as a result of the runs analysis. It is rare that things happen in trends. As in this case, interventions cause processes to exhibit more of a "step change" pattern. Since the system has changed, it must be subsequently monitored by its most current stable behavior.

Figure 7.23: FSH Run Chart Showing "Step" Change

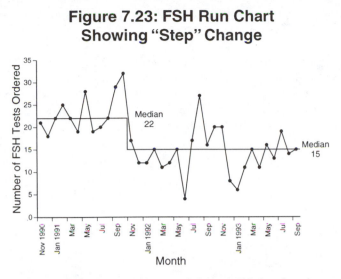

This plot recognizes the special cause in the data by showing separate medians for each system.

A runs analysis of the current FSH ordering process beginning with the intervention in November 1991 shows it to be stable. There are no trends, no runs of length eight, no alternating patterns of 14 points, and eight runs obtained from the 19 data points (Four of the original 23 were not counted since they were on the median of 15). Table 7.3 shows we would expect between eight and 16 runs. A control chart analysis (Figure 7.24) shows that the process is centered at 14, and, in any one month, common cause variation leads one to expect between two and 27 FSH tests to be ordered.

Figure 7.24: Control Chart of Current FSH Ordering "Process"

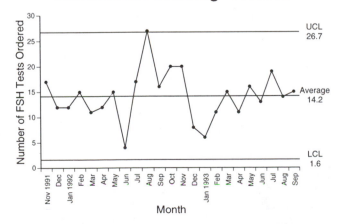

The common cause "window" for this process is 2 to 27 tests in any given month.

Observe that one month, August 1992, is right at the upper common cause limit of tests, 26.8. It is also interesting that the number of runs was the minimum that would be expected. Remember the fundamental question about data: How were these data collected? It turned out that the tabulated FSH value not only includes menopausal women, but also FSH tests given to check for infertility. An exceptionally high number of FSHs happened to be performed for infertility in August 1992. To get a "clean" number, i.e., one representing only tests given for menopause, chart reviews would have been necessary every month. The team concluded that the logistical difficulties of monthly chart reviews made the current aggregation sufficient for their objective of simply monitoring the process.

In assessing the current gains, the process has gone from a monthly average of 23, based on the data through October 1991, to the current monthly average—14—based on the subsequent data. Continued plotting of the monthly results monitors whether the gains are still being held.

"How Were These Data Collected?": The Venipuncture Data Example

Figure 7.25 shows a run chart of 25 data points collected by a lab supervisor to help her determine staffing requirements. There are no trends, no runs of length eight, and 12 runs for the 22 data points not on the median (with 7 to 16 runs expected). Hence, no special causes. Since this seems to statistically indicate that the process exhibited only one center, one may as well calculate the average (62) and staff based on that. Should any further questions be asked, e.g., *How were these data collected?* Since we appear to have a common cause process, we should look at a common cause strategy, such as stratification.

7

Figure 7.25: Run Chart of Venipunctures Performed

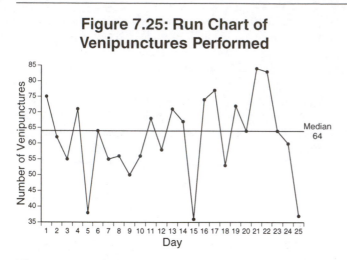

There are no obvious special causes in this process.

These 25 data points represent five weeks of data collected Monday through Friday. Does this spark any theories about special causes? Any ideas for stratification? Figure 7.26 shows the same run chart, but each data point is coded by the day of the week it represents: M=Monday, T=Tuesday, W=Wednesday, R=Thursday, F=Friday. Do any obvious special cause patterns make themselves clear?

(As these examples and analyses continue, is the value of displaying data graphically becoming more obvious?)

Figure 7.26: Coded Run Chart of Venipuncture Data

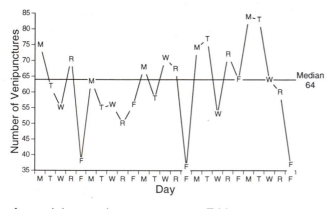

A special cause is now apparent. Fridays seem to have fewer venipunctures than other days of the week.

It appears that low counts consistently correspond to Fridays. In fact, this theory can be further tested by a technique known as "analysis of means" (ANOM), a more formal statistical analysis of stratification, to be

discussed in Chapter 8. ANOM is a very powerful tool for comparing strata.

Figure 7.27 shows the ANOM for the venipuncture data by day of the week. The first data point is the average of the five Mondays, the second data point the average of the Tuesdays, and so on. The centerline, 62, represents the average of *all* 25 data points.

Figure 7.27: Analysis of Means Comparing Day of the Week

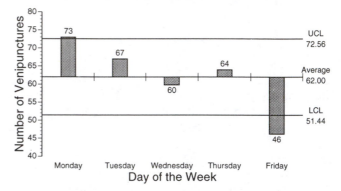

ANOM shows that both Fridays and Mondays have different venipuncture rates than other days of the week.

Note the two horizontal lines that, in essence, form a "dead band" around the average. These are calculated *from the data.* They represent the range of common cause variation expected around an average of five measurements taken from a process whose average is 62. Observations falling inside this dead band region should not be treated differently than one another, since they differ only due to common causes. Think back to Chapter 4's room of 50 people flipping coins. The average will be 25, but the expected "dead band" will range from 14 to 36.

Note that Friday is not the only day outside of the band; Monday falls out as well. Thus, Friday tends to have fewer venipunctures on average and Monday typically has more. Tuesday, Wednesday, and Thursday have different individual averages, but they are all within the band.

How can this be interpreted? Monday and Friday are special causes. Their differences from the overall average of 62 cannot be attributed merely to common cause. Monday and Friday each have their own unique averages, 75 for Monday and 40 for Friday. The chance that Monday and Friday differ from the average of 62 only due to common cause is less than 1 percent. Thus the risk of tampering is low.

On the other hand, the differences from 62 seen in the averages of Tuesday, Wednesday and Thursday (as well as their differences from each other) can be attributed to common cause because they all fall within the band of common cause variation around the average. Even though Tuesday has the highest value of the three and Wednesday the lowest, this difference is not enough to justify adjusting the staffing accordingly. Since the difference is due to common cause, the averages of the three days could reverse during a different time period, even if the process doesn't change. Staffing should be planned to expect 62 venipunctures on these days.

From the run chart, one could have näively concluded that staffing needed to be consistent for 62 venipunctures per day since that analysis indicated the presence of common causes only. However, that would have been a prediction assuming common cause when special causes were actually present. By asking questions about the data collection and process, special causes were exposed through stratification (studying the current process). This would allow *better predictions with less variation*: The supervisor should staff for 75 venipunctures on Monday, 62 on Tuesday through Thursday, and 40 on Friday. Or perhaps she shouldn't staff for the average. A typical Monday would range from 57 to 93, and a typical Friday would range from 27 to 53. Tuesday, Wednesday, and Thursday can be expected to range from 46 to 78. What would ensure good customer service?

Are there other questions which could refine the predictions even further? For example, are there certain peak times of the day? Are these times the same or different depending on the day? "Cutting new windows" by stratification across the time-of-day might be useful.

A large part of the management function is understanding variation for purposes of prediction!

Converting a Run Chart Into a Control Chart: The Computer Information System Percent Uptime Example

These data once again represent a major medical center's actual experience. Computer uptime was a very important index to one of the center's high level managers. To understand why uptime wasn't consistently reaching 100 percent, the data in Table

7.5 were collected over a 19 month period. Table 7.6 shows the data sorted in ascending order. Since there are 19 numbers, the median is established by calculating $\frac{19+1}{2}= 10$, and finding the 10th smallest (or largest) number. With these data the median is 99.3 percent.

Table 7.5: Computer Information System Percent Uptime Data

Month	Percent Uptime
January 1989	98.0%
February	98.7
March	98.7
April	99.2
May	99.2
June	100.0
July	99.7
August	99.5
September	99.0
October	98.6
November	100.0
December	99.3
January 1990	99.8%
February	99.8
March	98.5
April	100.0
May	100.0
June	98.6
July	99.7
Average	99.3%

Table 7.6: Computer Information System Percent Uptime Data Sorted in Ascending Order

Month	Percent Uptime	Order
January 1989	98.0	1st (Smallest)
March 1990	98.5	2nd
October 1989	98.6	3rd
June 1990	98.6	4th
February 1989	98.7	5th
March 1989	98.7	6th
September 1989	99.0	7th
April 1989	99.2	8th
May 1989	99.2	9th
December 1989	99.3	(Median) 10th
August 1989	99.5	11th
July 1989	99.7	12th
July 1990	99.7	13th
January 1990	99.8	14th
February 1990	99.8	15th
June 1989	100.0	16th
November 1989	100.0	17th
April 1990	100.0	18th
May 1990	100.0	19th (Largest)

When 100 percent was finally achieved in June 1989, the manager told the computer department to "Send out for pizza and send me the bill." However, the disturbing "trend" over the next four months made him feel the employees were taking advantage of the situation. It was time to get tough. After the disappointing 98.6 percent result in October, the manager strongly demanded 100 percent from his people. When 100 percent was achieved the following month, though, there was no pizza.

The manager's actions were based on data. However, those actions presumed all variation was due to special cause. *Columns of numbers say nothing!* A graph is required to properly interpret the data. What can be said about the *process* producing these data?

Figure 7.28 shows a run chart of the computer uptime results. A quick glance yields the following conclusions:

1) No trends. The initial trend of 6 months only counts as a trend of 4 because two points (March and May) repeat exactly their preceding values. The perceived managerial trend of 100 percent down to 98.6 percent was only length 5;

2) No runs of 8 either above or below the median;

3) Eight sets of runs in the 18 data points not on the median, with six to 13 expected.

Hence, a common cause system!

Figure 7.28: Run Chart of Percent Computer Uptime Data

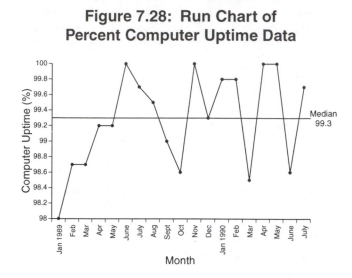

In spite of the apparent upward trend at the beginning of the plot, no special causes can be detected with these data.

Look again at the manager's actions. In treating the 100 percent month as unique, a common cause may have been treated as a special cause. In treating months 6-10 as a "trend", a probable common cause was treated as a special cause. By treating the change from 98.6 percent to 100 percent as if it were due to his strong-arm action, a common cause may have been treated as a special cause. What situations have you either observed or been in that were handled similarly? What were the results? Did things improve or stay the same? How did the people in those processes feel and subsequently behave? What should be done differently?

Figure 7.29 shows a control chart of these data. As shown in the MI telephone example, a control chart is a time plot of the data. It includes lines added for the average and the limits of common cause variation. These limits represent a *range* ("dead band") around the average where individual data points may be expected to fall *if the underlying process does not change*. (Once again, the process of 50 people flipping coins, although averaging 25 heads, will yield individual numbers between 14 and 36.)

Figure 7.29: Control Chart for Percent Computer Uptime Data

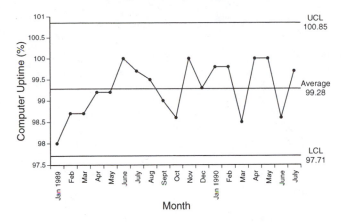

The control chart shows that given the current process, 100% uptime will be achieved in some, but not all months.

Since these data passed all the rules of the run chart, one can preliminarily conclude that a consistent process produced these data, i.e., it had one center. Because the run chart tells us the data all come from a single process, their average can represent the average of that process. (Note that if the run chart analysis had shown evidence of two or more processes during the time period, the average of all the numbers would have been meaningless. The cardiac mortality rates of Clinic 2, as plotted in Figure 4.5 were an example of taking the average of data from three processes. The Clinic 2 average was not an indication of the performance of Clinic 2.)

The average of the computer uptime process is 99.3 percent. Coincidentally, this is also the median.

Two questions remain:

1) What are the common cause, inherent limits of this process, i.e., what is the dead band around the average which indicate stable behavior?

2) How much difference between two consecutive data points is "too much"?

Table 7.7 once again shows the uptime data, but the next column contains a number known as the **moving range.** The moving range is calculated from the data and is a way of quantifying its variation. Intuitively, if most of the data represent a common cause system, it would seem safe to assume that two *consecutive* values in time would be a good estimate of common cause variation. It is immaterial whether the variation is positive or negative—it is just considered variation.

The box "Calculating the Moving Range" demonstrates the moving range calculation. For the computer uptime data in Table 7.7, the first moving range, 0.7, is obtained by subtracting the *first* data point from the *second* (98.7 - 98.0). The next moving range, 0, is obtained similarly by subtracting the *second* data point from the *third* (98.7 -98.7). This continues until the last moving range, 1.1, is obtained by subtracting the *eighteenth* observation from the *nineteenth* observation: (99.7 - 98.6).

7

Calculating the Moving Range

The moving range is a measure of the variation between two consecutive data points. It is calculated simply as the absolute value of their difference. In other words, one value is subtracted from the other. If the result is positive, it is the moving range between the two points. If the result is negative, delete the minus sign to make it positive. The new result is the moving range between the points.

A procedure for calculating the moving range of a set of data follows:
- A. List the data in time sequence.
- B. Subtract the first point from the second and ignore the sign. (Moving ranges are always positive)
- C. Return to Step B and use the second and third numbers, third and fourth, etc.

Example 1

Moving ranges will be calculated for the first seven months of the cardiac mortality data from Clinic 2 used to create Figure 4.5.

Month	Data	Moving Range Calculation	
1	4.06		
2	3.64	3.64 − 4.06 = -0.42	This is negative, so remove the minus sign. The moving range is 0.42.
3	3.50	3.50 − 3.64 = -0.14	This is negative, so remove the minus sign. The moving range is 0.14.
4	3.92	3.92 − 3.50 = 0.42	
5	3.78	3.78 − 3.92 = -0.14	This is negative, so remove the minus sign. The moving range is 0.14.
6	3.22	3.22 − 3.78 = -0.56	This is negative, so remove the minus sign. The moving range is 0.56.

Reprinting the data and moving ranges,

Month	Data	Moving Range
1	4.06	*
2	3.64	0.42
3	3.50	0.14
4	3.92	0.42
5	3.78	0.14
6	3.22	0.56

Note that there are six measurements in the data but only five moving ranges. There will always be one less moving range than there are data points.

Table 7.7: Percent Computer Information System Uptime Data

Time Order	Percent Uptime	Moving Range
January 1989	98.0%	*
February	98.7	0.7
March	98.7	0.0
April	99.2	0.5
May	99.2	0.0
June	100.0	0.8
July	99.7	0.3
August	99.5	0.2
September	99.0	0.5
October	98.6	0.4
November	100.0	1.4
December	99.3	0.7
January 1990	99.8%	0.5
February	99.8	0.0
March	98.5	1.3
April	100.0	1.5
May	100.0	0.0
June	98.6	1.4
July	99.7	1.1

Table 7.8: Percent Computer Information System Median Moving Range Calculation

Sorted Moving Range	Order
0.0	1st (Smallest)
0.0	2nd
0.0	3rd
0.0	4th
0.2	5th
0.3	6th
0.4	7th
0.5	8th
0.5	Median is average 9th
0.5	of 9th and 10th 10th
0.7	11th
0.7	12th
0.8	13th
1.0	14th
1.3	15th
1.4	16th
1.4	17th
1.5	18th (Largest)

Once the moving ranges have been determined, calculate the Median Moving Range (MMR). **This is the key number for understanding the common cause variation. All subsequent calculations will involve it.** This is the median of the moving ranges as calculated from the data *in their naturally occurring time order, not in their sorted order.* When calculating the MMR, be sure to remember that the number of moving ranges is always one less than the number of data points.

Table 7.8 contains the sorted moving ranges for the computer data. The 19 data points yield 18 moving ranges. Since 18 is even and N/2 = 9, the MMR is the average of the ninth and tenth sorted moving ranges. In this case, they both happen to be 0.5, so the MMR is also 0.5.

Multiplying the MMR by 3.865 (a constant derived from statistical theory) yields the *maximum difference between two* **consecutive** *data points which could be attributable to common cause.* If a moving range exceeds the upper limit of MMR x 3.865, (MRMax), it indicates the presence of a special cause. The factor 3.865 is valid for any time sequence where the *median* (not the average!) moving range is calculated, regardless of the sequence length.

A special cause as indicated by this test could indicate one of two possibilities. The first is that the process exhibited a significant shift in its average. Figure 7.30 contains a control chart of the Clinic 2 cardiac mortality data used in Figure 4.5. (As will be discussed subsequently, a control chart is not the recommended first strategy; but this data set will make that point.) The data and moving ranges are listed in Table 7.9. The moving range between Months 23 and 24 exceeds MRMax of 1.62, indicating a special cause.

Figure 7.30: Control Chart of Cardiac Mortality Data from Clinic 2.

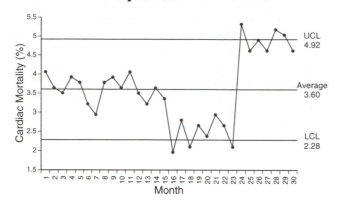

The second shift in the process average corresponds with a moving range which exceeds MRMax in Table 7.9. The MRMax is not sensitive enough to detect the first shift.

Table 7.9: Clinic 2 Cardiac Mortality Data and Moving Ranges

Month	Cardiac Mortality	Moving Range
1	4.06	*
2	3.64	0.42
3	3.50	0.14
4	3.92	0.42
5	3.78	0.14
6	3.22	0.56
7	2.94	0.28
8	3.78	0.84
9	3.92	0.14
10	3.64	0.28
11	4.06	0.42
12	3.50	0.56
13	3.22	0.28
14	3.64	0.42
15	3.36	0.28
16	1.96	1.40
17	2.80	0.84
18	2.10	0.70
19	2.66	0.56
20	2.38	0.28
21	2.94	0.56
22	2.66	0.28
23	2.10	0.56
24	5.32	3.22*
25	4.62	0.70
26	4.90	0.28
27	4.62	0.28
28	5.18	0.56
29	5.04	0.14
30	4.62	0.42

The median moving range is 0.42, making MRMax = 3.865 x 0.42 = 1.62. The Moving Range with the asterisk exceeds MRMax

Note that while the special cause is obvious from Figure 7.30, it would not be as obvious if we were looking at the plot in Month 24 and did not have the benefit of the subsequent six months of data. What if there was no plot? How would we assess this process via a typical "this month/last month/12 months ago/year-to-date" summary?

Figure 7.30 also shows a shift in the process average beginning in Month 16. The moving range between Months 15 and 16 is 1.40, which is below MRMax. The MRMax is not as sensitive to changes as the control limits around the average. In fact, the data point for Month 16 falls below the lower common cause limit on the control chart in Figure 7.30 and would have been immediately detected as a special cause. However, if the shift is large enough, the MRMax can be useful in early detection of process changes. The synergistic use of special cause tests rarely allows a true special cause to escape.

The second type of special cause indicated by the MMR is one unusual data point. This will be the case if the very next moving range is *also* a special cause. This is illustrated in Figure 7.31 and Table 7.10, which are based on the computer uptime data from Table 7.5. However, in Table 7.10, the value for March 1990, (98.5) has been mistyped as 89.5. The moving range between February and March 1990, 10.3, is well above the MRMax of 1.93, as is the moving range between March and April.

Figure 7.31: Computer Uptime Data with March 1990 Entered Incorrectly

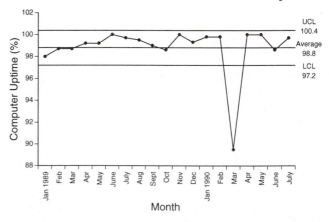

The outlier in March 1990 (due to the typing error) corresponds with two consecutive moving ranges which exceed MRMax in Table 7.10.

Table 7.10: Computer Uptime Data with "Typo"

Time Order	Percent Uptime	Moving Range
January 1989	98.0%	*
February	98.7	0.7
March	98.7	0.0
April	99.2	0.5
May	99.2	0.0
June	100.0	0.8
July	99.7	0.3
August	99.5	0.2
September	99.0	0.5
October	98.6	0.4
November	100.0	1.4
December	99.3	0.7
January 1990	99.8%	0.5
February	99.8	0.0
March	89.5	10.3*
April	100.0	10.5*
May	100.0	0.0
June	98.6	1.4
July	99.7	1.1

The two consecutive points with extremely large Moving Ranges indicate a single unusual point. In this case it was caused by a typo; the value for March 1990 should be 98.5.

For the actual computer uptime data in Table 7.5, MRMax = 0.5 x 3.865 = 1.93. Note that no moving range exceeds this value. The previously discussed change from 98.6 percent (the end of the 5 point "trend") to 100 percent (Moving Range = 1.4) could have been a natural event occurring randomly in this process. It probably had nothing to do with the manager's exhortation.

The next step is to obtain the common cause limits. This involves two calculations. First, the MMR is multiplied by 3.14. Then this quantity is added to the average to obtain the **upper control limit**. The same quantity (MMR x 3.14) is subtracted from the average to give the **lower control limit**. Once again, the 3.14 is derived from statistical theory and is valid for any time sequence where the *median* moving range has been calculated. The box "Calculating Control Limits" describes the sequence in more detail.

Calculating Control Limits

Control limits cover the region around the process average where data should fall if the process has no special cause variation. Control limits are calculated as follows:

A) Calculate the Median Moving Range (MMR)
B) Calculate the average of the data
C) Multiply the MMR by the factor 3.14
D) The Upper Control Limit = Average + (MMR x 3.14)
E) The Lower Control Limit = Average - (MMR x 3.14)

The Clinic 2 data from Table 7.9 will be used to demonstrate the calculation.

A) Calculate the Median Moving Range (MMR)
       The MMR of the data from Table 7.9 is 0.42

B) Calculate the average of the data
       The Average of the Clinic 2 data in Table 7.9 is 3.60

C) Multiply the MMR by the factor 3.14
       0.42 x 3.14 = 1.32

D) The Upper Control Limit = Average + (MMR x 3.14)
       UCL = 3.60 + 1.32 = 4.92

E) The Lower Control Limit = Average - (MMR x 3.14)
       LCL = 3.60 - 1.32 = 2.28

Note that control limits are sometimes referred to as "3 standard deviations", "3 sigma" or, using the Greek letter, "3σ" limits. This is **NOT** the same as taking the standard deviation of the data (as defined in most statistical texts) and multiplying it by three. The presence of a special cause in the data will *inflate* this typical estimate and mask chances of finding the special causes in the process. The MMR will minimize the effect of special causes, give a more realistic estimate of the common cause variation, and allow the special causes to be properly detected.

Note that the standard deviation as calculated from the MMR can be determined from Step C. In this case it is 1.32/3, or 0.44. Had the data been put through the "traditional" calculation of standard deviation, the result would have been 0.94—over twice as large. Why the difference? Because the traditional calculation includes common cause variation *and* the two special causes in the process.

7

Returning again to the computer data MMR x 3.14 = 0.5 x 3.14 = 1.57. The control limits are 99.3 + 1.6 = 100.9 percent and 99.3 - 1.6 = 97.7 percent. All the observations fall within this range.

Do not be troubled by the fact that the upper control limit is greater than 100 percent. The process does not understand that it is not possible to obtain a number greater than 100 percent. What this does suggest is that *100 percent is not an unusual event for this process*. Achieving 100 percent is within the common cause, inherent variation of this process. It is not necessarily a significant event. One also notices that the 98.6 result was not necessarily atypical of this process. In fact, somewhere, although it is impossible to say when, a "terrible month" of 97.7 lurks. Why? Because!

How will improvement take place? If one steps back and looks at this as a process, it is currently stable and operating at 99.3 percent. Until there is a significant change, this is the number that should be used for planning purposes. Reacting to the individual monthly results will result only in tampering.

A common cause strategy is needed to improve. One would need to aggregate the data for the 19 months and ask questions to suggest stratifications. When did the downtime occur? Was it certain times during the day? Certain days of the week? Certain times in the month? What were the causes of downtime? Was there any pattern to when different causes occurred? Who was the system operator during downtime? A Pareto analysis of these may expose a special cause. As with the venipuncture data, there may be a *consistent* special cause to explain the months where 100 percent was obtained: The 100 percent months should not be treated and scrutinized individually. Despite the low figure of 0.7 percent downtime, 0.7 percent of 19 months is a non-trivial chunk of hours! Scrutinizing an individual month's downtime would be a very deceptive, low-yield strategy.

There seems to be a dilemma. The goal of 100 percent is contained within the common cause variation. It can be achieved in individual months without any improvement to the system. How could interventions be evaluated?

Once a control chart has determined that a system is stable, the rules used with the run chart can still be applied as more data are obtained. So, if an improvement team makes an intervention and the control chart has:

1) a trend of 6 or 7 ascending months
2) a run of 8 above the current average, or
3) less than the expected number of runs,

it could be assumed that the intervention created a special cause with a beneficial effect.

A Warning about Arbitrary Numerical Goals

This example shows another danger with arbitrary numerical goals, especially when they lie within a process's common cause variation. Immediate reaction to individual data points then becomes tampering. This usually makes things worse. The common cause variation in subsequent data is used to evaluate the effects of this tampering. Random patterns are misinterpreted as special causes according to interpreter biases. To complicate matters, tampering often becomes a "normal" input to the process and actually inflates the underlying, inherent, existing common cause variation. The difference is that variation due to tampering is created. It is inappropriate variation in addition to the normal process variation. As a matter of fact, some forms of tampering can increase the inherent common cause variation of a process by approximately 40 percent. This further masks the problem with no resulting improvement.

Processes do not understand goals. Processes can only perform at the levels allowed by their inputs. One must study a process to understand its *capability* with respect to the goal. After this, one must learn whether observed variation, i.e., failure to meet the goal, is due to special or common causes. *Focus on the process, not its output, but allow the output to serve as an indicator of assessment and measurement of the progress of process improvement.*

Table 7.11 summarizes where we have been so far in this chapter. The first thing to do with data is plot it in time sequence. Applying run charts and control charts allow for proper interpretation of the variation in the data.

Table 7.11: How to Convert a Time Ordered Sequence of Data into a Control Chart

1) Use at least 15 data points. A minimum of 20 points is ideal.

2) Plot the data in their naturally occurring time order. If there are no obvious special causes, find the median and refer to the run chart rules in Figure 7.20.

3) If there are special causes at this point (trends, shifts, too few or too many runs), try to identify the reasons for them. The presence of special causes, if not accounted for, could invalidate the use of Steps 7–10, resulting in a control chart with a meaningless average.

4) Compute the moving ranges (MR) between adjacent points in time. Recall that "N" data points produce "N-1" moving ranges.

5) Sort these moving ranges in ascending order and determine the **Median Moving Range** (MMR).

6) Determine MRMax by multiplying the MMR by 3.865.

   If any individual moving range exceeds MRMax, chances are your process exhibited a significant shift (special cause) at that point. Two consecutive special cause moving ranges typically signal the presence of an outlier.

7) *If the runs analysis in 2) showed no special causes*, calculate the average of all the data. Otherwise, depending on your objectives, calculate the appropriate average of the data based on your runs analysis. Typically this will be the most recent stable system.

8) Multiply MMR by 3.14.

9) The upper control limit is the average + (3.14 x MMR).

10) The lower control limit is the average – (3.14 x MMR).

   The area between the upper and lower control limits represents the *region* where you *expect* your data to fall if only common causes are present. These limits are based on minimizing the risk of mistakenly believing common cause variation to be special cause. With the limits set this way this risk is typically less than 0.5 percent. Any point outside the limits represents a special cause (different process) acting on the system.

11) Look for any obvious patterns or peculiarities in the pattern such as cycles, clusters close to the limits, or any other direct process influences such as known interventions. Keep using runs analysis when subsequent data points are plotted.

The Need for Both the Run Chart and the Control Chart

Many books teach control charts but very few talk about run charts. Generally, the only rule people remember is that any data points outside the control limits are special causes. This is a natural human tendency since it is easier to investigate a specific point in time and take a one-time, local action on a special cause rather than go through the more complicated process of understanding and fundamentally changing a process. However, this is also a hidden trap which can tend to cause a narrow focus on individual data points while missing the larger picture.

To illustrate this, we will revisit the FSH data previously plotted as a run chart in Figure 7.22. The chart had shown the presence of two systems due to implementation of a project team's recommendations in November 1991. This time, though, the control chart procedure will be applied without the initial runs analysis. The resulting chart is shown in Figure 7.32.

October 1991 and June 1992 fall outside the control limits. Without the insight from the runs analysis that two different systems are present, it might be tempting to treat those two months as unique, special causes. They would be investigated and, no doubt, a reason (albeit incorrect) would be found why point October 1991 was "high" and June 1992 was "low". Action would be taken. Yet, this would be missing the major finding in the data: The process itself changed in November 1991! October 1991 was a *common cause* in the *old* system, and June 1992 was a *common cause* in the *new* system. The special cause in the second system in July 1992, when an unusually large number of FSH tests were performed for infertility, would also be missed.

The control chart in Figure 7.30 demonstrates this danger also. Six points exceed the control limits, but they were all the result of two special causes: one at Month 16, and the other at Month 24.

It is permissible to use the moving range of *all* the data (unless observation suggests otherwise). However, the presence of multiple averages as suggested by runs analysis demands multiple control charts, the most important of which is suggested by *the most recent stable history* (in the case of Figure 7.30, observations 24 through 30).

Figure 7.32: Control Chart for FSH Data Using All Data for Calculations

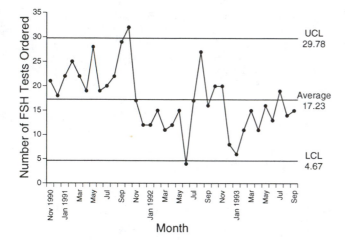

A naïve interpretation of this chart would find special causes at October 1991 and June 1992 instead of the true special causes in November 1991 and July 1992.

These simple examples demonstrate that one should *always* do a run chart first. Run charts provide an extremely helpful visual aid when making the best decisions as to where significant special causes may have occurred to change the process average. This helps fight the natural tendency to single out and react to pseudo special causes. This is especially useful in the early stages of a project where analysis of process history helps obtain valuable clues about past special causes and allows the creation of a current baseline.

In fact, routine use of control charts can overcomplicate a situation. The objective of improvement is the creation of beneficial special causes. One is trying to change the average of the current process, i.e., "move the needle," for which the run chart is perfectly designed.

The run chart information allows the appropriate averages to be calculated when constructing the control chart. If multiple processes are found to exist in the time period, they need to be separated before doing further analysis. With the FSH data, the most recent stable system (from November 1991 through the end of the data) was analyzed separately with a run chart in Figure 7.23. Analyzing the systems individually helps identify further special causes unique to the separate processes. Once a control chart of a stable system has been calculated, the runs analysis rules should also be used in addition to the common cause limits as subsequent data points are plotted.

A final word: One must not become a slave to statistical rules. Consider them as complementary elements to a team's master knowledge of a situation. When using the rules, however, always use them in the context of a chart and become dogmatic about their use only in the absence of knowledge. *The objective of proper use of the rules is to be able to ask the right questions about the observed variation and plan appropriate subsequent data collection.*

Reconsideration of QA Data Presentation: Cesarean Section Data

Let's pause for a moment and see how run charts and control charts can be applied to provide more insight into a typical QA presentation. Table 7.12 contains four years of cesarean section data tabulated monthly. The calculations for the median cesarean section rate and the Median Moving Range are in Table 7.13.

Table 7.12: Cesarean Section Data

Month	Cesarean Section	Total # of Births Births	Percent Cesarean Section Births	Moving Range
Jan. '90	47	257	18.29	*
Feb.	48	265	18.11	0.18
March	50	298	16.78	1.33
April	50	294	17.01	0.23
May	62	351	17.66	0.65
June	47	245	19.18	1.52
July	54	336	16.07	3.11
August	55	281	19.57	3.50
Sept.	62	294	21.09	1.52
Oct.	49	285	17.19	3.90
Nov.	46	269	17.10	0.09
Dec.	51	247	20.65	3.55
Jan. '91	60	285	21.05	0.40
Feb.	40	258	15.50	5.55
March	43	280	15.36	0.14
April	44	293	15.02	0.34
May	57	346	16.47	1.45
June	38	304	12.50	3.97
July	56	346	16.18	3.68
August	47	311	15.11	1.07
Sept.	44	276	15.94	0.83
Oct.	46	283	16.25	0.31
Nov.	44	267	16.48	0.23
Dec.	39	265	14.72	1.76
Jan. '92	50	595	17.12	2.40
Feb.	46	373	12.33	4.79
March	45	269	16.73	4.40
April	48	285	16.84	0.11
May	39	300	13.00	3.84
June	50	289	17.30	4.30
July	31	282	10.99	6.31
August	47	275	17.09	6.10
Sept.	42	299	14.05	3.04
Oct.	49	286	17.13	3.08
Nov.	38	244	15.57	1.56
Dec.	39	249	15.66	0.09
Jan. '93	38	237	16.03	0.37
Feb.	32	224	14.29	1.74
March	37	260	14.23	0.06
April	40	277	14.44	0.21
May	41	296	13.85	0.59
June	40	272	14.71	0.86
July	42	267	15.73	1.02
August	34	288	11.81	3.92
Sept.	42	241	17.43	5.62
Oct.	37	268	13.81	3.62
Nov.	32	232	13.79	0.02
Dec.	40	231	17.32	3.53

Table 7.13: Median Calculations for Cesarean Section Rate and Moving Range

Sorted Data	Order	Sorted Moving Range	Order
10.99	1st	0.02	1st
11.81	2nd	0.06	2nd
12.33	3rd	0.09	3rd
12.50	4th	0.09	4th
13.00	5th	0.11	5th
13.79	6th	0.14	6th
13.81	7th	0.18	7th
13.85	8th	0.21	8th
14.05	9th	0.23	9th
14.23	10th	0.23	10th
14.29	11th	0.31	11th
14.44	12th	0.34	12th
14.71	13th	0.37	13th
14.72	14th	0.40	14th
15.02	15th	0.59	15th
15.11	16th	0.65	16th
15.36	17th	0.83	17th
15.50	18th	0.86	18th
15.57	19th	1.02	19th
15.66	20th	1.07	20th
15.73	21st	1.33	21st
15.94	22nd	1.45	22nd
16.03	23rd	1.52	23rd
16.07	24th	1.52	24th
16.18	25th	1.56	25th
16.25	26th	1.74	26th
16.47	27th	1.76	27th
16.48	28th	2.40	28th
16.73	29th	3.04	29th
16.78	30th	3.08	30th
16.84	31st	3.11	31st
17.01	32nd	3.50	32nd
17.09	33rd	3.53	33rd
17.10	34th	3.55	34th
17.12	35th	3.62	35th
17.13	36th	3.68	36th
17.19	37th	3.84	37th
17.30	38th	3.90	38th
17.32	39th	3.92	39th
17.43	40th	3.97	40th
17.66	41st	4.30	41st
18.11	42nd	4.40	42nd
18.29	43rd	4.79	43rd
19.18	44th	5.55	44th
19.57	45th	5.62	45th
20.65	46th	6.10	46th
21.05	47th	6.31	47th
21.09	48th		

7

There are 48 values of cesarean section rates. The median is the average of the 24th and 25th sorted values (the numbers in the boxes). Since there is always one less moving range than there are data values, only 47 numbers go into the calculation of the median moving range. The median is the 24th sorted value.

Figure 7.33:
Run Chart of C-Section Data

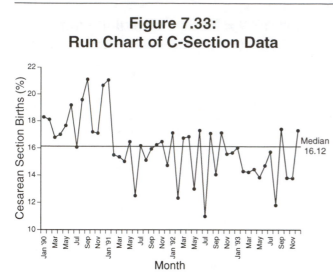

Ten consecutive points (November 1992 – August 1993) fall below the median, signaling a special cause. However, since the first 13 months (January 1990 – January 1991) seem to have an average above the rest of the data, the special cause is likely to have occurred between January and February 1991.

A run chart (Figure 7.33) shows a run of length 10 below the median from November 1992 through August 1993. We can conclude that the process exhibited more than one average. Is it possible to determine where the special cause occurred? The simplest explanation comes from looking at the plot. The first 13 months (January 1990 - January 1991) clearly had a higher average than the rest of the data. Even though these 13 months did not provide the special cause signal, pursuing the simplest explanation is usually the best strategy.

Figure 7.34: Run Chart of Current
C-Section "Process"

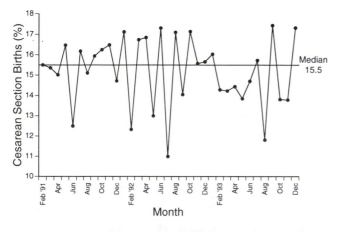

This plot shows the second system (February 1991 – December 1993) to have no special causes.

A subsequent runs analysis of the second system, February 1991 through December 1993 (Figure 7.34) confirms that it indeed seems to exhibit common cause behavior (no trends, no runs of length 8; 22 runs obtained, with 12 to 23 expected). Since the run chart shows this system to be stable, we can legitimately determine the common cause limits. Figure 7.35 shows the control chart. The center line of 15.17 was calculated from data taken in February 1991 and beyond.

Figure 7.35: Control Chart of Current
C-Section Process

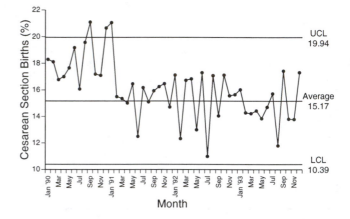

Even though all the data are shown, the average is based on the data from February 1991 – December 1993 (the current process).

Statistically a good argument can be made that the previous conclusion that "the first 13 months are a special cause" is valid. These 13 months are all above the current average. So, a good summary of this period is that the C-section rate has gone from 18.4 percent (through January 1991) to 15.2 percent (February 1991 and beyond). A new intervention is being planned, and the current baseline of 15.2 percent plus or minus 4.8 percent will be used to assess its effect. The runs rules can be used as well as noting whether a month falls below 10.39% (providing that neighboring data visually support the theory that a shift has occurred).

Note that the median moving range of **all** the data was used for the calculations. Since the median is robust (not affected by outliers) to the special cause of the process shift, it is not necessary to recalculate it. This "one-stop shopping" aspect of the median moving range is what makes it so desirable for control chart calculations.

A quick glance at a run chart can be a good indication of whether the variation of the process changed during the period of study. If the common cause variation seems to have changed, the MMR could need recalculation. For example, Figure 7.36 shows a run chart of a hospital's myocardial infarction survival data. It can be seen that not only did the average change after the first year, but the variation also increased. This is a rare case when the median moving range should be recalculated.

Figure 7.36: Run Chart for Myocardial Infarction Survival Rate

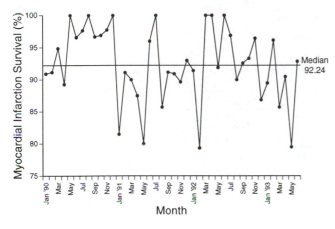

This plot shows a rare case where the process variation changed (as well as the process average). A control chart of these data should be based on the moving ranges beginning with January, 1991.

A Word About Bar Graphs

Bar graphs are frequently misused. The baseline of the bars in such graphs is usually arbitrary (or zero), or the bars are shown as deviations from a numerical goal. This contributes to organizational tampering by giving an incorrect interpretation of variation, i.e., anything on the wrong side of the goal is the result of a special cause.

It is particularly misleading to see a time plot presented as a series of bars sprouting from an arbitrary baseline, once again deceiving the eye. *Isn't the basic issue here where the bar ends*? If so, couldn't this sequence of numbers be turned into either a run or control chart to measure the process's stability and capability? Doesn't this seem like a higher yield strategy?

The bar graph in Figure 7.1 is presented again in Figure 7.37. How could this be done differently?

People intuitively seem to want to group the data by month and plot all the Januarys together, all the Februarys together, etc. This occurs because people feel strongly that it is only "fair" to compare similar months. What is the theory?

They are assuming the presence of "seasonality" in the data, i.e., certain months are consistently different from other months. Isn't seasonality another type of special cause? If someone theorizes it to be present, what are the odds of finding it? Pretty high – even if it isn't there! Suppose that there is only common cause? The potential for tampering exists again. How could one use *theory* to decide, instead of intuition?

Figure 7.38 shows a simple run chart of the data. This chart never fails to elicit an audible reaction when presented to an audience. It is virtually impossible to intuit the downward pattern when the data are presented as a series of bar graphs. Yes, there are special causes, but what are they? Differences from year to year? True seasonality? How could one know?

7

Figure 7.37: Bar Graph of Patient Counts
Patient Counts

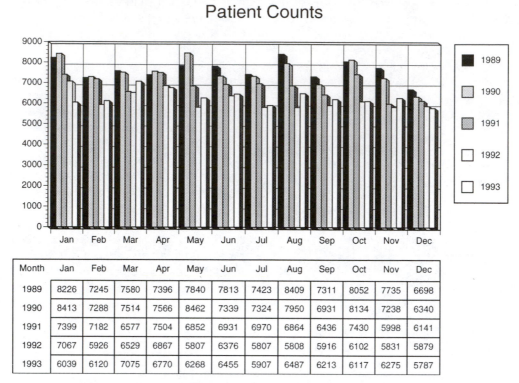

Month	Jan	Feb	Mar	Apr	May	Jun	Jul	Aug	Sep	Oct	Nov	Dec
1989	8226	7245	7580	7396	7840	7813	7423	8409	7311	8052	7735	6698
1990	8413	7288	7514	7566	8462	7339	7324	7950	6931	8134	7238	6340
1991	7399	7182	6577	7504	6852	6931	6970	6864	6436	7430	5998	6141
1992	7067	5926	6529	6867	5807	6376	5807	5808	5916	6102	5831	5879
1993	6039	6120	7075	6770	6268	6455	5907	6487	6213	6117	6275	5787

Bar graphs are a poor tool for plotting data over time.

Figure 7.38: Run Chart of Patient Counts

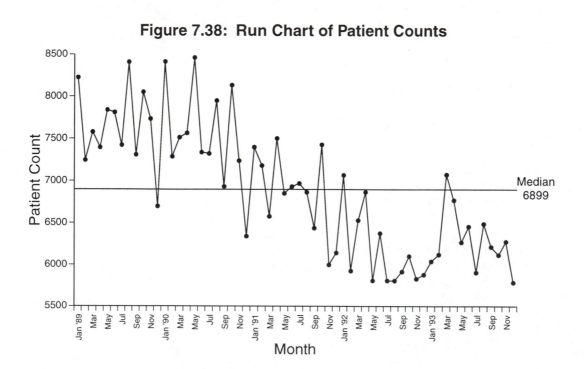

The perspective of a run chart is dramatically different than that of a bar chart.

As with the venipuncture data in Figure 7.27, analysis of means can determine whether a difference exists between the years. (Again, ANOM calculations will be demonstrated in Chapter 8.) Figure 7.39 shows this analysis comparing the averages for each year with the appropriate common cause limits drawn in (and calculated from the data themselves). The conclusions are:

1) The years 1989 and 1990 were similar

2) There was a significant drop in 1991

3) Another significant drop occurred in 1992

4) There was no change from 1992 to 1993.

Figure 7.39: Analysis of Means of Patient Count by Year

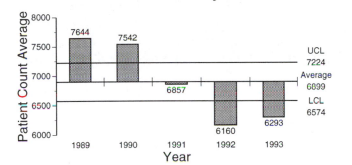

The ANOM shows significant changes between 1990, 1991 and 1992.

In making a direct comparison from one year to the next we are making an assumption that there is the potential for a special cause "shock" to the system every January. This could easily be due to changes in health insurance enrollments. A further assumption is that their effect on the process is constant throughout the rest of the year.

Once the differences between years have been uncovered, a natural follow-up question would regard seasonality over and above the yearly changes. While the process average may change from one year to the next, are any months *consistently* different from the others *regardless of the year?* Are there any predictable patterns from month to month?

Again ANOM is useful here because it can adjust for the differences from year to year and just look at variation from month to month. The plot is in Figure 7.40, where each point represents the average of each month over the five year period. In other words, the first point is the average of the five January results for each year, the second point is the average of the five February results, etc.

Figure 7.40: Analysis of Means of Patient Count by Month

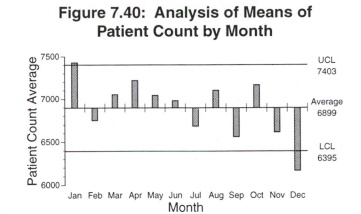

The ANOM shows that December has consistently lower patient counts and January has consistently higher patient counts than other months in the year.

The common cause bands calculated from the data suggest that seasonality is evident only in January, which tends to be above average, and December, which tends to be below average. Since the averages for February through November all fall within the band, *there is no statistical evidence of any differences between them.* People are usually surprised at the seeming lack of statistical seasonality. What causes such initially strong intuitive (albeit incorrect) perceptions?

One final graph that would be useful would be the status of the current "process" relative to previous process history. Since the last two years, 1992 and 1993, seem to be operating with the same process, they can be considered the most recent stable system.

Figure 7.41 contains a control chart of all the data, but the limits are calculated based on data only from 1992 and 1993. In addition, Januarys and Decembers, because they are special causes, are plotted on the graph but omitted from the calculations. Had they been included, the common cause band would be inflated. From the common cause limits, one can see that the natural swing in the patient counts is plus or minus 1100 for any one month! Is it any wonder that looking only at a table of numbers would make one think there is a pattern of seasonality?

7

Figure 7.41: Control Chart of Current Process

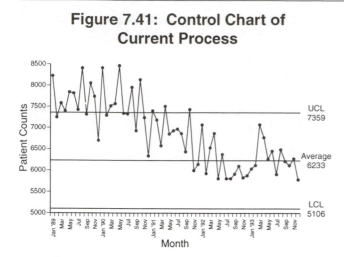

The limits are calculated with data from the current process, i.e., 1992 and 1993. January and December data are omitted from the average since they are special causes as indicated by Figure 7.40.

One More Useful Test for Special Causes

The following data (Figure 7.42) were obtained from a major medical center that was trying to improve its phone service. It is presented in the proverbial bar graph format and ... is not very useful.

Figure 7.42: Telephone Data in a Bar Graph Format

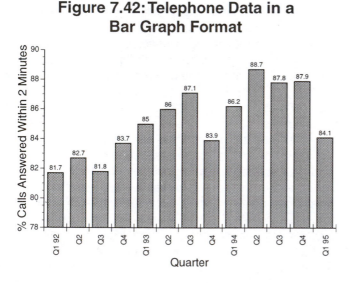

The data are presented in Table 7.14. How about a run chart? (Figure 7.43)

Table 7.14 - Telephone Data

Month	% Answered in 120 sec.	MR	Sorted Data	Sorted MR
1	81.7	*	81.7	0.1
2	82.7	1.0	81.8	0.9
3	81.8	0.9	82.7	0.9
4	83.7	1.9	83.7	1.0
5	85.0	1.3	83.9	1.0
6	86.0	1.0	84.1	1.1
7	87.1	1.1	85.0	1.3
8	83.9	3.2	86.0	1.9
9	86.2	2.3	86.2	2.3
10	88.7	2.5	87.1	2.5
11	87.8	0.9	87.8	3.2
12	87.9	0.1	87.9	3.8
13	84.1	3.8	88.7	*

Figure 7.43: Run Chart of Telephone Data

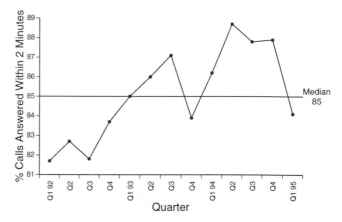

None of the special cause tests are triggered (no trends; no runs of length 8; five runs observed when three to ten are expected). So far, there are no signs of improvement.

Next let's try a control chart (Figure 7.44).

Figure 7.44: Control Chart of Telephone Data

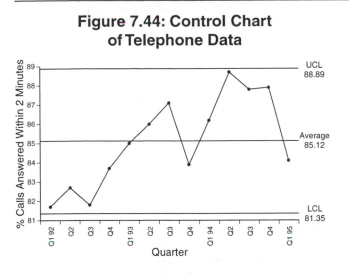

There is no special cause moving range to indicate a significant shift toward better service. Neither is there a data point outside the upper common cause band that might also indicate a shift. So, given one's current arsenal of rules, one could conclude that no progress has been made in improving phone service. What does your intuitive observation of the plot suggest?

Regardless of your intuitive conclusion, there is one more important statistical rule that can be used to determine the presence of special causes. The control chart is shown again in Figure 7.45, but this time, two additional lines have been drawn 2/3 of the distance between the average and the usual common cause limits.

Figure 7.45: Control Chart of Telephone Data Incorporating Two Standard Deviation Limits

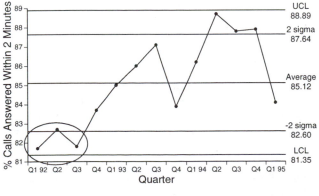

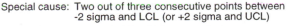

Special cause: Two out of three consecutive points between -2 sigma and LCL (or +2 sigma and UCL)

Walter Shewhart, inventor of the control chart, originally designated that common cause limits should be drawn at three standard deviations on either side of the average. This is the policy the authors have

followed thus far in this book. Astonishingly, Shewhart did not rely on elegant mathematical or statistical proofs. Instead it is rumored that he merely stipulated "three standard deviations seem to work very well" in balancing the risk of two errors. The two error types are: Type I: Treating a deviation as a special cause when it is common cause, and Type II: Failing to recognize a deviation as a special cause and treating it as common cause.

As a little math will tell you, 2/3 of the distance between the average and the upper and lower common cause limits means that these additional lines are drawn at a distance of two standard deviations from the average (sometimes called "two sigma limits"). Two standard deviations has become such a rule of thumb (alleged 5 percent risk of treating a common cause as if it were a special cause) in statistics that many people use two standard deviations *instead* of three when they construct their control charts. The analogy is not without risk. It seriously increases the probability of incurring a Type I error as discussed above. The authors' feeling is that two standard deviation limits should be used *in addition to* the traditional three standard deviation limits.

(These next four paragraphs are a bit more mathematical–it's ok to skip them.) People seem to forget that when they are taught decision-making in a typical statistics course, they are applying a decision rule to *one decision only* from a data set. In this case, the "95% confidence" strategy implicit in two standard deviations makes the error of treating a common cause as if it were special a 5 percent risk. It is the only decision being made.

However, consider the current data set of 13 observations. Isn't an implicit decision being made as each data point is considered, resulting in 13 independent decisions? If two standard deviations are used as a cutoff for special cause *and if no special causes are present*, what is the probability of observing 13 data points *all* between two standard deviations? This probability is approximately $(0.95)^{13} = 0.513$.

Thus, using a two standard deviation criterion on a time sequence of 13 data points would incur a risk of $(1 - 0.513) = 0.487$ of observing *at least one* point out of the 13 exceeding the two standard deviation limits! This translates into a 50% risk of tampering.

Using Shewhart's recommended three standard deviations, the probability is approximately $(0.997)^{13} =$

0.962 of observing all 13 observations between the three standard deviation limits *if no special cause is present.* Thus, the risk of tampering becomes (1 - 0.962) = 0.038. So, the *overall rate of protection* in using three standard deviation limits is close to 5%, which is what Shewhart discovered and recommended. Since the risk of each error type comes at the expense of the other, the three standard deviation criterion seems to be a healthy balance of the risks.

This may seem unduly conservative to some. The authors agree. In recent years, a rule has been developed that incorporates the sensitivity of the two standard deviation criterion and balances it with the conservative nature of the three standard deviation criterion. The rule becomes: When an observation is between two and three standard deviations on a control chart, a special cause is indicated *if* either of the next two points also falls in this range. This is sometimes called the "two out of three" rule, and is demonstrated beautifully by the first three data points of the phone data (Figure 7.45). Observation 1 is in the two to three standard deviation range; the next observation is not. Yet, the second subsequent observation returns to the range of the initial point. Combined with the master knowledge that interventions were taking place, it seems reasonable to conclude that the phone answering rate has indeed increased. Note that observations 10-12 also exhibit this rule. As with runs analysis, the observations signaling the special cause may or may not be where the special cause actually occurred.

Figure 7.46 shows a control chart where observations 1-3 are not included in the average, since logic would seem to dictate that these represent a different process. Since the variation does not seem to have changed, all the data are used to determine the median moving range. Note that although observation ten is in the two to three standard deviation range, neither observation 11 nor 12 is. The conclusion is that stable behavior has been exhibited by this system from observations 4-13, and the current average is 86.0%. This is an improvement from the 82.1% of the process that generated the first three observations.

Since the typical three standard deviation limits can be quite wide, a further advantage of two standard deviation limits is that they indicate where the process output will fall 90-98% of the time. (This is part of The Empirical Rule, developed by Wheeler and Chambers.[3]) For the current example, given an average of 86.0%, 90-98% of the quarters will fall between 83.5 and 88.6%.

A Clinical Example: Hypertension Management

The implications of applying control charts to routine clinical practice is profound, but the surface has barely been scratched. Clinical professionals typically react to one number, e.g., test result, and take an action. Any number exhibits variation (or has uncertainty associated with it) even if it is measured only once. However, in the professional's mind, the current number is compared to either its predecessor or some standard, and an action is taken. Remember the fundamental question: Is the *process* that produced this current data point the same as the *process* that produced the previous data point? Is it the same as the process that produced the standard?

A general internist was treating a patient for hypertension. This patient was very motivated and took his blood pressure quite often. Run charts of the systolic and diastolic readings from 55 blood pressure measurements taken over the course of three years are shown in Figures 7.47a and 7.47b, respectively. Run rules aren't needed to see that there is a problem.

It seems obvious that there have been two processes at work. The change seems to have occurred around observation 26, and the two processes have been separated there in Figures 7.48 and 7.49. Figures 7.48a and 7.48b show the control charts for "Process 1" and Figures 7.49 show the control charts for "Process 2." They exhibit remarkably stable behavior, but look at the range of common cause variation! One

Figure 7.46 Control Chart of Telephone Data Excluding First Three Quarters

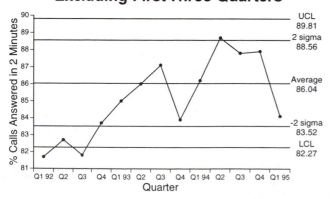

may not like this inherent range, but "it is what it is" and reflects the current process, which also includes the measurement process. How much variation is inherent in the actual measurement of blood pressure regardless of the patient? In addition to charting the process, calculation of MRMax shows that, for the current processes, it would take a difference of greater than 31 between two consecutive systolic or diastolic readings to consider it a special cause.

Medication interventions were made following observations 46 and 54, but the disturbing run of eight points above the average in the systolic chart at the end of Figure 7.48a makes one question their success. Is there some way to reduce the inherent variation so that special causes can be diagnosed and reacted to more quickly? The authors have no additional information, but it is tempting to ask, "How were these data collected?" and "How could these data be collected to minimize common cause variation?" Control charts could be used to test effectiveness of such strategies.

7

Figure 7.47a: Run Chart of Systolic BP Readings

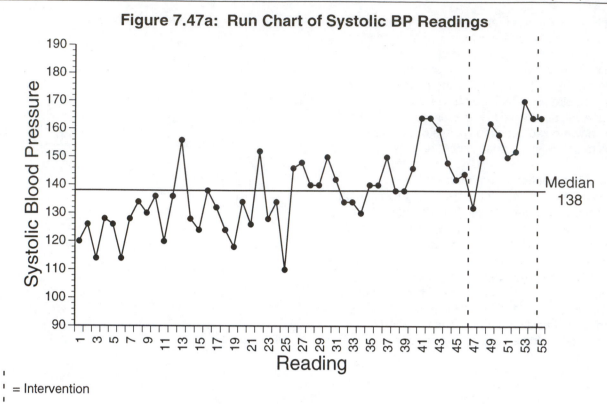

= Intervention

Figure 7.47b: Run Chart of Diastolic BP Readings

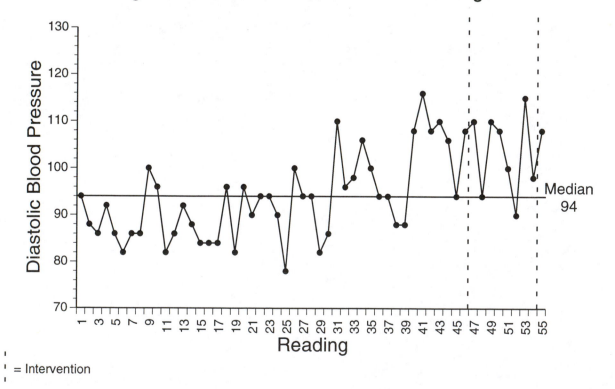

= Intervention

Both systolic and diastolic readings show evidence of special causes – too few runs and eight consecutive points on the same side of the median.

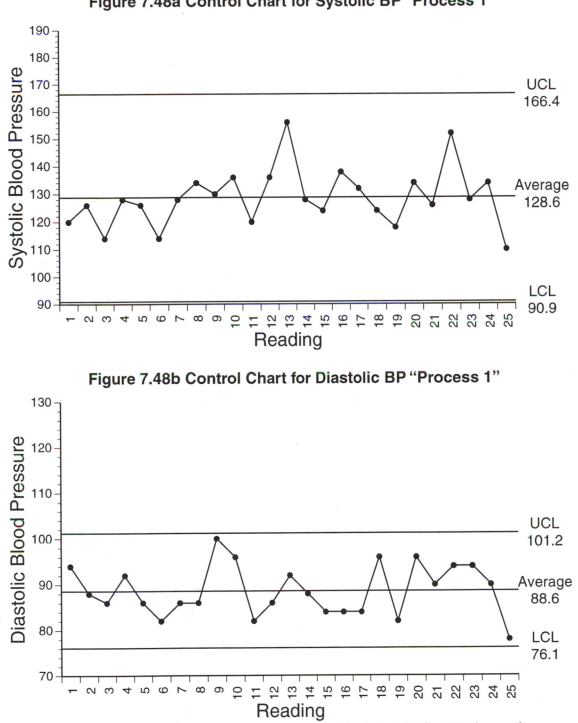

Figure 7.48a Control Chart for Systolic BP "Process 1"

Figure 7.48b Control Chart for Diastolic BP "Process 1"

Both the systolic and diastolic processes were stable during the first 25 observations

Additional data were recently received and run charts of this new history (Figures 7.50a and 7.50b) are plotted relative to the previous most stable history represented by observations 26-55.

Interventions were made following observation 55, 60, 76, 81 (medication was stopped), 87, 90, 99. Quite the appearance of a roller coaster ride! However, note that Figure 7.50a ends with a run of 10 below the median. Since these seem to represent a new process, control charts for diastolic and systolic readings with limits based on the last 10 observations are shown in Figure 7.51. The maximum common cause difference between two consecutive observations is currently 31 for systolic and 23 for diastolic.

Figure 7.49a Control Chart for Systolic BP "Process 2"

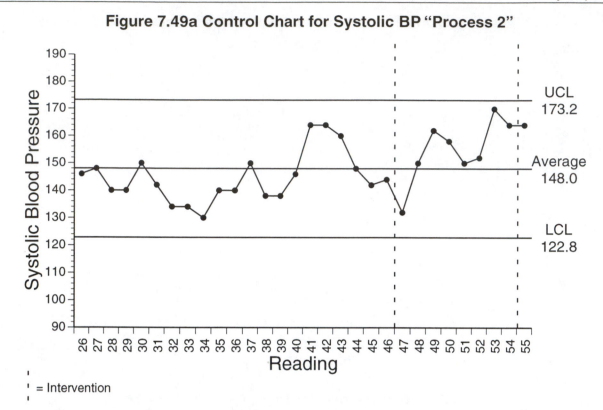

The systolic process increased after the 25th measurement, (Figure 7.48a), and increased again beginning around observation 48.

Figure 7.49b: Control Chart for Diastolic BP "Process 2"

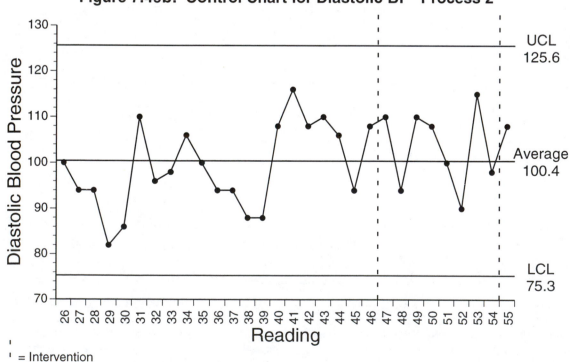

The diastolic process appears stable during observations 27 – 55, but at a higher level than the first 25 observations.

Figure 7.50a: Run Chart of Subsequent Systolic BP Relative to Baseline

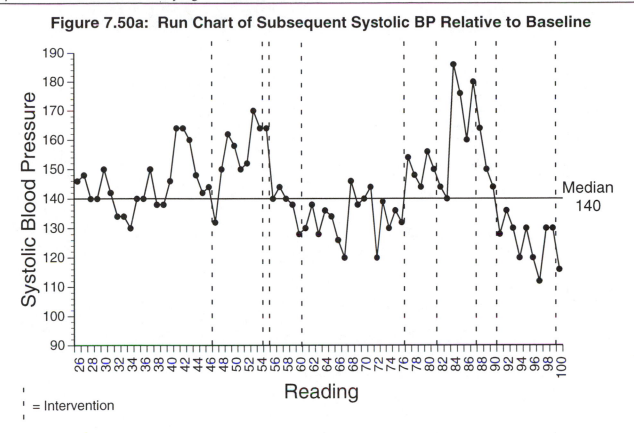

= Intervention

Figure 7.50b: Run Chart of Subsequent Diastolic BP Relative to Baseline

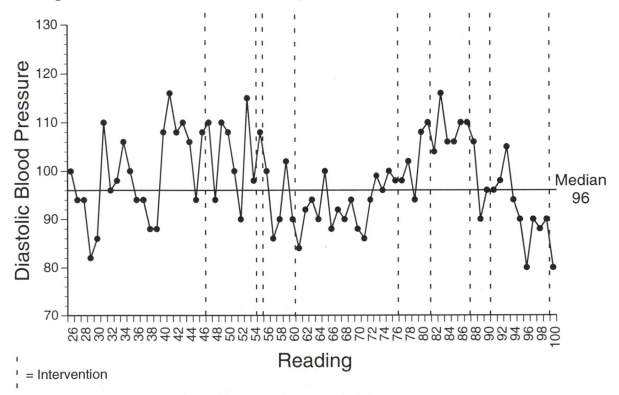

= Intervention

This runs analysis uses observations 26-55 as a starting point for the analysis of new data.

Figure 7.51a: Control Chart of Most Current Systolic "Process"

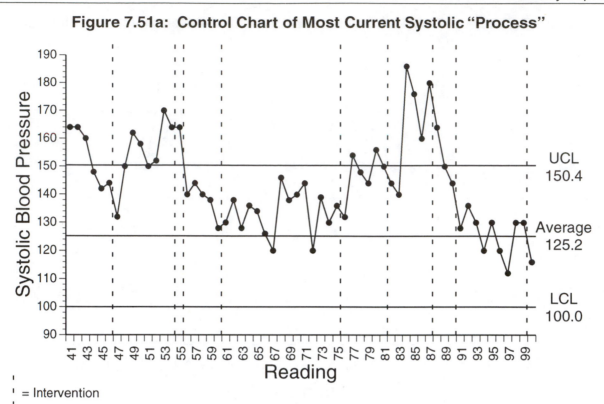

= Intervention

Figure 7.51b: Control Chart of Most Current Diastolic "Process"

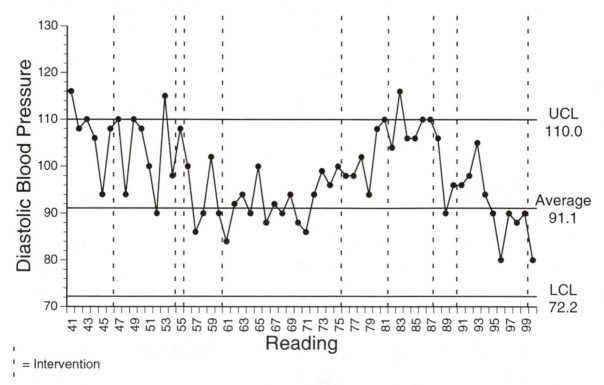

= Intervention

The limits are based on observations 91 – 100, the most recent stable system.

These control charts are quite similar both in their average and control limits to those originally presented in Figure 7.47. The patient seems to have settled back into his original, healthy process capability. The current chart can be used to "hold the gains" and raise an alert when further change is needed.

Does this example suggest changes in processes for handling chronic diseases: hypertension, diabetes, depression, psychiatric indicators of behavior, use of blood thinning agents, etc.? Wouldn't it be useful to have some information as to the inherent, common cause variation in numbers commonly used to monitor disease? How could one not want to know?!

A Lurking Managerial Trap

Figures 7.52a-d show run charts of data from four processes. Runs analysis would indicate that process 1 exhibits stable behavior. Runs analyses of processes 2, 3, and 4, on the other hand, indicate significant special cause variation. Once again, this demonstrates the power of plotting data over time and applying runs analysis based on statistical theory. But, wait... how were these data collected?

7

Figure 7.52a: Run Chart for "Process 1"

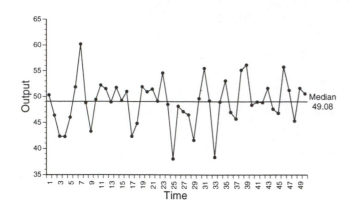

Figure 7.52b: Run Chart for "Process 2"

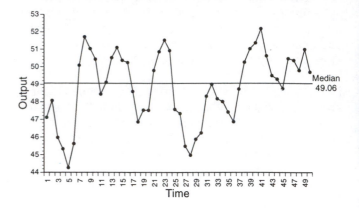

Figure 7.52c: Run Chart for "Process 3"

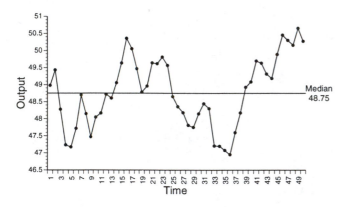

Figure 7.52d: Run Chart for "Process 4"

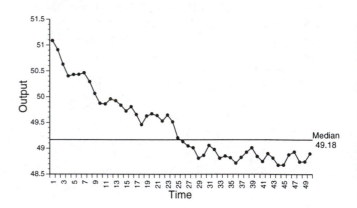

These plots are all different manifestations of the same random process.

Actually, these four plots show the **exact** same data! As hard as it is to believe, this is indeed true. The difference is in the process of creating these numbers from the original data.

The data began as 101 random numbers generated from a Normal distribution with an average of 50 and a standard deviation of 5. The individual numbers vary between approximately 35 to 65. Observations 52-101 are plotted as a run chart in Figure 7.52a. This represents the true process. It shows stable, common cause behavior.

Observations 52-101 are also plotted in Figures 7.52b-7.52d, but three common techniques have been used to "smooth" some of the variation in the data. They are all variations on what is commonly known as a "rolling" average, sometimes called a "moving" average.

In Figure 7.52b, each data point is averaged with its three immediate predecessors, making it a rolling average of four. Thus the first point 47.1, is the average of observations 52, 51, 50 and 49. (For these data, the numbers 50.3, 44.9, 50.7 and 42.5 were averaged.) The second point, 48.1, is the average of observations 53, 52, 51 and 50, (In this case, 46.4, 50.3, 44.9 and 50.7) etc. The final point in Figure 7.36b is the average of observations 101, 100, 99 and 98. Why would anyone do this? If numbers reported in a given quarter are actually the average of the last four quarters, they are rolling averages of four. *Four quarter* rolling averages are very popular as management indicators.

Figure 7.52c uses rolling averages of 12 in which each data point is averaged with its eleven immediate predecessors. The first point is the average of observations 52 through 41, the second is the average of observations 53-42, etc., The final point on this graph is the average of observations 101-90. Where might one encounter rolling averages of 12? *Twelve month* rolling averages are very common indicators and used in many financial calculations such as days per 1000 and outstanding accounts receivable.

Figure 7.52d uses rolling averages of 52 in which each data point is averaged with its fifty-one immediate predecessors. The first point averages observations 52-1, the second 53-2, etc., and the final 101-50. *Fifty-two week* rolling averages are very commonly used as economic indicator summaries.

These graphs are examples of a sort of "reverse tampering", i.e., creating the appearance of a special cause when the true process is actually common cause. Due to the fact that each number in Figures 7.52b-7.52d is not independent (because they all contain a large amount of overlap with their predecessors) commonly used *statistical techniques become inappropriate and invalid*. In fact, the figures show that the larger the amount of overlap, the more severe the appearance of special cause.

Why do people use such techniques as "rolling" averages? Because they are uncomfortable with variation. These techniques are based on intuition and not theory. Arbitrary averages are rolled until the person feels the data are "smoothed" sufficiently to his or her liking. They have not smoothed the process, however; the variation still exists whether they like it or not. It is much better to plot the data as independent numbers and quantify the variation inherent in the observed process. It is only then that improvement can begin.

Summary

Once again, whether or not people understand statistics, they are already using statistics. This chapter has presented the heart of what seem to be the common, well-meaning errors in perceptions when people use and analyze data. Tampering, though unintentional, is rampant, and the losses caused by it are incalculable. These are good people doing their best.

Variation is everywhere. Only through statistical thinking and the use of basic statistical theory can variation be understood so that appropriate action can be taken. Many concepts were presented.

The major change is to move away from using highly aggregated summaries of data. In designing data studies, substitute more frequent, smaller samples in time for huge, "one shot" studies and *plot* the results over time. Our recommendation is to plot the data first as a run chart; then, if there are no special causes, as a control chart of all the data. If the run chart shows signs of special causes, it is better to plot control charts of each process represented in the data.

Much of the discussion in this chapter concerned control charts. While there are other types of control charts, the authors have found that in a medical environment, identifying special causes with the control chart taught here ("Individuals" control chart) will serve *most* purposes. Most books which talk about control charts are aimed at a manufacturing audience and typically get bogged down in "sampling" and "rational subgrouping". This tends to overwhelm people and cause them to lose sight of original purpose of the charts.

In analytic statistics, sample size is not an issue since one is always studying the stability of a process. The choice of how frequently in time to sample, not the total number of samples, is the issue. Other factors include the source of variation currently being studied and the time frame within which one desires to be alerted to special causes. It is different than designing a "one-shot", controlled research study. Objectives tend to be fluid in an atmosphere of continuous improvement. Also, in tracking many normal process outputs, they are not strictly "designed" data collection: they are routinely produced daily, weekly, monthly, or whatever. So the individuals chart is almost always appropriate for tracking a process over time.

Donald Wheeler and John Dowd[2], two prominent statisticians of international reputation for whom the authors have great respect, feel that in most cases, when studying a process over time, the Individuals chart is the best choice. In most circumstances, it is a very close approximation to what the "correct" chart would have given. Note that in plotting the cesarean-section data, the individuals chart was chosen because the data was *plotted over time.* If a subsequent comparison were to be made between hospitals, doctors, etc., the *most recent stable history* of cesarean-sections for each system would be *aggregated,* and stratification then would be used to compare individual performances (no time involved except for deciding what period to aggregate). A more statistical form of stratification, Analysis of Means, is the subject of the next chapter.

Finally, if the thought of calculating common cause limits makes you "sweat", plotting routine data over time and then just using simple run charts will stop untold tampering. After you become more comfortable with this technique, then try adding control limits.

Chapter 9 will summarize the basic points regarding data presented thus far. It is intended to serve as a quick reference on the key principles and supply a road map for truly using "data skills" as a conduit to transformation.

Notes to Chapter Seven

1.   Mills JL. *Data Torturing.*

2.   Wheeler DJ. *Understanding Variation: The Key to Managing Chaos.*

3.   Wheeler DJ and Chambers DS. *Understanding Statistical Process Control.*

Chapter Seven Exercises

The following exercises are based on real data. The attempt is to take you through the thought process you should use when faced with a set of data. You will also note the wide variety of types of data used. These show how opportunities for tampering are rampant in everyday work. You may also notice that several of the solutions aren't necessarily black-and-white—an ever present issue in the real world. Solutions appear in Appendix C.

1. The Aggregated Medication Error Data

The following table shows monthly medication error data for a typical medical center.

Month	Medication Errors
3/92	82
4/92	81
5/92	55
6/92	65
7/92	113
8/92	77
9/92	75
10/92	79
11/92	70
12/92	87
1992 Total	1002
1/93	90
2/93	69
3/93	65
4/93	66
5/93	65
6/93	64
7/93	52
8/93	80
9/93	72
10/93	70
11/93	58
12/93	56
1993 Total	807
1/94	50
2/94	77
3/94	72
4/94	81
5/95	74
6/94	74
7/94	71
8/94	73
9/94	82
10/94	93
11/94	69
Thru 12/15	18
1994 Total	834

a) Sketch a run chart and perform a runs analysis.

You know from your own facilities how much attention medication errors get. Based on your runs analysis, how much improvement has this facility seen to justify all this attention? Do you think they have been using a common cause or a special cause strategy in reaction to errors (variation)? What might you recommend?

b) Calculate the moving ranges, find the median moving range, and determine the current state of its medication error process. Are you surprised by the month-to-month variation one must live with despite the process's stability? Should a common cause or a special cause strategy be used to improve it? Any ideas? How would you know if they worked?

2. The Adverse Drug Event Data

A hospital joined a major initiative for reducing adverse drug events. It was well-known that these errors were underreported. So early in the project, there was a substantial education effort to increase awareness of such errors, reduce fear of punitive consequences, and set up a reliable process for reporting errors. It was believed that with this support an honest assessment of the current state of the process would be obtained.

The data below were collected after a dramatic rise was observed on a run chart. This indicated that the new process had indeed taken hold.

Day	Adverse Drug Events	Day	Adverse Drug Events
2/26	11	3/29	6
2/27	11	3/30	0
2/28	6	3/31	3
2/29	10	4/1	1
3/1	6	4/2	4
3/2	4	4/3	10
3/3	11	4/4	3
3/4	8	4/5	2
3/5	6	4/6	3
3/6	6	4/7	0
3/7	4	4/8	3
3/8	9	4/9	4
3/9	5	4/10	6
3/10	8	4/11	2
3/11	2	4/12	0
3/12	6	4/13	0
3/13	11	4/14	2
3/14	5	4/15	3
3/15	6	4/16	3
3/16	8	4/17	2
3/17	3	4/18	1
3/18	3	4/19	1
3/19	1	4/20	5
3/20	8	4/21	2
3/21	3	4/22	12
3/22	5	4/23	4
3/23	0	4/24	3
3/24	1	4/25	5
3/25	3	4/26	6
3/26	4	4/27	3
3/27	9	4/28	8
3/28	4	4/29	1

a) Does it seen stable? Or is the reporting process still "growing"? Or have the number of errors decreased? If so, does this necessarily indicate improvement? If you determine the process is not stable, take your best guess as to how much of the most recent stable history represents the current state of the process.

Another major education effort was initiated. The data for the subsequent month is shown below.

Day	Adverse Drug Events	Day	Adverse Drug Events
5/1	7	5/17	2
5/2	5	5/18	0
5/3	4	5/19	0
5/4	3	5/20	3
5/5	6	5/21	8
5/6	10	5/22	4
5/7	7	5/23	12
5/8	1	5/24	1
5/9	1	5/25	14
5/10	1	5/26	4
5/11	5	5/27	1
5/12	4	5/28	3
5/13	5	5/29	10
5/14	5	5/30	5
5/15	7	5/31	2
5/16	5		

b) What was the effect of the education? How could you construct a run chart to demonstrate this? How could one use the data at this point for improvement of the process?

3. **The Newspaper Bar Graph Problem**

Shown below are two bar graphs taken from the business section of a major metropolitan newspaper. The intent is supposedly to shed insight on productivity changes coupled with changes in wages and benefits.

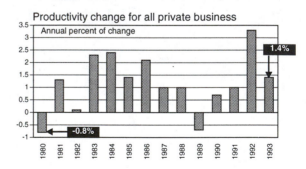

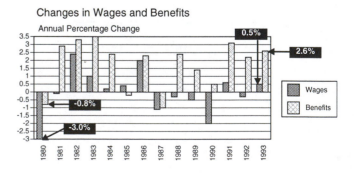

a)   What are your comments on the display of this data? What kinds of questions would you like to ask? If such a set of data were presented at your facility, how long could such a meeting last and how would these graphs be discussed?

The actual data points were approximated from the graphs and are listed below:

Year	Productivity	Wages	Benefits
1980	-0.8	-3.0	-0.8
1981	1.3	-0.1	2.9
1982	0.1	2.4	3.3
1983	2.3	1.0	3.5
1984	2.4	0.2	2.4
1985	1.4	0.4	-0.2
1986	2.1	2.0	2.3
1987	1.0	-1.1	-1.0
1988	1.0	-0.3	2.4
1989	-0.7	-0.5	1.4
1990	0.7	-2.0	0.5
1991	1.0	0.6	3.1
1992	3.3	-0.3	2.2
1993	1.4	0.5	2.6

b)   Sketch a run chart for each indicator and assess the process stability from 1980-1993.

c)   Calculate the common cause limits for each process. What have you discovered?

d)   How do you compare this process of analysis to your initial intuitive "ouija board" analysis?

4.   The Patient Satisfaction Survey Data

A medical center had a process in place whereby a patient, if desired, could fill out a comment card on their way out. They rank various aspects of their visit on a scale of 1 (Poor) to 5 (Excellent). These were sent back to marketing and the averages tabulated every month. Various groups were given their results, judged, and told to "do something about it."

Nineteen months of data for one group's "overall satisfaction" are shown below.

Month	Overall Satisfaction	Month	Overall Satisfaction
1	4.29	11	4.51
2	4.18	12	4.49
3	4.08	13	4.35
4	4.31	14	4.21
5	4.16	15	4.42
6	4.33	16	4.31
7	4.27	17	4.36
8	4.44	18	4.27
9	4.26	19	4.30
10	4.49		

a)   What are your comments on the data collection process, analysis process, and feedback/action processes?

b)   Sketch a run chart for these data. How would you judge the process performance over the last nineteen months?

c)   Calculate the moving ranges for this data. How much of a difference between two consecutive months is normal? Based on this criterion, have any significant shifts been observed? Are any results excessively high or low (i.e., two consecutive special cause moving ranges)?

d)   What are the common cause limits for this process? If the current process continues, where will the data fall 90-98% of the time? Do you find the inherent common cause "shocking"? What does this data indicate about the effectiveness of the current process for using this data? Are you surprised?

5. The Transcription Productivity Data

After taking a quality improvement course, a supervisor decided to use run and control charts to assess her group's productivity "process." The following data represent calculation of overall department productivity and are reported every two weeks starting in 1995. So, observations 1-26 represent 1995 and 27-34 represent 1996.

Two Week Period	Avg. Minutes Transcribed / Hour	Two Week Period	Avg. Minutes Transcribed / Hour
1	9.3	18	10.3
2	11.4	19	10.6
3	11.1	20	11.7
4	10.8	21	11.1
5	11.2	22	11.0
6	11.4	23	11.2
7	12.0	24	10.6
8	10.9	25	12.1
9	12.0	26	11.9
10	10.8	27	10.0
11	11.2	28	11.9
12	10.4	29	11.6
13	10.9	30	11.9
14	10.8	31	11.5
15	10.0	32	11.3
16	10.9	33	11.6
17	11.4	34	11.6

a) Find the median and sketch a run chart. Does this data "pass" the run chart analysis? What is your intuition telling you? How could you confirm your intuitive thoughts?

b) Calculate the moving ranges and find the median moving range. Does the quantity (3.865 x MMR) help to confirm some of your intuition? What theories does this analysis suggest? Does this make you want to reconsider your runs analysis?

c) Is calculating the average for this data a clear cut process? How would you assess the current state of its performance? How much improvement, if any, have you noticed since 1995?

6. The Overtime Data

A supervisor in a particular department was getting a lot of "heat" regarding her overtime costs. She received a labor report every two weeks that consisted of the proverbial "rows/columns/this month/last month/YTD/vs. last year/variance" summary. Almost two years of her overtime data is given below.

Pay Period	Overtime	Pay Period	Overtime
1	1.98	23	0.75
2	0.67	24	0.96
3	0.49	25	0.57
4	0.74	26	0.39
5	0.21	27	0.82
6	0.64	28	0.29
7	0.90	29	0.58
8	0.45	30	1.30
9	1.03	31	0.42
10	0.18	32	0.27
11	0.13	33	1.51
12	0.70	34	1.20
13	0.47	35	0.83
14	0.70	36	2.99
15	2.21	37	1.30
16	0.34	38	1.51
17	0.59	39	1.12
18	1.00	40	1.68
19	0.59	41	0.54
20	0.58	42	0.48
21	0.69	43	0.70
22	1.41		

a) Do a run chart of this data. Does "plotting the dots" give clearer insight than a list of raw data? Do any special causes seem apparent?

b) Calculate the moving ranges, find the median moving range, and see whether utilizing (3.865 x MMR) helps to confirm some of your suspicions in (a).

c) Suppose you are told ("How were these data collected?") that periods 1, 15, & 36 were two-week periods that contained Monday holidays. Are these necessarily the only special causes present? Suppose you are also told that two receptionists quit during period 33 and that their replacements were not hired until period 41. Did this period seem atypical to the process? What implications do these events have in calculating the average for the control chart?

d) Aside from the issues mentioned in (c), has her process been behaving relatively consistently over the last two years? How would you characterize the current process performance, i.e., where is it "centered" and what is the *range* of overtime she can *expect* in any one two-week period? What about 90-98% of the time?

e) Given the current state of her process, is it reasonable to expect her to get by with zero overtime consistently? Currently, is the occurrence of zero overtime a special or common cause? Has she been doing the best she can with her process? Has management "heat" resulted in improvement?

f) If all management does is apply "heat," what are the budgetary implications? Can this process be improved? How? Special cause strategy? Common cause strategy? Both?

g) Could the reporting of overtime to managers be improved? From the results of your analysis, what are the limitations of month/YTD/Last Year/Variance reporting? How is this supervisor especially handicapped regarding her YTD figures?

b) Is the fact that they seem to have a tendency toward positive variances a common or special cause?

    (Hint: Even though the data is limited, it's all you've got. Do a control chart of the "variance days." What do all of the tests tell you?)

c) Is it possible that the process is really on budget? What might be a way to tell?

d) Given the current process, what are the implications in terms of budgeting? What other actions should be considered? Should they be based on a common cause or special cause strategy?

e) From your analysis, where will the process fall 90-98% of the time? What would the "month of horrors" look like? Is it a number that your "ouija board" would even consider? What would the reaction be if people had no knowledge of statistical theory?

7. The Utilization Management Data

A certain consultant came into covert possession of the following graph. People seemed to think that their minds were being "messed with." Look familiar?

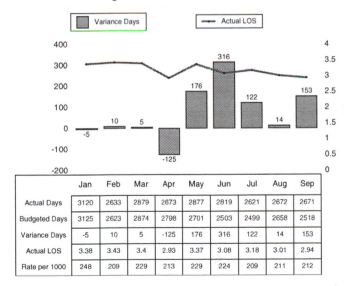

	Jan	Feb	Mar	Apr	May	Jun	Jul	Aug	Sep
Actual Days	3120	2633	2879	2673	2877	2819	2621	2672	2671
Budgeted Days	3125	2623	2874	2798	2701	2503	2499	2658	2518
Variance Days	-5	10	5	-125	176	316	122	14	153
Actual LOS	3.38	3.43	3.4	2.93	3.37	3.08	3.18	3.01	2.94
Rate per 1000	248	209	229	213	229	224	209	211	212

a) Given this current method of presentation, what could you do? (Hint: The consultant was baffled!)

All right, then...What *should* you do?

8. Patient Transfer Time Data

A multi-disciplinary team at a hospital wanted to improve the process of transferring patients from the ICUs to non-critical care units. A measurement was obtained by subtracting the time the patient left the unit from the time the data were transferred in the computer system. Sixty-two patients were transferred in one week and the data are shown in their time order below:

Patient	Time to Transfer Data	Patient	Time to Transfer Data
1	22	32	55
2	27	33	28
3	12	34	39
4	-4	35	75
5	30	36	16
6	24	37	28
7	22	38	8
8	-12	39	13
9	56	40	6
10	38	41	46
11	306	42	38
12	0	43	-3
13	39	44	2
14	293	45	38
15	-21	46	7
16	38	47	47
17	117	48	-3
18	150	49	-15
19	230	50	76
20	17	51	90
21	28	52	18
22	29	53	54
23	23	54	-58
24	0	55	67
25	3	56	56
26	-4	57	123
27	80	58	180
28	26	59	26
29	70	60	43
30	-6	61	30
31	28	62	-3

a) Do a run chart of the data. Does the runs analysis indicate any special causes? Do any data points appear to be suspicious?

b) Calculate the moving ranges and find the median moving range. Does the quantity (3.865 x MMR) help to resolve some of your suspicions from (a)?

c) Construct the control chart using all the data for the average. Does this further confirm some of your suspicions about certain data points? What seems to be the "typical" time and what is the range any individual patient's transfer may expect, given the current process?:

d) Recalculate the control chart average and resulting common cause limits by eliminating the high special causes. Also add the two standard deviation limits. Where does the process seem to be centered and what is the range of time any individual transfer would experience in 90-98% of the instances? Do you see this range as a possible compromise to patient care?

e) Would a special cause or a common cause strategy be necessary to improve this process? In collecting the data, the nurses developed an ad hoc data sheet that only obtained the transfer times. What other information may have been useful in "studying the current process"? What tool could be useful to gain insight into understanding the wide variation?

9. The Critical Pathway Data Problem

A critical pathway for a certain DRG was implemented, and data was obtained on individual patients both before and after implementation. The lengths of stay (LOS) and charges were obtained for the last 29 patients prior to implementation of the pathway as a baseline and 50 patients subsequent to implementation. They are sorted by admit date order and are listed below:

Admit Order	LOS	Charges	Admit Order	LOS	Charges
1	4	11687	41	3	8839
2	5	10434	42	4	10841
3	11	20992	43	4	11053
4	3	9499	44	3	10847
5	4	9281	45	5	10714
6	3	8794	46	5	10863
7	7	12824	47	3	9228
8	4	10415	48	5	11610
9	4	11130	49	2	8983
10	6	17536	50	3	9949
11	5	12872	51	4	9933
12	6	14332	52	2	8543
13	5	11227	53	3	8296
14	4	12946	54	4	9071
15	5	11154	55	3	8552
16	5	10737	56	4	13262
17	7	13647	57	3	8611
18	7	19602	58	4	10531
19	4	8765	59	7	15164
20	3	11869	60	4	11047
21	12	20117	61	5	16455
22	3	9381	62	3	10505
23	5	12506	63	5	12161
24	4	9287	64	3	9988
25	4	12978	65	2	8153
26	4	12820	66	3	9649
27	4	14037	67	3	10266
28	5	12353	68	5	13310
29	5	12497	69	3	10240
30	3	10167	70	3	12651
31	3	9914	71	4	9760
32	4	12486	72	2	7990
33	3	10336	73	3	9757
34	4	10282	74	4	10501
35	4	11225	75	3	8775
36	3	10224	76	3	12824
37	3	10222	77	3	10193
38	3	9703	78	3	8704
39	4	11417	79	3	11111
40	4	12578			

a) Do a run chart of both LOS and Charges and use runs analysis to determine whether the critical pathway caused a change in the LOS and/or total charges.

b) Calculate the common cause limits for charges separately in the pre- and post-test periods. Are there any outliers, i.e., "train wrecks" contained within each period? What savings, if any, per patient have been realized by implementation of the critical path? Do you have any comments about the variation observed in the pre- vs. post-pathway periods?

c) The insurers were pleased that savings were realized on this DRG and felt the average cost to be "relatively reasonable." In order to "hold the gains" they are now going to require an explanation of any individual case that comes in more than $1000 above the average. Does this represent a common cause or special cause strategy? Given the data, what kind of strategy is needed for further improvement? Do you have any suggestions on how to "slice and dice" the data to expose further improvement opportunity?

7

Chapter Eight
Statistical Stratification: Analysis of Means

Key Ideas

- When looking at improvement opportunities, the mindset must change from "comparisons of individual performances" to "comparison of individual performances to the inherent 'system'"

- Analysis of means (ANOM) is a powerful, objective technique that assesses a current system and exposes potential opportunity

- By identifying an individual as "outside" the system, we know that they have a different process than others. Collegial discussion and data are needed to determine whether the special cause is inappropriate or unintended

- The control charts used to assess individual performance and obtain averages for the ANOM are also powerful individual feedback tools that can assess an individual's efforts to improve

- Common cause limits for a system are obtained *from the data*. There is no guarantee of finding special causes. One should not approach a problem with an a priori assumption that there should be a given percentage of special causes.

- Rankings are ludicrous as a means for motivating improvement. People "inside" the system are indistinguishable and *cannot be ranked*.

- Typical displays of percentage data are extremely deceptive.

- Any graphical display of numbers needs a context of common cause variation for proper interpretation.

Revisiting QA vs. QI

Wouldn't traditional QA data be more helpful if presented in control chart form, rather than its usual aggregate summaries, bar graphs and rankings? Rankings usually don't help to understand variation and root causes. On the other hand, they frequently result in tampering. Management may automatically assume the people with the highest and lowest rankings of that time period are special causes. Furthermore, people falling within a common cause

band of the system average are statistically indistinguishable: *They cannot be ranked!*

A common defensive reaction to ranking (particularly among those ranked near the bottom) is "it can't be me-the data are obviously at fault." It may be useful to start with Professor Tukey's strategy of finding out what's wrong with the numbers by examining their operational definitions. Are these fair comparisons? Even if they are, how should the observed variation be interpreted? What represents true special cause? What is the process for using these data? What variation is appropriate? Unintended? What should people do differently?

Guess what: In any ranking, someone has the biggest number and someone else has the smallest number!! *There is no common cause to provide a context of interpreting the observed variation.* The numbers are being viewed in a vacuum. They cannot be viewed in the proper context because we do not know the common cause variation. Without knowledge of common cause variation, we cannot determine special causes. Even when presented "graphically" in a bar graph format, the bar graph is virtually useless unless it has the *specific* objective of either a Pareto analysis or stratified histogram to expose hidden special causes in *inputs*. The rankings are generally based on reported results, which are *outputs*.

Presentations of traditional "95 percent confidence intervals" around each individual's average are also inaccurate and not helpful. This presentation may be appropriate for research, but not for an improvement objective. The purpose of improvement studies is to *expose* hidden special causes. However, they are often analyzed as though the special causes are not there i.e., in an enumerative framework. As a result, the standard deviation is usually inflated. All the overlapping confidence interval presentation format seems to do is create nodding heads, no discussion, and rampant confusion. Does anything really ever change from these presentations?

Analysis of Means (ANOM) is a technique for assessing a current system and exposing improvement opportunities. It was invented by Ellis Ott. It is quite simple. It can be used appropriately either with data reported in percents, with proportional data, or with continuous data.

8

Analysis of Means for Data Reported in Percents: The Antibiotic Protocol

Much of QA data presentation reports percent conformance, such as the percent of patient records with documented Pap smears. ANOM for percent data is an alternative way to report QA results.

First, we must clarify what is meant by "percent data". Percent data is a count of events, divided by another count. The counts used are the total number of events that could be observed for specific event A, divided by the observed count of the specific event A where it would have been possible to observe A's occurrence. In equation format, the percent data fraction is:

$$\frac{\text{Observed number of specific event A: X}}{\text{Total number of events where it might have been possible to observe specific event A: Y}}$$

Without the detailed definitions, the equation would be:

$$\text{Percent data fraction} = \frac{\text{Observed X}}{\text{Observable Y}}$$

One such example is the cesarean section data. It is relatively easy to count the number of cesarean section births and the total number of births. However, even with something which appears this simple, operational definitions of "birth" and "cesarean section birth" are still required. For example, do you count all births in the total Y, or only live births?

Analysis of means for proportions should *not* be used when the ratio of two continuous variables is used in percent form. An example is financial dollar ratios, such as accounts receivable collected / accounts receivable billed. In this case, they are considered "continuous" data, and a different ANOM technique is needed. This will be discussed later on in this chapter.

Analysis of means is not to be confused with time plots. Its intent is to expose special causes between individual performances or processes. It is a more formal, statistical version of stratification. In this context the word "individual" could mean person, department, day of the week, or any other input that could serve as a basis for stratification. In essence, we collect data over a long time period. If the process is stable, the data are aggregated over time, and then disaggregated by the input of interest. The horizontal axis no longer represents time. Instead, positions on the axis are arbitrarily assigned to the various individual components of that input. Prior to aggregating data it is critical to be able to answer "Yes"

to the question: Would a plot of these aggregated data in their time order indicate a stable process?

The example which will demonstrate ANOM is based on the experience of one of the authors. In addition to demonstrating the use of computation of ANOM for percent data, it takes a critical look at an actual conformance protocol.

In a class of drugs, certain specific drugs are deemed more acceptable than others for reasons of cost, effectiveness, etc. An antibiotic managed care protocol was received by a group of physicians. While designed with the best intentions, it bore no resemblance to any theoretically sound statistical methodology. In this protocol, a class of drugs was chosen and the percent of use of a specific drug within the class was studied among physicians. A certain target percent was considered "desirable".

The protocol is given below, with commentary on each chapter indicated by [brackets]. All italics have been added by the authors for emphasis.

> "For any given diagnosis or for any therapeutic class of drugs, there are usually several choices of drug therapy. This study is designed to compare physician's selection of antibiotics when several choices are available. This is accomplished by comparing the antibiotic-specific prescribing behavior of physicians who see similar types of patients and identifying those physicians that deviate from the established norm or standard."

"Identification of outliers"

1) "Data will be tested for normal distribution"

   [Many statistics courses impart to their students an obsession with the normal distribution. In this case, *it is not relevant* because each individual prescription is evaluated and can only fall into one of two classes. It is either a member of the target population, i.e., "yes," or it is not, i.e., "no." Technically speaking, these data should be considered from a *binomial* distribution. In this protocol the test for normality is moot.]

2) "If distribution is normal—Physicians whose prescribing deviates greater than *one or two* standard deviations from the mean are identified as outliers."

[By definition of the normal distribution approximately 1/3 of the individuals will be further than one standard deviation away from the mean, and approximately five percent will be beyond two standard deviations. They are not outliers, it is just common cause variation. Thus, if the data passed the test for normality, the existence of outliers couldn't be proven!

The previous paragraph assumes that the standard deviation is calculated correctly. A common but incorrect method of calculation (as in this case) seriously inflates the standard deviation. As a result, people arbitrarily use lower thresholds to determine alleged significance. Calculating the traditional standard deviation of the 51 percentages is inappropriate for this type of data. The presence of special causes, even on the correct type of data, seriously inflates the traditional calculation.]

3) "If distribution is not normal—Examine distribution of data and establish an *arbitrary* cutoff point above which physicians should receive feedback (this cutoff point is *subjective and variable* based on the distribution of ratio data)."

[Sound familiar? How about using some theory? We will soon see how analysis of means can provide a more objective view.]

"Intervention"

1) Report results to local P & T Committee and/ or Medical Director

2) Provide feedback to outlier physicians in the form of the following material:

- summary details of the physician's antibiotic prescribing sorted by antibiotic class

- summary of study results and brief explanation of how they were identified as an outlier

- patient antibiotic medication profiles for those patients receiving target antibiotics

- educational document reviewing the standard antibiotic therapy for disease states for which the target antibiotics are commonly prescribed."

[For physicians reading this, have you ever received such "helpful" feedback? Did it truly motivate you to want to change your behavior? When this example is presented to audiences of physicians, they often respond with a collective pantomime of what appears to be throwing something in the garbage.]

Given this data collection and analysis process, what are the odds of tampering? What are the results of this type of process?

To show how the analysis would be performed, the protocol included an example, based on real data. Figure 8.1 presents the analysis graphically as suggested in the protocol. Lines have been drawn at one, two and three standard deviations. The percentages are sorted in ascending order.

Figure 8.2 shows the proper statistical analysis using ANOM for proportions. Each point along the horizontal axis represents a specific physician. Unlike control charts, this axis has nothing to do with time. The vertical axis represents the number of target prescriptions written by each individual physician divided by the total number of prescriptions in that class of drugs written by that physician. Each physician's result is plotted. Then the average of *all* of the physicians' results (number of target prescriptions written by all physicians divided by the total number of prescriptions in that class of drugs by all physicians) is drawn in as a center line.

A vertical band of common cause is calculated for each physician and placed around the overall average. This is to see whether, given the proportion that seems *inherent* to this process (process capability), this physician's individual result is truly "inside the system" (common cause) or "outside the system" (special cause). The formula for computing the common cause limits will be presented shortly. However, some readers will have noticed that the bands do not have the same width for all physicians.

Figure 8.1: Analysis of Drug Data as Proposed by Protocol

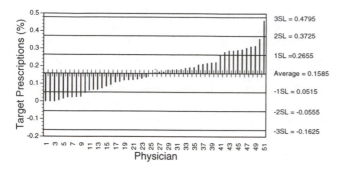
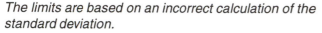

The limits are based on an incorrect calculation of the standard deviation.

Figure 8.2: Correct Statistical Analysis of Drug Data

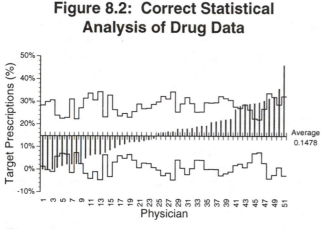

The limits are based on the common cause variation.

The vertical bands differ because each physician wrote a varying number of prescriptions (the denominator of the proportion). If a coin is flipped four times and no heads are obtained, do you really want to call the coin "unfair?" On the other hand, if the same coin is flipped 16 times without obtaining any heads, how do you feel about calling the coin "unfair?" With more flips we become more confident of the coin's fairness or lack thereof. We can estimate the coin's "true probability" better with more flips. In other words, assuming a fair coin, zero heads obtained from a "window of opportunity" of four flips could be common cause. However, zero heads obtained from a "window of opportunity" of 16 flips is a special cause.

Similarly, we will be more certain whether physicians' deviations from the system average represent common cause variation if they wrote more prescriptions. This variation in certainty is reflected by variation in the widths of the common cause bands.

The individual limits in Figure 8.2 are quite variable. They are based on using three standard deviations to detect outliers. (While readers may be more familiar with comparisons based on two standard deviations, the reasons for using three standard deviations are briefly discussed at the end of this example). Isn't it interesting to note that the three standard deviation limits, when calculated correctly, seem to be as narrow as the one standard deviation limits in the proposed protocol analysis?

We can then say with low risk of being wrong, that anyone outside his or her individual common cause band is a special cause. In other words, these physicians are truly "above average" or "below average."

What should one conclude? Only that these physicians have a different "process" for prescribing this particular drug than their colleagues. By examining the "inputs" to those individual processes (people, methods, machines, materials, environment and measurements), this special cause of variation can be understood. Maybe some of the variation is appropriate because of the type of patient (people) they treat. However, some of it may be inappropriate due to their "methods" of prescribing it. Remember, improved quality relates to reducing *inappropriate and unintended* variation. One can't just tell them, "Do something!" without answering the natural resulting question, "Well, what should I do differently from what I'm doing now?" As always, this will take data.

Most of the physicians (about 75 percent) fall within their common cause bands. Therefore this seems to be a stable process representing majority behavior. A good summary of the process of prescribing the targeted drug seems to be that its use within its class has resulted in a process capability of 14.8 percent. The majority process average then is that of the drugs in this class, this specific drug is prescribed about 15 percent of the time.

Approximately 15 percent of the physicians exhibit "above average" behavior in prescribing this particular drug and 10 percent exhibit "below average" behavior. (Note from Figure 8.1 that the memo's proposed analysis would not detect any "below average" prescribing behavior since the lower limit is less than 0. Insight into these could be quite beneficial or might find inappropriate prescribing behavior). It is interesting to note that physicians 48 and 49 have high proportions, but not outside their individual common cause bands. Given the number of total prescriptions they wrote, it is still possible that they exhibited a behavior of 15 percent use of the target drug.

One more word about goals. Suppose a goal had arbitrarily been set that "The target drug should not be more than 15 percent of prescriptions in this class!" Since Figure 8.2 captures the *actual process capability*, the effect of this goal can be assessed. *The process is meeting the goal* with the exception of the "above average" physicians who are outside their common cause limits.

But, in addition to the "above average" physicians who were special causes, 20 physicians are "above the goal" BUT within the common cause band. If just the "no more than 15 percent" goal were used, 40 percent(!) of the all the physicians in the study would *inappropriately* receive feedback. They are statistically no different from the goal *nor* are they different from the 18 physicians (35 percent) who happened to "win the lottery" and ended up in the common cause band below the average.

Suppose the goal had been set at 10 percent. The process wouldn't have changed, since processes don't understand goals. However, even *more* tampering (albeit well-meaning) would result. *This process, as it currently exists and operates, would not be capable of meeting a goal of 10 percent. There would need to be a fundamental change in **all** physician behavior.* This is a case where studying the physicians who are special causes "below average" could yield some appropriate behaviors that could lead to such improvement. This could be summarized with one more statistical theorem: "A process is what it is. The first task is to find out what it is."

Calculating the Limits

The calculation of these limits is relatively simple. As indicated before, this method applies only when one has an aggregated set of data in percent form. The calculation is described in detail in the box, "Calculating Common Cause Limits for ANOM for Proportions or Percent Data." Recall that this type of data is a fraction with a numerator and denominator. Before calculating the limits, one must know the numerator and denominator making up each individual percentage. The numerator and denominator must represent counts of individual events. In this example, the numerator is a count of the prescriptions written for the targeted drug, and the denominator is a count of the total number of prescriptions written in the class of drugs.

For this group of physicians, the 51 numerators, i.e., the number of target prescriptions, were added and divided by the sum of the 51 denominators, i.e., the total number of prescriptions in this class, which yielded a proportion of 0.148 (14.8 percent). This is the average and is also the center line on the graph.

To obtain the *common cause band* for each individual physician, the formula described in the box gives an upper common cause limit of:

$$0.148 + 3 \times \sqrt{\frac{0.148 \times (1 - 0.148)}{n_i}} \,.$$

The lower common cause limit is:

$$0.148 - 3 \times \sqrt{\frac{0.148 \times (1 - 0.148)}{n_i}} \,.$$

n_i is the denominator for the individual physician. "3" represents the desired width of the common cause band, i.e., three standard deviations.

The individual variation in limits makes this an extremely cumbersome set of calculations to do by hand. However, there are many computer software packages which can do these calculations. Minitab, SAS, JMP, and Statgraphics are such packages.[1]

8

Calculating Common Cause Limits for ANOM for Proportions or Percent Data

The data must be in the form of a fraction. The numerator represents counts of target events that occurred and the denominator represents total counts of events that could have occurred. The numerator and denominator for each individual data point are also required. The formulas are based in statistical theory for percentage data.

A. Add all the numerators
B. Add all the denominators
C. Calculate the average proportion by dividing the result in "A" by the result in "B". Note this is *not* the same as taking the average of the proportions themselves.
D. The upper common cause limit for an individual $= \text{Average} + 3 \times \sqrt{\dfrac{\text{average} \times (1 - \text{average})}{n_i}}$

E. The lower common cause limit for an individual $= \text{Average} - 3 \times \sqrt{\dfrac{\text{average} \times (1 - \text{average})}{n_i}}$

where n_i is the denominator of the proportion for that individual.

This will be demonstrated using four physicians from the Antibiotic Protocol example. Note that the values obtained here will be slightly different from the values in Figure 8.2, because those values are based on all the data. The values here are based on only four physicians. The data are:

Physician	Total Number of Prescriptions in the Class	Number of Target Prescriptions	Percent of Target Prescriptions
46	217	64	0.295
8	202	5	0.025
45	192	56	0.292
5	190	3	0.016

What are the common cause limits for these physicians? The ratio is formed as:

$$\frac{\text{Number of Target Prescriptions}}{\text{Total Number of Prescriptions in the Class}}$$

A. Add all the numerators
   The sum of the numerators is $64 + 5 + 56 + 3 = 128$

B. Add all the denominators
   The sum of the denominators is $217 + 202 + 192 + 190 = 801$

C. Calculate the average proportion by dividing the result in "A" by the result in "B". Note this is *not* the same as taking the average of the proportions themselves.
   $$\text{Average} = \frac{128}{801} = 0.160$$

Calculating Common Cause Limits for ANOM for Proportions or Percent Data (continued)

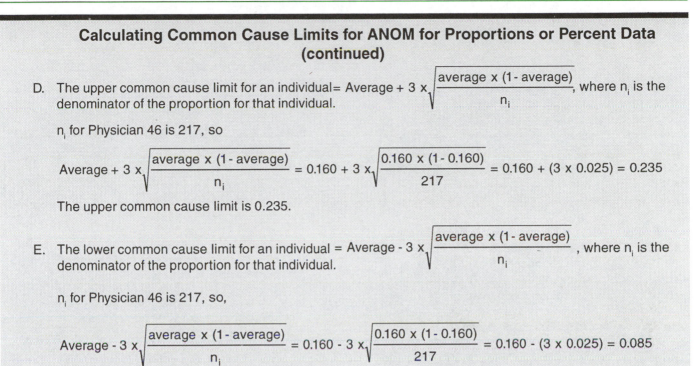

D. The upper common cause limit for an individual $= \text{Average} + 3 \times \sqrt{\dfrac{\text{average} \times (1 - \text{average})}{n_i}}$, where n_i is the denominator of the proportion for that individual.

n_i for Physician 46 is 217, so

$$\text{Average} + 3 \times \sqrt{\frac{\text{average} \times (1 - \text{average})}{n_i}} = 0.160 + 3 \times \sqrt{\frac{0.160 \times (1 - 0.160)}{217}} = 0.160 + (3 \times 0.025) = 0.235$$

The upper common cause limit is 0.235.

E. The lower common cause limit for an individual $= \text{Average} - 3 \times \sqrt{\dfrac{\text{average} \times (1 - \text{average})}{n_i}}$, where n_i is the denominator of the proportion for that individual.

n_i for Physician 46 is 217, so,

$$\text{Average} - 3 \times \sqrt{\frac{\text{average} \times (1 - \text{average})}{n_i}} = 0.160 - 3 \times \sqrt{\frac{0.160 \times (1 - 0.160)}{217}} = 0.160 - (3 \times 0.025) = 0.085$$

The lower common cause limit is 0.085.

The common cause limits for the other physicians are calculated similarly. The only difference is the value of n_i, the total number of prescriptions in the class. Their common cause limits can be calculated to be:

Physician	Percent of target prescriptions	Lower common cause limit	Upper common cause limit	Interpretation
46	0.295	0.085	0.235	Above the system
8	0.025	0.083	0.237	Below the system
45	0.292	0.081	0.239	Above the system
5	0.016	0.080	0.240	Below the system

None of these physicians fall inside their common cause region. Physicians 45 and 46 seem to operate in a different system than Physicians 5 and 8.

The text used an example of flipping a coin four or sixteen times. The common cause limits for the probability of obtaining heads can be calculated as follows. If the coin is fair, the average or probability of obtaining a head is 50 percent or 0.50. For four flips the limits are $0.5 \pm 3 \times \sqrt{\dfrac{(0.5) \times (1 - 0.5)}{4}}$, covering the interval from -0.25 to 1.25.

In other words, four flips could result in any combination of heads or tails. It is impossible to assess the fairness of the coin from just four flips. Four heads in four flips (100 percent or 1.00) is not an indication of a special cause.

On the other hand, if the coin was flipped 16 times, the common cause limits are $0.5 \pm 3 \times \sqrt{\dfrac{(0.5) \times (1 - 0.5)}{16}}$, covering an interval from 0.125 to 0.875. With 16 flips, a result of 1.00 (all heads) is not in the common cause range, and should be considered a special cause.

A Brief Note on the Use of Three Versus Two Standard Deviations

A comparison against two standard deviations has traditionally been the "gold standard" in research. Two standard deviations represent an approximate five percent risk of tampering, i.e., treating a result as "significant" or from special cause when it is not. Most trials are well-designed toward making a specific conclusion, and that conclusion is the *only one made* at the end of the trial. Thus a five percent risk is usually reasonable.

In everyday work, literally *hundreds* of decisions are made daily. If *each one* were made with a five percent risk of tampering, the chances of making at least one of those decisions incorrectly is quite high. If a five percent threshold were used, considerable inappropriate action would be taken routinely in daily work. By raising the risk threshold to three standard deviations (approximately 0.3 percent risk of tampering), one's *overall risk* of tampering on any one day or any one data set used to compare multiple performers, is one to five percent. As can be seen by the examples, there is plenty of "low hanging fruit" in any organization. Three standard deviations is a virtual assurance that the largest opportunities will be found and that most action taken will be correct and productive.

In the improvement paradigm, using three standard deviations as the "gold standard yardstick of common cause" seems to balance these two risks:

- the risk of taking inappropriate action when none is required (tampering)

- the risk of taking no specific action when action is required (treating observed variation as common cause when it is special).

Also, as noted from the antibiotic protocol, incorrect calculation of the standard deviation is common, which results in an inflated estimate. It has incorrectly necessitated the arbitrary use of two and sometimes even one standard deviation as a threshold for action.

Based on the risk one is willing to accept, if more statistical rigor is desired, Table 8.1 can be used to determine the width of the common cause band around the system average. Because *simultaneous* decisions are being made, the table adjusts the common cause band based on the number of averages being compared to one another. The

constants are given for *overall* error rates (risk of treating common cause as if it were special; i.e., falsely believing that any of the averages are different from any of the others) of 10%, 5%, and 1%. These constants were derived from the theory developed by Ott.

Table 8.1 - Factors for Analysis of Means

Number of Groups Being Compared	10% Risk	5% Risk	1% Risk
2	1.16	1.39	1.82
3	1.73	1.95	2.40
4	1.93	2.16	2.62
5	2.07	2.30	2.76
6	2.18	2.41	2.87
7	2.26	2.49	2.95
8	2.33	2.55	3.02
9	2.39	2.61	3.07
10	2.44	2.66	3.12
15	2.61	2.83	3.29
20	2.73	2.94	3.39
30	2.88	3.09	3.53
40	2.98	3.18	3.62
50	3.05	3.25	3.68
60	3.11	3.31	3.73

The theory is very similar to the discussion about Shewhart's recommendation for the routine use of three standard deviations on an individuals control chart. The difference is in the specific number of comparisons being made. In ANOM, the number of comparisons is known, and a constant can be theoretically derived. In a typical control chart, data points are constantly being added and the number of comparisons is theoretically "infinite". Given the "infinite" number in control charts, from Shewhart's experience three standard deviations represents the best insurance for balancing the two risk types when plotting data over time.

Look again at the physician drug data just presented (comparing 50 physicians). One can observe from the table that the use of three standard deviations gives the analysis an overall risk of about 10% for treating common cause as if it were special. To increase the protection to 5%, a multiplier of 3.25 would have to be used. If even a more conservative criterion is desired, 3.68 standard deviations would decrease the risk to 1%. Looking at the table, one can observe that three standard deviations is quite robust for a "relatively safe" level of risk. Brian Joiner, a student of Ott's, has said that Ott himself used three most of the time.[2] Heero Hacquebord, one of the world's leading Deming disciples, has said to one of the authors, "I use three...what the heck?"[3]

One other hidden advantage is implicit in ANOM. In deciding whether someone is a special cause, the authors have seen many analyses that literally delete every individual, recalculate the average with the individual deleted, then compare the individual's result to the deleted average. In his genius, Ott designed this technique right into ANOM *without having to delete individuals!* The standard deviation limits have been statistically adjusted, a priori, by a "shrinking" factor so the data point can be compared as if it had been deleted.

With fewer levels of comparison (especially five or less) it may be advantageous to use the actual widths suggested by Table 8.1 because the number "three" may be too conservative. The exercises at the end of the chapter will demonstrate the judicious use of this table.

More About The Deceptiveness of Percentages

The following bar graphs were used to shed insight into how pre-existing conditions may affect research outcomes. Seven facilities were being used to obtain data. The bar graphs for two such conditions are shown, along with the bars for the seven clinics' aggregate averages. Presumably, if the variation were deemed "excessive," the results could be case-mix-adjusted, typically by linear regression.

Figure 8.3a: Bar Graph of Pre-existing Condition 1

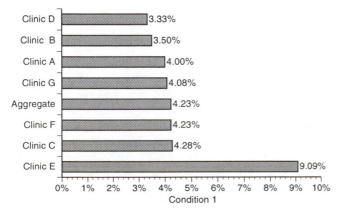

Figure 8.3b: Bar Graph of Pre-existing Condition 2

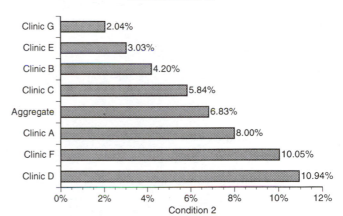

Bar graphs of percentages present misleading perspectives about differences between the clinics.

In figure 8.3, it seems "obvious" that the percent incidence of pre-existing Condition 1 is much higher at Clinic E, probably necessitating some type of adjustment for that clinic's results. For pre-existing Condition 2, the overall variation among clinics is quite excessive, once again probably necessitating an adjustment. In addition, 13 other pre-conditions were studied.

By digging through many sheets of "rows and columns" the actual data used to obtain the percentages were compiled. They are listed in Table 8.2. The bar graph format was converted into an ANOM format using a control chart for percentages. The resulting chart for each set of data is shown in Figure 8.4.

Table 8.2: Data For Pre-Existing Condition Data

Clinic	Condition 1	Condition 2	Total Cases
A	4	8	100
B	5	6	143
C	11	15	254
D	2	7	60
E	3	1	33
F	8	19	189
G	2	1	49
Total	35	57	828

The limits for pre-existing Condition 1 are calculated as follows: The average value is the total incidences of Condition 1 divided by the total cases over all the clinics, i.e., $\frac{35}{828}$, or 4.23%.

Referring to Table 8.1, there are seven clinics being compared. If we wish to use 5% and 1% risks, the appropriate factors are 2.49 and 2.95, respectively. The limits for 5% are:

$$0.0423 \pm 2.49 \times \sqrt{\frac{0.0423 \times (1 - 0.0423)}{\text{Total cases for the clinic}}}$$

The corresponding limits for a 1% risk are:

$$0.0423 \pm 2.95 \times \sqrt{\frac{0.0423 \times (1 - 0.0423)}{\text{Total cases for the clinic}}}$$

For Clinic A, the 5% limits are:

$$0.0423 \pm 2.49 \times \sqrt{\frac{0.0423 \times (1 - 0.0423)}{100}}$$

$$= 0.0423 \pm 2.49 \times \sqrt{\frac{0.0405}{100}}$$

$$= 0.0423 \pm 0.0501$$

These translate to 0.0924 for an upper 5% limit, and a lower limit that is less than 0. For ANOM with proportions, a limit less than 0 should be considered 0.

If the value 2.49 is replaced with 2.95 (from Table 8.1), the upper 1% limit can be shown to be 0.0594, or 5.94%. In other words, to declare Clinic A outside the common cause system, its result would have to be greater than 5.94%. The lower 1% limit for Clinic A is less than 0, and should be considered 0.

Limits for the other clinics and for Condition 2 are calculated similarly.

Figure 8.4a: ANOM Charts of Pre-existing Condition 1

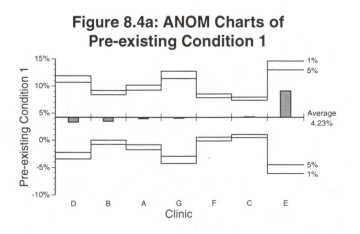

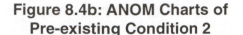

Figure 8.4b: ANOM Charts of Pre-existing Condition 2

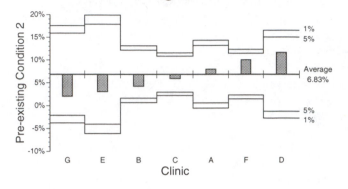

The correct Analysis of Means shows that the differences between the clinics are all common cause.

Quite a different interpretation—the seven clinics represent a common cause system for *both* conditions! Actually, this was true for almost all the pre-existing conditions. Any routine "adjustments" would be treating common cause as special, ultimately overcomplicating the interpretation. An initial ANOM has the potential to prevent this tampering which, unfortunately, is probably part of a "standard" analysis of such data. Such well-meaning analyses tend to be overly-complicated PARC analyses and create spurious results. In the process, there will have been many non-value meetings that are just reactions to the *data* process and not the *actual* process being improved. If, even after the ANOM, a relationship between the outcome and pre-condition is theorized, a simple scatter plot may be quite informative. Beware of "packaged" analysis programs that don't take a simple, visual approach.

Refer back to Figure 8.3. Why didn't Clinic E's "obvious" high percentage get flagged by the ANOM? Look at the number of cases for Clinic E. There were only 33. Look at the formula for calculating the limits of the ANOM. As the number of cases decreases, the width of the limits increases. We are more confident of the results when we have more data from which to draw. It is entirely possible that a clinic with an average of 4.23% could produce 3 occurrences out of 33 opportunities, for a 9% rate. However, if the 9% rate continued for more than about 100 cases, it would be evidence that the clinic is outside the system.

Thus, a small denominator caused the deceptive result in Condition 1. A discomfort with variation, coupled with a need to "explain" it, caused overreaction to Condition 2.

Bar graphs of percents are relatively useless unless they are used to do Pareto analysis through stratification. As can be seen from both this data and the pharmacy data, it is virtually impossible to interpret percent data unless the denominators are known.

Another Example of Percentage Deceptiveness in Continuous ANOM

The following proportional chart (p-chart) was presented to a hospital's upper management. It describes the fraction of patients who were successfully treated and discharged following a primary procedure of coronary artery bypass. The data represent four years of monthly data. The limits are calculated by the p-chart procedure described earlier in this chapter, even though this is not a formal ANOM. Technically, the p-chart is the "correct" chart to use for this kind of data. But when the denominators are "large" (>50 starts to give a good approximation), the individuals' chart as presented in Chapter 7 becomes a good approximation. In the C-section data where we used an individual's chart, the denominators were in the 250-300 range. In this case, the denominators ranged from the teens to low thirties, which would make use of the individuals chart technique suspect. (Wheeler argues in his book, *Understanding Variation*, that the p-chart may not necessarily be correct even in this situation. The argument is subtle, but is irrelevant to the point of this example.[4])

Figure 8.5: P-Chart of Bypass Survival Rate

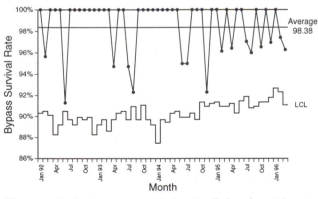

The survival rate appears to be declining (or at least more variable) toward the end of this time period. Note that the lower limit varies due to the different number of procedures performed in a given month.

A member of the executive team was familiar with run and control charts and became concerned when looking at the graph. Even though all the data points

were between the limits, he felt that somewhere in 1994 the survival rate started to worsen, with the trend continuing until the present. What do you think?

There is another special cause rule that has not been mentioned, and it seems to apply here. A special cause exists if one observes *at least seven-in-a-row of the same data value*. Note in this case that it happens twice: Observations 7-15 are all 100% as are observations 21-29. This test can sometimes signal an issue in the *data collection process*. Since the data are percentages, with both numerators and denominators, a run chart of the denominators can sometimes provide further insight. Figure 8.6 contains the run chart for the survival rate denominators.

Figure 8.6: Run Chart of Bypass Survival Rate Denominators (Number of Procedures Performed)

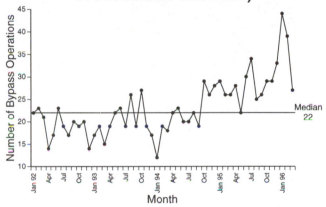

The number of operations increased beginning in month 34.

It is clear that the process had indeed changed, *but not necessarily the percent survival*. With a 98.4% survival rate and a "window of opportunity" of typically 13-26 (expected 90-98% of the time from 2 sigma limits on a control chart) it was unusual to see any deviant events in a given month–virtually everyone survived. In other words, given the current survival rate and typical number of operations performed, *monthly data are not discriminating enough for meaningful analysis of process stability*. However, as of month 34, the typical number of operations increased by 10 per month. The new "window" of 22 to 37 operations, combined with a survival rate of 98.4%, is indeed sufficient to allow monthly data to assess the ongoing stability of the process.

If you still have any doubts about the process being stable for the entire 51 months, look at the ANOM in Fig. 8.7. It compares the results of months 1-33 (637 survivals out of 646 operations) versus months 34-51 (520 survivals out of 530 operations). There is no evidence nor hint of a statistical significant difference.

Figure 8.7: ANOM Comparing Time Frame with Fewer Procedures Against Time Frame With More Procedures

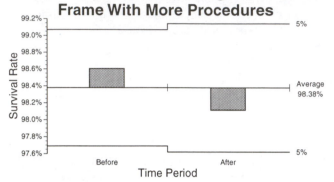

There is no evidence of a change in survival rate when the number of procedures increased.

Analysis of Means for Continuous Data

(Although ANOM for continuous data is the most complex technique discussed in this book, it is extremely powerful, and we felt that it must be addressed. However, to be used properly, one must be aware of the "prickly" subtlety inherent in its use. Despite this, the following description is useful when the challenge is an initial, macro exposition of hidden improvement opportunities. The data sets used will illustrate its enormous versatility.)

Many times, comparisons need to be made among individuals in a work process. The goal should be to identify the current state of the process and find hidden special causes to study for improvement opportunities. As shown earlier in this chapter, analysis of means of percentages is a very powerful technique for doing this. Due to the nature of much of the quality data available, it is applicable for many current data collections. However, the data in Table 8.3 are also quite typical in many situations. As can be seen, they are hardly amenable to percentage type analysis. They represent monthly productivity data for three physicians in a practice as measured in total RVUs per month. The clinic administrator was interested in predicting future productivity for budgeting purposes. She also wondered whether there were differences among the physicians. The first two data points are missing for Physician 2 because he was new at the clinic as of March 1994. The moving ranges are also shown.

Table 8.3: RVU Data

Month	MD1	MR	MD2	MR	MD3	MR
Jan-93	482	*	*	*	529	*
Feb	402	80	*	*	421	108
Mar	424	22	321	*	417	4
Apr	380	44	353	32	565	148
May	287	93	304	49	425	140
Jun	438	151	266	38	565	140
Jul	525	87	359	93	482	83
Aug	388	137	432	73	426	56
Sep	507	119	439	7	506	80
Oct	510	3	370	69	476	30
Nov	418	92	407	37	464	12
Dec	592	174	330	77	343	121
Jan-94	526	66	342	12	498	155
Feb	459	67	325	17	390	108
Mar	367	92	479	154	393	3
Apr	456	89	413	66	344	49
May	486	30	476	63	415	71
Jun	385	101	378	98	404	11
Jul	370	15	471	93	398	6
Aug	478	108	468	3	401	3
Sep	427	51	381	87	490	89
Oct	453	26	550	169	338	152
Nov	489	36	350	200	618	280
Dec	584	95	392	42	413	205
Jan-95	546	38	617	225	383	30
Feb	401	145	444	173	437	54
Mar	468	67	606	162	451	14
Apr	430	38	620	14	432	19
May	404	26	503	117	488	56

Using what you have learned so far in this book, an assessment must be made as to whether each physician's process is stable. So, the run chart for each is shown in Figure 8.8.

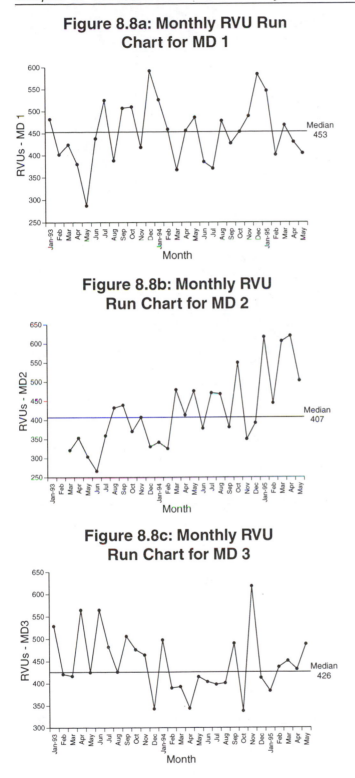

Figure 8.8a: Monthly RVU Run Chart for MD 1

Figure 8.8b: Monthly RVU Run Chart for MD 2

Figure 8.8c: Monthly RVU Run Chart for MD 3

All charts pass the run rules, even though the charts look suspicious for MDs 2 and 3.

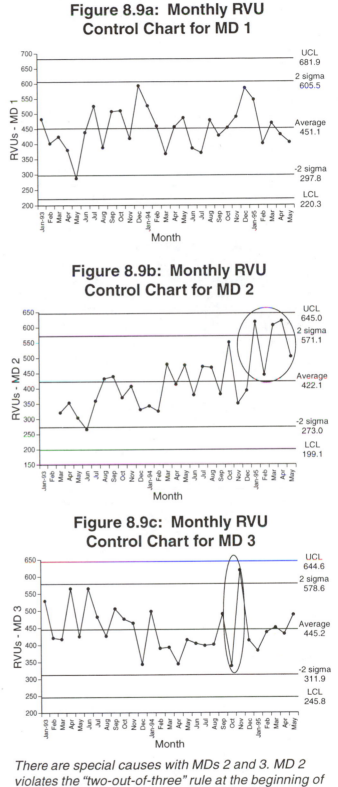

Figure 8.9a: Monthly RVU Control Chart for MD 1

Figure 8.9b: Monthly RVU Control Chart for MD 2

Figure 8.9c: Monthly RVU Control Chart for MD 3

There are special causes with MDs 2 and 3. MD 2 violates the "two-out-of-three" rule at the beginning of 1995, and MD 3 had a moving range that exceeded MRMax.

8

Despite the suspicious look of the charts for MD 2 and MD 3, they pass all the run test rules. So far, we cannot prove the presence of special causes. What should be done next? Maybe control charts of each MD with both two and three standard deviation limits drawn in will help to clarify the situation (Fig. 8.9).

MD 2 shows a special cause. January-March 1995 demonstrate the "two out of three" rule (two out of three consecutive data points falling between two and three standard deviations). So do the February-April 1995 data. A reasonable theory might be that, being a new doctor in a group, it takes time to build a practice. It seems that he has finally "found his rhythm." The best approximation of the current state of his process would be the average of observations 25-29, i.e., 558 RVU per month.

(Note: The analysis is not so clear cut. March 1993 - February 1994 seem to form a clear system and are consistent with the "growing the practice" theory. The question for this analysis becomes, Does the current process begin in March 1994 or January 1995? After much hand-wringing, we decided to use just the 1995 data, with the final factor being that this happens to coincide with the calendar year. Maybe there were changes in the definitions of RVU, maybe he received a new panel of patients. Who knows? There doesn't seem to be a similar 1995 "phenomenon" for his partners.)

The only special cause shown by MD 3 is the special cause moving range from observation 22 to 23. Some may think that "something doesn't look quite right about his pattern," and we agree. But, it is not so clear which particular observations, if any, should be deleted. Until further data are obtained, it is probably best to be conservative and use all the data in the subsequent analysis. Deletion of observations probably wouldn't change the assessment of the situation in any appreciable way.

So, we have three averages: MD 1=451.1, MD 2=558, MD 3=445.2. Are they different? There could be as many different interpretations as there are people reading this, so let's use some statistical theory to reduce the "ouija board" factor. One of them, MD 2, happens to be the "biggest" and one of them, MD 3, happens to be the "smallest." Are any differences real or can they all be explained by common cause?

First, as in a p-chart ANOM, one calculates the average of the system. The system is the aggregated monthly average of the three physicians. In this case, the average of the 63 observations (29 each for MDs 1 & 3 and 5 for MD 2), is 456.9 RVU per month. One would draw a chart with 456.9 as a center line and then plot each physician's average along the horizontal axis (Figure 8.10)

Figure 8.10: Physician Averages Plotted Without Common Cause Limits

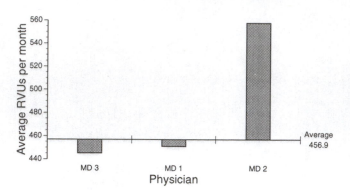

This is the first step in constructing an ANOM plot for continuous data.

The next question becomes, How does one calculate the common cause band around the average to see whether each physician is in, above, or below the system? This is where things start to get a little tricky.

In looking at the three control charts, one notices that the common cause limits are about the same for each physician: plus or minus 200. As it turns out, since the variation of each physician is relatively similar, it is statistically advantageous to combine the three sets of moving ranges into one set and determine the median moving range of *all* of these. In other words, the 28 moving ranges of MD 1 are combined with the 26 moving ranges of MD 2 and the 28 moving ranges of MD 3 as shown in Table 8.4. These 82 moving ranges are then sorted and the median found. In this case, the overall MMR is 70.

Next, this overall median moving range is converted to a standard deviation by dividing it by 0.954. As in the control chart calculations with the constants 3.865 and 3.14, the 0.954 is derived from statistical theory and used to convert a *median (not* average*)* moving range to the process standard deviation *regardless* of how many moving ranges were calculated in the original data. So, for our system, the standard deviation of an individual monthly observation is 73.4.

Table 8.4: Moving Ranges of all MDs Combined

MD1 Moving Range	MD2 Moving Range	MD3 Moving Range	Sorted Moving Range	Sorted Order	Sorted Moving Range	Sorted Order	Sorted Moving Range	Sorted Order
80	32	108	3	1st	44	29th	93	55th
22	49	4	3	2nd	49	30th	93	56th
44	38	148	3	3rd	49	31st	95	57th
93	93	140	3	4th	51	32nd	98	58th
151	73	140	4	5th	54	33rd	101	59th
87	7	83	6	6th	56	34th	108	60th
137	69	56	7	7th	56	35th	108	61st
119	37	80	11	8th	63	36th	108	62nd
3	77	30	12	9th	66	37th	117	63rd
92	12	12	12	10th	66	38th	119	64th
174	17	121	14	11th	67	39th	121	65th
66	154	155	14	12th	67	40th	137	66th
67	66	108	15	13th	69	41st	140	67th
92	63	3	17	14th	71	42nd	140	68th
89	98	49	19	15th	73	43rd	145	69th
30	93	71	22	16th	77	44th	148	70th
101	3	11	26	17th	80	45th	151	71st
15	87	6	26	18th	80	46th	152	72nd
108	169	3	30	19th	83	47th	154	73rd
51	200	89	30	20th	87	48th	155	74th
26	42	152	30	21st	87	49th	162	75th
36	225	280	32	22nd	89	50th	169	76th
95	173	205	36	23rd	89	51st	173	77th
38	162	30	37	24th	92	52nd	174	78th
145	14	54	38	25th	92	53rd	200	79th
67	117	14	38	26th	93	54th	205	80th
38		19	38	27th			225	81st
26		56	42	28th			280	82nd

As in the p-chart analysis, the people being compared may have differing numbers of observations making up their individual average. More data in the calculation of the individual average mean more confidence in the actual number obtained. In our current example, averages for MDs 1 & 3 are based on 29 values, while MD 2's is based only on five. So despite the fact that MD 2 seems higher, his large number could be an artifact of a small number of observations.

Similar to the p-chart, to obtain the common cause limit for each individual, divide the system standard deviation,

$$\frac{MMR}{0.954} = \frac{70}{0.954} = 73.4,$$

by the square root of the number of observations in that particular individual's average. This quantity is then multiplied by three (for three standard deviations) and added and subtracted from the *system* average (center line). In this example, the limits are:

$$456.9 \pm 3 \times \frac{73.4}{\sqrt{n}}$$

where "n" represents the number of individuals in the stratum of interest. Individual physicians are judged based on whether they fall in or outside of the common cause band. The ANOM Chart for RVU is in Figure 8.11. Figure 8.12 contains a summary of the ANOM process.

Figure 8.11: ANOM of RVUs

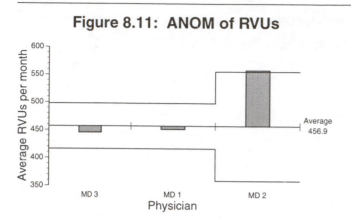

The ANOM analysis shows MD 2's average to be slightly outside the system.

So, the common cause band for MD 1 & MD 3 is

$$456.9 \pm 3 \times \frac{73.4}{\sqrt{29}} = 456.9 \pm 40.9$$

or 416.0-497.8. They both fall in the system. Despite the fact that their averages happen to fall below the system average, neither is a "below average" performer.

MD 2's common cause band is

$$456.9 \pm 3 \times \frac{73.4}{\sqrt{5}} = 456.9 \pm 98.5$$

or 358.4-555.4. He is a special cause (barely). His productivity is "above" the system, i.e., he seems to be truly "above" average. There is something different about his process. The question now becomes, By studying MD 2's practice "process," can we learn anything that would help improve the productivity of MDs 1 & 3? Or, given the inputs to MD 2's process, is the current state of system variation appropriate?

If any interventions are made, each physician can now measure his progress toward new goals by continuing to plot data on his control chart (Figure 8.9). These could also aid the clinic administrator in budgeting, comparing projected income to financial goals (to determine feasibility) as well as determining when to revise budgetary forecasts if special causes are observed.

Figure 8.12 A Process for Continuous Analysis of Means

1. Decide which factor will be used to stratify the data. Sort the data for each stratum. Within each stratum, sort the data in its naturally occurring time order.

2. Compute the moving ranges within each strata and combine them into one column. Find the overall median moving range of the data set. Convert it to the system standard deviation by dividing it by 0.954, i.e., $\dfrac{MMR}{0.954}$.

3. For strata with 10 or more observations, plot a run chart and/or control chart. You can choose whether to use the system standard deviation as calculated in (2) and/or use the standard deviation for the individual stratum being plotted. Delete obvious individual special causes from the subsequent ANOM analysis. Then, assess the period of data that represents the *most recent stable history* of the stratum. Use that stable system to determine the current process average in the ANOM.

4. Calculate the "grand" average of all the individual data points being used in the ANOM (this corresponds to the weighted average of all the strata). This represents the "system" average.

5. Plot the averages of each stratum on a chart and draw the system average as a centerline.

6. Calculate the common cause band by which each stratum average will be judged versus the system average as:

$$3 \times \frac{\text{system standard deviation}}{\sqrt{\text{number of observations in the stratum}}}.$$

7. Add and subtract the quantity calculated in (6) to the centerline where the particular individual stratum average is plotted.

$$\text{system average} \pm 3 \times \frac{\text{system standard deviation}}{\sqrt{\text{number of observations in the stratum}}}.$$

8. If the stratum average falls within its common cause band around the centerline, it is considered "in" the system and no different from the system average. *The stratum averages that fall inside the common cause band are considered statistically indistinguishable.* Any attempt at a ranking would be incorrect.

9. Observations outside of the common cause band on either side can be considered truly "above" or "below" average.

A Note on the Use of Three Standard Deviations in Continuous ANOM

It is important to note that Table 8.1 (used in p-chart ANOM to determine the number of standard deviations to use for common cause) does **not** necessarily apply to continuous ANOM. The explanation of why this is true is somewhat complicated. The median moving range provides only a very approximate estimate of the standard deviation, and the ANOM objective is an exposition of the big hidden special causes. As a result, it is probably best to stick with using three standard deviations regardless of the number of comparisons being made. Most of the time, three is good enough. The ANOM procedure as described is approximate, but its intent is to bring a sanity based in theory to the proverbial "fishing expedition."

The MI Nurse Phone Productivity Data

A new system of centralized phone care delivered by specially trained registered nurses is being implemented at a large clinic. Phone data are available for each of the 64 nurses. The nurses log on at the beginning of each shift. A computer tracks how much time they spend talking to patients; making outside calls to patients; waiting for an incoming call; and with their phone in "not ready" status. "Not ready" means that the phone cannot accept an incoming call, mostly due to documentation of the previous call, but also for miscellaneous other reasons.

An initial attempt to analyze productivity showed the data to be badly contaminated. This was due to rampant variation among the nurses as to when to put their phones on "not ready." Subsequently, better operational definitions and standardized processes were established. The following analysis was the first attempt to compare productivities for purposes of system education. Instead of blaming and finger-pointing, the intent was to expose special causes, discuss the appropriateness of the variation, and reduce the unintended variation. The goal was to increase productivity. It was agreed that an ANOM analysis would be presented in a blinded fashion to the nurses. In other words, each nurse would know who she was on the macro analysis, but would not be able to identify others. Each nurse would also receive the control chart of her own data. It was hoped that healthy, productive, collegial discussion would ensue.

Another objective was to assess the current system's actual productivity. The supervisor wanted to staff based on the assumption that 80% of the typical nurse's staffed time is spent either talking, making outside calls, or waiting for a call. The 80% was also their ultimate goal for this system. She wanted to know how they were doing relative to the goal.

Data were taken for ten shifts for each nurse during July. The number of data points for each nurse ranged from 2 to 11. Forty nurses had exactly 10 data points, 50 had in the range of 9 to 11. The term "% Work" was defined as the sum of "talk" time, "outside call" time, and "wait" time divided by the "total staffed" time.

Some readers may wonder why continuous ANOM is being used and not the percentage version. This is because, despite the number being a percent, it is not collected by measurement of discrete events. It is not as if each minute of staffed time is *individually assigned* as either "work" or "not ready". Minutes are continuous in nature and can take on any value.

A control chart was plotted for each nurse to see whether the data formed a stable system and also to look for outliers. Fifty-two nurses' data exhibited common cause behavior with no outliers. Examples of two charts containing special causes are shown in Figure 8.13.

Figure 8.13a: Control Chart of Nurse 29's "Work Time"

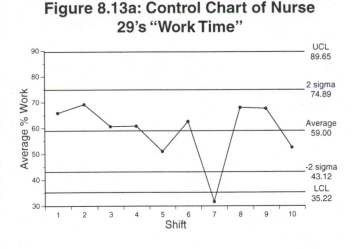

Figure 8.13b: Control Chart of Nurse 59's "Work Time"

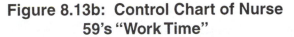
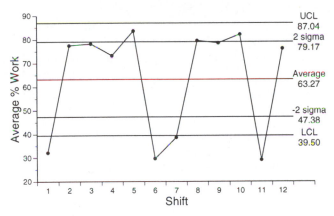
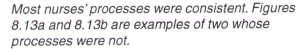

Most nurses' processes were consistent. Figures 8.13a and 8.13b are examples of two whose processes were not.

(After excluding Shift 7, Nurse 29's average becomes 62.03. After excluding Shifts 1, 6, 7, and 11, Nurse 59's average becomes 78.70.)

When special causes were present, obvious outliers, e.g., observation 7 in Figure 8.13a, were deleted from the subsequent ANOM. Figure 8.13b shows quite a different problem. This seems to be the classic problem of combining "boiling" water and "ice" water for an average. Observations 1, 6, 7, and 11 were eliminated from the ANOM analysis, but the reason for this odd pattern needs to be found!

This database of 64 nurses originally contained 601 data points. Ultimately, 20 data points were eliminated as outliers from the subsequent ANOM analysis. However, they were plotted and identified on the individual nurses' graphs so as to discuss possible reasons for them.

In analyzing each individual nurse's data, two "passes" were conducted. The first used the standard deviation based on each nurse's individual data. However, since each nurse had approximately 10 data points, the limits could vary quite a bit from nurse-to-nurse due to the lack of numerical information. (Recall Table 7.11, which recommended trying to have at least 15 points, and preferably 20.)

Second, the moving ranges for all 64 nurses were combined and sorted (537 moving ranges–Thank goodness for computers!). The overall MMR was 7.57. Then, the system standard deviation was calculated. Each nurse's control chart was replotted using this common standard deviation. These charts seemed to do a much better job of assessing each nurse's data, especially for finding outliers. With only 10 observations, outliers can exert quite an influence on the individual's common cause limits. The system standard deviation provides a better estimate for the "yardstick" used to compare the nurses.

In any case, the 64 averages (with individual special causes deleted) are shown in Figure 8.14 along with the system average of 61.43%.

Figure 8.14: Plot of Average Work Time for Each Nurse

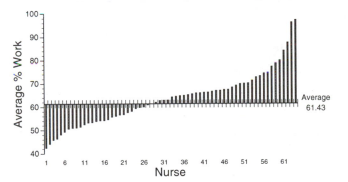
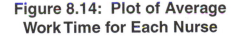

While there is variation, it is hard to say where the common cause limits fall.

Once again, there are probably as many interpretations of this graph as there are people reading this. The 64 individual averages along with the number of data points used to obtain the average are listed in Table 8.5.

Table 8.5: Phone Productivity Averages by Nurse

Nurse	% Work Time	Number of Shifts	Nurse	% Work Time	Number of Shifts
1	42.49	10	33	64.29	8
2	44.22	10	34	64.53	10
3	45.93	11	35	64.81	10
4	46.50	7	36	64.94	9
5	48.27	10	37	65.20	10
6	49.41	9	38	65.60	9
7	50.70	10	39	65.97	10
8	51.08	4	40	66.08	9
9	51.17	10	41	66.23	10
10	51.49	10	42	66.31	10
11	52.52	8	43	66.64	8
12	53.32	9	44	66.98	8
13	53.42	10	45	67.10	6
14	53.96	10	46	67.39	10
15	54.24	11	47	67.48	10
16	54.30	10	48	68.42	10
17	54.74	4	49	69.28	10
18	55.80	8	50	69.90	10
19	56.16	10	51	70.10	10
20	56.70	6	52	70.18	9
21	56.82	10	53	71.39	10
22	57.74	10	54	72.78	10
23	58.25	9	55	73.25	10
24	59.41	10	56	74.46	10
25	59.92	10	57	74.79	6
26	60.10	10	58	77.31	10
27	60.99	10	59	78.70	8
28	61.39	10	60	80.02	10
29	62.03	9	61	84.10	2
30	62.76	10	62	87.62	10
31	62.94	10	63	96.27	4
32	63.00	10	64	97.30	10

Based on the overall median moving range of 7.57, the system standard deviation is

$$\frac{7.57}{0.954} = 7.94.$$

Hence the common cause band for most of the data (40 nurses containing 10 data points) is:

$$61.43 \pm 3 \times \frac{7.94}{\sqrt{10}} = 61.43 \pm 7.53$$

or 53.90 - 68.96%.

Nurses with more shifts will have slightly narrower limits, and those with fewer shifts will have wider limits. In other words, given these data, the current process seems to be operating at 61.43% Work time relative to the goal of 80%. Thirty-six of the nurses are "in" the system. If they are working at this rate and 10 data points are collected, they will obtain an average between 53.90-68.96%. Any number in this range is indicative of a work process of 61.43%. Twelve nurses

seem to be "below" average and 16 nurses seem to be "above" average. This is shown visually with the ANOM chart below.

Figure 8.15: ANOM of MI Nurse Phone Productivity

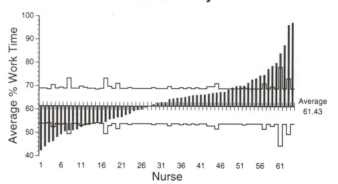

Thirty-six nurses are operating "in" the system, 12 are "below," and 16 are "above."

It could be worth studying the work processes of the 16 nurses who are above average. Changes to the current standard process based on these nurses could bring it closer to the goal of 80%.

Informal scanning of the data showed that many nurses with high % Work also had high % Wait times. Since this is a 24-hour service, it would be interesting to note the typical times these nurses work, e.g., after midnight.

Does increased talk time create more "Not ready" time due to the time required to document the calls? Is 80% a realistic goal for this process? As you can see, the ANOM is the tip of the iceberg, but leads to healthy questioning of the process. How have data like this been treated in the past at your organization? It probably resulted in lots of action, but did it give sustained results?

After collegial discussion of appropriateness, the 12 below average nurses need to at least be brought "into the system" and demonstrate 61% behavior. Ongoing plotting will be useful to assess progress of individual nurses and the overall system. Any subsequent data will be appended to the current data set.

The ER "Unpredictable Admit" Data

The supervisor of inpatient admissions at a hospital was troubled. From 6 PM to 11 PM, her people also had to handle "unexpected" admissions to the emergency room. This was a disturbance to the other work they also had to do. (Does this supervisor see "unexpected" admissions as a common cause or a special cause to her system of inpatient admissions? What do you think?)

She decided to collect some data on the situation i.e., study the current process. Her staff worked Mondays-Fridays. She collected hourly data (6-7 PM, 7-8 PM, 8-9 PM, 9-10 PM, 10-11 PM) for approximately six weeks. The data are shown in Table 8.6. They are coded by day of the week.

Table 8.6: Emergency Room Admissions Data

Day of Week	6-7	7-8	8-9	9-10	10-11
Wed	2	8	7	8	8
Thu	8	4	11	6	5
Fri	5	6	5	6	2
Mon	3	5	7	9	11
Tue	3	5	7	7	8
Wed	9	4	5	8	1
Thu	2	3	7	10	3
Fri	1	2	5	6	3
Mon	5	4	10	11	6
Tue	4	2	3	7	6
Wed	1	3	8	9	6
Thu	4	4	8	6	6
Fri	3	5	6	8	6
Mon	4	1	5	13	6
Tue	9	7	9	7	6
Wed	4	6	11	9	6
Thu	3	4	9	8	4
Fri	2	3	5	5	6
Mon	7	10	10	12	6
Tue	1	5	8	6	5
Wed	2	5	1	11	8
Thu	5	2	7	4	5
Fri	4	3	9	8	6
Mon	2	5	4	5	4
Tue	6	2	8	7	5
Wed	3	5	1	9	10
Thu	3	1	5	4	7
Fri	4	5	6	9	9
Mon	3	2	3	11	3
Tue	4	7	6	15	4
Wed	6	5	12	3	8

Figure 8.16a:
Stratified Histogram by Day

Figure 8.16b: Stratified Histogram
by Time of Night

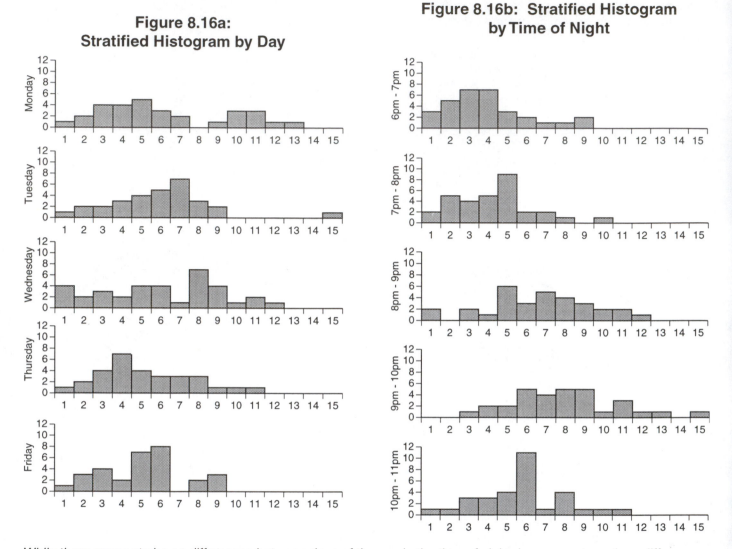

While there appear to be no differences between days of the week, the time of night does seem to make a difference.

Before doing any more formal statistical analysis, a few simple macro-level pictures might answer some natural questions about this process. First, do there seem to be any special causes by day of the week? Second, are there any special causes by hourly period? Two stratified histograms are shown in Figure 8.16. The first separates the data by day. The second separates the data by hourly interval.

Giving each a quick perusal, there seem to be no glaring differences by day of the week. However, there is an interesting "clump" of nine observations containing high values in the Monday data. This observation could be useful in subsequent analysis.

The second histogram is far more interesting. Distinct differences can be observed. The first two time periods seem indistinguishable from each other and, on the average, lower than the other three. It also looks as if the 9-10 PM hour has, on average, a much higher rate of ER admissions.

Analysis of means will now be used to statistically gain more insight into the situation. After the ANOM, any conclusions will be confirmed (or disputed) by time plotting of the original data as suggested by the analysis. As stated previously, any data set has an implicit time element, which must be considered sooner or later.

The first ANOM will compare totals by day of the week. In other words, at this point, there is no concern for the hourly pattern. The question is a "macro" one, Do some weekdays tend to have more admissions than other days?

The hourly totals were added to get a daily total. Table 8.7 shows the data for each day of the week grouped with its corresponding and subsequent weekly data. (Note that there are seven observations for Wednesdays.) Each group yields five moving ranges (Wednesday yields six) and these are shown next to the data columns. The median for these 26 moving ranges is seven (yielding a process standard deviation of $\frac{7}{0.954} = 7.34$).

Multiplying this by 3.865 yields the maximum moving range observable by common cause, MRMax. The MRMax is 27, which no point exceeds.

Table 8.7: ER Admission Data Sorted by Day

Week	Mon	MR	Tue	MR	Wed	MR	Thu	MR	Fri	MR
1	35	*	30	*	33	*	34	*	24	*
2	36	1	22	8	27	6	25	9	17	7
3	29	7	38	16	27	0	28	3	28	11
4	45	16	25	13	36	9	28	0	21	7
5	20	25	28	3	27	9	23	5	30	9
6	22	2	36	8	28	1	20	3	33	3
7					34	6				

The ANOM chart is shown below. A "typical" night yields 28.7 unexpected ER admissions. How do the days of the week compare in this system?

Figure 8.17: ANOM by Day of Week

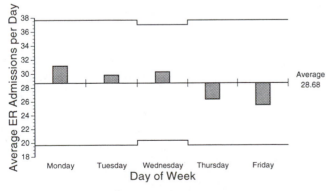

There are no statistically detectable differences between days of the week.

The five daily averages are plotted and all fall within the common cause band of the "system" of

$$26.68 \pm 3 \times \frac{7.34}{\sqrt{6}}$$

The band is slightly tighter for Wednesday because its average contains seven observations. Thus, the ANOM analysis confirmed our intuitive analysis via the stratified histogram. Even though Mondays have the "highest" average and Fridays the "lowest", there is no statistical difference between them.

Given this analysis, the daily totals are rearranged in their natural time order in Table 8.8 along with the corresponding moving ranges. The median moving range when calculated from the data in their time order is 7.5, which in essence agrees with the previous ANOM MMR of 7. The resulting control chart is also shown.

Table 8.8: Daily Data

Week	Day of Week	Daily Admissions	MR
1	Wed	33	*
1	Thu	34	1
1	Fri	24	10
1	Mon	35	11
1	Tue	30	5
2	Wed	27	3
2	Thu	25	2
2	Fri	17	8
2	Mon	36	19
2	Tue	22	14
3	Wed	27	5
3	Thu	28	1
3	Fri	28	0
3	Mon	29	1
3	Tue	38	9
4	Wed	36	2
4	Thu	28	8
4	Fri	21	7
4	Mon	45	24
4	Tue	25	20
5	Wed	27	2
5	Thu	23	4
5	Fri	30	7
5	Mon	20	10
5	Tue	28	8
6	Wed	28	0
6	Thu	20	8
6	Fri	33	13
6	Mon	22	11
6	Tue	36	14
7	Wed	34	2

Figure 8.18: Control Chart of Daily Totals

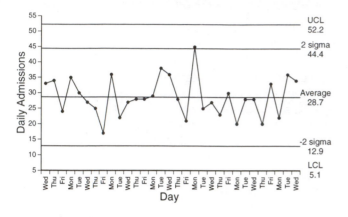

There are no special causes in the process. Thus the data can be used to make predictions.

Could a process appear more stable?

To conclude so far, this "unpredictable" process is actually quite predictable. On any given weekday night, this process averages 29 "unexpected" ER admits. How does this translate to any future individual weeknight reality? 90-98% of the nights will see between 13-44 unexpected admits. Occasionally, one may have as few as 5, but there may also be the night everyone dreads, with 53 unexpected admits. Why? Because! Such a night shouldn't be reacted to with an immediate adjustment for the following night, given the evidence of the chart. After such a night, subsequent plotting would be useful to either confirm whether it was just a common cause event or that a process change has really taken place. The "two out of three" rule along with the "eight observations above the average" rule should be watched closely. Study of this process now allows the luxury of prediction for this supervisor.

Now let's consider the more interesting question of differences among the five hourly periods. Similar to the daily data, the 31 individual daily observations for each time period were grouped together in their individual natural time order (5 x 31=155 observations). The moving range was found within each group, yielding 150 moving ranges. The data appear in Table 8.9.

Table 8.9: Hourly Data by Day

Day	6-7	MR	7-8	MR	8-9	MR	9-10	MR	10-11	MR
1	2	*	8	*	7	*	8	*	8	*
2	8	6	4	4	11	4	6	2	5	3
3	5	3	6	2	5	6	6	0	2	3
4	3	2	5	1	7	2	9	3	11	9
5	3	0	5	0	7	0	7	2	8	3
6	9	6	4	1	5	2	8	1	1	7
7	2	7	3	1	7	2	10	2	3	2
8	1	1	2	1	5	2	6	4	3	0
9	5	4	4	2	10	5	11	5	6	3
10	4	1	2	2	3	7	7	4	6	0
11	1	3	3	1	8	5	9	2	6	0
12	4	3	4	1	8	0	6	3	6	0
13	3	1	5	1	6	2	8	2	6	0
14	4	1	1	4	5	1	13	5	6	0
15	9	5	7	6	9	4	7	6	6	0
16	4	5	6	1	11	2	9	2	6	0
17	3	1	4	2	9	2	8	1	4	2
18	2	1	3	1	5	4	5	3	6	2
19	7	5	10	7	10	5	12	7	6	0
20	1	6	5	5	8	2	6	6	5	1
21	2	1	5	0	1	7	11	5	8	3
22	5	3	2	3	7	6	4	7	5	3
23	4	1	3	1	9	2	8	4	6	1
24	2	2	5	2	4	5	5	3	4	2
25	6	4	2	3	8	4	7	2	5	1
26	3	3	5	3	1	7	9	2	10	5
27	3	0	1	4	5	4	4	5	7	3
28	4	1	5	4	6	1	9	5	9	2
29	3	1	2	3	3	3	11	2	3	6
30	4	1	7	5	6	3	15	4	4	1
31	6	2	5	2	12	6	3	12	8	4

The overall median moving range was two (yielding a standard deviation of $\frac{2}{0.954} = 2.1$).

The maximum moving range between any two consecutive daily totals for the same time period is 2 x 3.865, which is approximately 8. One special cause of 12 was found in the 9-10 PM data from day 30 to day 31 (Day 31 happened to have the lowest total of all 31 days). Once again, the conservative approach is being taken and it will be left in. It will be reconsidered in the plot subsequent to the ANOM. The ANOM chart is shown below.

Figure 8.19: ANOM by Time of Night

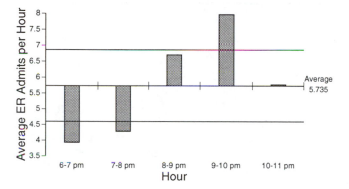

There are distinct difference in admissions at different times of the evening.

The overall average for a "typical" time period is 5.7. However, this again it appears to be made up of boiling water and ice water. The common cause band around which each time period is judged is:

$$5.7 \pm 3 \times \frac{2.1}{\sqrt{31}} \, ,$$

since all the time periods had the same number of data points (31). Our initial impression that the 6-7 PM and the 7-8 PM periods were indistinguishable and lower than the other three periods is confirmed. Period 4 (9-10 PM) also seems to be truly "above" average in terms of the number of ER admits handled. Period 3 (8-9 PM) and Period 5 (10-11 PM) are truly "average" and statistically indistinguishable from one another.

So, even though weeknight totals are indistinguishable, there is a special cause, predictable pattern *within* each night that could have staffing implications. Let's rearrange the original data and plot it with the information gained from the ANOM analysis to study this model's predictive ability.

The data were rearranged in their literal time order for each group of time periods. To do this, we take the data as presented in Table 8.9 and put it into three columns. These three columns are presented in Table 8.10. They are those suggested by the ANOM by time of night:

A. the data for 6-7 PM & 7-8 PM (62 observations: 2 data points per day x 31 days),

B. the data for 8-9 PM & 10-11 PM (62 observations), and

C. the data for 9-10 PM (31 observations: 1 observation per day x 31 days).

8

Table 8.10: Time of Night Data Sorted into Three Systems

Day	Time	Admissions	Day	Time	Admissions	Day	Time	Admissions
1	6-7 PM	2	1	8-9 PM	7	1	9-10 PM	8
1	7-8 PM	8	1	10-11 PM	8	2	9-10 PM	6
2	6-7 PM	8	2	8-9 PM	11	3	9-10 PM	6
2	7-8 PM	4	2	10-11 PM	5	4	9-10 PM	9
3	6-7 PM	5	3	8-9 PM	5	5	9-10 PM	7
3	7-8 PM	6	3	10-11 PM	2	6	9-10 PM	8
4	6-7 PM	3	4	8-9 PM	7	7	9-10 PM	10
4	7-8 PM	5	4	10-11 PM	11	8	9-10 PM	6
5	6-7 PM	3	5	8-9 PM	7	9	9-10 PM	11
5	7-8 PM	5	5	10-11 PM	8	10	9-10 PM	7
6	6-7 PM	9	6	8-9 PM	5	11	9-10 PM	9
6	7-8 PM	4	6	10-11 PM	1	12	9-10 PM	6
7	6-7 PM	2	7	8-9 PM	7	13	9-10 PM	8
7	7-8 PM	3	7	10-11 PM	3	14	9-10 PM	13
8	6-7 PM	1	8	8-9 PM	5	15	9-10 PM	7
8	7-8 PM	2	8	10-11 PM	3	16	9-10 PM	9
9	6-7 PM	5	9	8-9 PM	10	17	9-10 PM	8
9	7-8 PM	4	9	10-11 PM	6	18	9-10 PM	5
10	6-7 PM	4	10	8-9 PM	3	19	9-10 PM	12
10	7-8 PM	2	10	10-11 PM	6	20	9-10 PM	6
11	6-7 PM	1	11	8-9 PM	8	21	9-10 PM	11
11	7-8 PM	3	11	10-11 PM	6	22	9-10 PM	4
12	6-7 PM	4	12	8-9 PM	8	23	9-10 PM	8
12	7-8 PM	4	12	10-11 PM	6	24	9-10 PM	5
13	6-7 PM	3	13	8-9 PM	6	25	9-10 PM	7
13	7-8 PM	5	13	10-11 PM	6	26	9-10 PM	9
14	6-7 PM	4	14	8-9 PM	5	27	9-10 PM	4
14	7-8 PM	1	14	10-11 PM	6	28	9-10 PM	9
15	6-7 PM	9	15	8-9 PM	9	29	9-10 PM	11
15	7-8 PM	7	15	10-11 PM	6	30	9-10 PM	15
16	6-7 PM	4	16	8-9 PM	11	31	9-10 PM	3
16	7-8 PM	6	16	10-11 PM	6			
17	6-7 PM	3	17	8-9 PM	9			
17	7-8 PM	4	17	10-11 PM	4			
18	6-7 PM	2	18	8-9 PM	5			
18	7-8 PM	3	18	10-11 PM	6			
19	6-7 PM	7	19	8-9 PM	10			
19	7-8 PM	10	19	10-11 PM	6			
20	6-7 PM	1	20	8-9 PM	8			
20	7-8 PM	5	20	10-11 PM	5			
21	6-7 PM	2	21	8-9 PM	1			
21	7-8 PM	5	21	10-11 PM	8			
22	6-7 PM	5	22	8-9 PM	7			
22	7-8 PM	2	22	10-11 PM	5			
23	6-7 PM	4	23	8-9 PM	9			
23	7-8 PM	3	23	10-11 PM	6			
24	6-7 PM	2	24	8-9 PM	4			
24	7-8 PM	5	24	10-11 PM	4			
25	6-7 PM	6	25	8-9 PM	8			
25	7-8 PM	2	25	10-11 PM	5			
26	6-7 PM	3	26	8-9 PM	1			
26	7-8 PM	5	26	10-11 PM	10			
27	6-7 PM	3	27	8-9 PM	5			
27	7-8 PM	1	27	10-11 PM	7			
28	6-7 PM	4	28	8-9 PM	6			
28	7-8 PM	5	28	10-11 PM	9			
29	6-7 PM	3	29	8-9 PM	3			
29	7-8 PM	2	29	10-11 PM	3			
30	6-7 PM	4	30	8-9 PM	6			
30	7-8 PM	7	30	10-11 PM	4			
31	6-7 PM	6	31	8-9 PM	12			
31	7-8 PM	5	31	10-11 PM	8			

Fortunately, since there was no difference by day of the week, these did not need to be further subdivided by a special cause pattern inherent in the week. The control chart for each "process" is shown below.

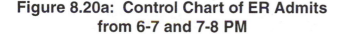

Figure 8.20a: Control Chart of ER Admits from 6-7 and 7-8 PM

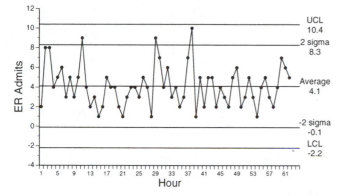

Figure 8.20b: Control Chart of ER Admits from 8-9 and 10-11 PM

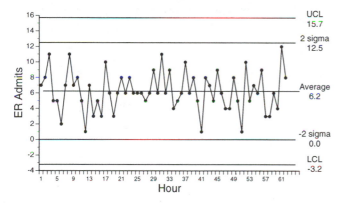

Figure 8.20c: Control Chart of ER Admits from 9-10 PM

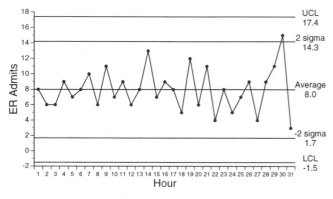

While the averages vary among the different hour groupings, the admissions within the time periods are consistent and predictable.

This heretofore allegedly "unpredictable" system has been shown to be quite predictable! The data fit the model proposed by the two ANOMs perfectly. Reconsider the possible special cause for the last data point of the 9-10 PM process. Even though it previously contained a special cause moving range, the median moving range of this particular process's data is 3. Multiplying 3 x 3.865=11.6, which is approximately 12, there seems to be no reason for declaring it a special cause. There is a statistical reason why this could happen, but the authors choose not to bore you with it. It is partially explained by the "Note" below.

(Note: Some purists may disagree with this analysis. It is not "technically" correct because these data are not truly continuous data. They are discrete "counts." Given such data, systems with higher averages also have higher standard deviations, which is the explanation for the disappearance of the moving range of 12 as a special cause. However, as stated at the beginning of this chapter, under most conditions, what has been done here is a *legitimate* approximation. The objective was a macro exposition of special causes in a vague situation, *which subsequent plotting of the data confirmed*. People desiring more information on specific techniques and when to use them are referred to the Executive Learning videos on variation and control charts (see Bibliography) and Donald Wheeler's books, *Understanding Statistical Process Control* and *Advanced Statistical Process Control*, both published by SPC Press.)

This analysis was a relatively straightforward one and simplified by the fact that the relationships between the hourly patterns were statistically identical regardless of the day of the week. However, in many cases, this is not so. There can be what is called a "statistical interaction" between the "slicing" and "dicing" factors. In the case of the current data set, this would mean that the hourly pattern relationships would be *different* for *some* days of the week. For example, in analyzing incoming phone call data, Mondays especially seem to have their own hourly pattern "finger print" that is unique from those of Tuesday through Friday. In analyzing Emergency Room admit data, weekends have their own unique patterns relative to weekdays.

It is beyond the scope of this book to show how to statistically identify such interactive relationships. However, if one has a theory as to a certain inherent relationship in the data, judicious use of plotting and identifying the suspected factors on the plot may allow one to see the pattern. For example, when the data were plotted at the end of the previous analysis to

8

confirm the predictive ability of the suggested ANOM model, identification of the days of the week or hourly intervals on the plots would have shown a random pattern (The author statistically tested this data set for the presence of interaction. There was none suggested.). Suppose that Fridays for some reason had a consistently heavier flow of patient ER traffic than Monday through Thursday. In that case, the Friday data points would virtually always appear to be "above average" on the combined 6-7 PM / 7-8 PM and the 8-9 PM / 10-11 PM plots because the Friday pattern was different and typically higher than the Monday-Thursday pattern. Ellis Ott would always insist that his students "Plot the data." It's important when possible to complement the statistical analysis with one's "master knowledge" of a situation through some type of plotting.

The Lab & X-Ray Utilization Data

A department head wanted a utilization analysis of the 29 members regarding their lab and x-ray charges. The costs were operationally defined on a "per office visit" basis. The aggregated 1994 and 1995 charges were obtained for each physician (2 data points per physician) along with the following bar graphs supplied by the utilization department with good intentions. Are the bar graphs helpful?!

Figure 8.21a: Bar graph of 1995 Lab Charges

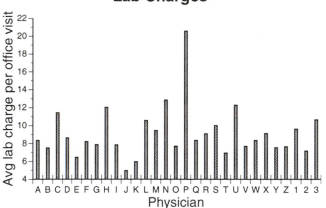

Figure 8.21b: Bar graph of 1995 X-ray Charges

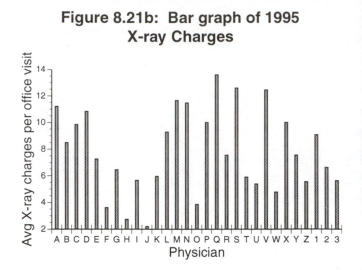

The bar graphs aren't useful for comparing physician performance since they do not contain any system information.

Unlike the previous examples, we do not have the luxury of doing either run charts or control charts since we have only two data points per physician. Might it still be possible to apply analysis of means? Absolutely!

If the data are in constant dollars and price increases factored out (questions that must be asked), in theory shouldn't the difference between 1995 and 1994 for each physician be common cause variation? Can you see that due to the time element in the data, the absolute value of the difference between 1995 and 1994 can be treated as a moving range? The data along with the resulting moving ranges are shown in Table 8.10. Note that with the layout of this table, the moving ranges are calculated across the columns instead of down the rows. We are taking the difference between the 1994 (second and fifth columns) and 1995 (third and sixth columns).

(Note: For those with the skill or those who have access to a statistician, it may be a good idea to do a paired T-test on the year-to-year differences. One could also do the easier non-parametric sign test to see if there are a disproportionate number of either positive or negative differences. If there is a significant difference between the years, the median moving range method will yield an inflated estimate of the standard deviation. This can be an important issue that often arises in comparing year-to-year data. Just be forewarned. It is not a factor in this example.)

Table 8.11: Data and Moving Ranges

MD	Lab94	Lab95	MR	XRay94	XRay95	MR
A	9.82	8.34	1.48	8.98	11.20	2.22
B	9.07	7.50	1.57	6.94	8.48	1.54
C	10.35	11.42	1.07	9.96	9.84	0.12
D	8.68	8.61	0.07	8.56	10.84	2.28
E	6.10	6.46	0.36	6.68	7.26	0.58
F	7.96	8.20	0.24	4.30	3.62	0.68
G	7.00	7.87	0.87	6.54	6.46	0.08
H	6.88	12.03	5.15	6.94	2.74	4.20
I	6.44	7.84	1.40	5.48	5.66	0.18
J	3.93	4.96	1.03	4.18	2.20	1.98
K	5.37	5.97	0.60	4.94	5.96	1.02
L	8.03	10.58	2.55	7.02	9.28	2.26
M	10.20	9.45	0.75	11.96	11.66	0.30
N	10.82	12.85	2.03	9.56	11.48	1.92
O	7.46	7.71	0.25	4.66	3.86	0.80
P	13.31	20.58	7.27	7.70	10.00	2.30
Q	*	8.35	*	*	13.60	*
R	7.74	9.09	1.35	9.04	7.54	1.50
S	8.08	10.00	1.92	7.06	12.60	5.54
T	6.07	6.94	0.87	5.48	5.90	0.42
U	9.54	12.28	2.74	6.14	5.38	0.76
V	7.48	7.68	0.20	10.88	12.46	1.58
W	8.17	8.35	0.18	5.56	4.78	0.78
X	9.17	9.11	0.06	9.76	10.00	0.24
Y	5.76	7.55	1.79	7.80	7.54	0.26
Z	7.09	7.65	0.56	3.68	5.54	1.86
1	11.25	9.61	1.64	8.38	9.08	0.70
2	9.16	7.17	1.99	8.48	6.62	1.86
3	*	10.66	*	*	5.64	*
Med.			1.07			1.02

Do some of the data points disturb you? The MRMax of the lab data is 1.07x3.865 = 4.14. Note that physicians H and P's 1994-1995 differences exceed this amount. Obviously this is some type of special cause that requires investigation. However, all the remaining moving ranges are well within common cause. In the subsequent ANOM, one can plot the averages for physicians H and P. However, it may be wise to omit them from the system average since it is not clear exactly what their averages mean.

In like manner, the X-Ray data yield 3.865 x 1.02 = 3.94 as the MRMax, which is exceeded by physicians H and S. Once again, these need to be investigated and will be omitted from the system average in the subsequent ANOM.

Omitting physicians H and P from the Lab data yields a system average of $8.33. Since most physicians have two data points, their averages are calculated and plotted vis-a-vis this average. To calculate the common cause limits for an average of two data points:

The standard deviation is $\frac{1.07}{0.954}$ =1.12.

So, the common cause band is

$$8.33 \pm 3 \times \frac{1.12}{\sqrt{2}} , \text{ or } 5.95 - 10.70 .$$

Note that physicians Q and 3 were new to the department in 1995, so they have only one data point in their calculation, resulting in a wider common cause band. The ANOM chart is shown in Figure 8.22.

Figure 8.22: ANOM of Lab Charges by Physician

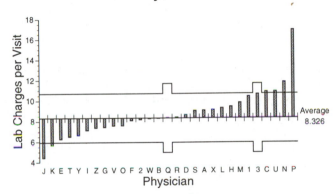

Five physicians fall outside the system. Physicians H and P are plotted but not included in the calculation of the average due to their large MRMax values.

Of the 27 physicians being analyzed, 22 are "in" the system, 2 are "below" the system, and 3 are "above" the system. It appears to be a relatively stable process. Collegial discussion may be useful in finding out if the those above the system have process inputs that justify their figures. Meanwhile, are Physicians J and K underutilizing? If improvement is needed, the lab costs for the physicians in the system can be aggregated. They could then be and "sliced" and "diced" via Pareto analysis to discover the 20% of the tests accounting for 80% of the costs. Discussion should follow as to whether this pattern is appropriate. If you wanted to predict charges for the subsequent year, it may be necessary to obtain quarterly or even monthly data to test the stability assumption prior to projecting the yearly figures.

The X-Ray analysis is shown in Figure 8.23. As with the Lab charges, physicians H and S are plotted, but omitted from the average. The system average is $7.59. From the MMR of 1.02, the standard deviation is 1.07. Thus, the resulting common cause band is

$$7.59 \pm 3 \times \frac{1.07}{\sqrt{2}} , \text{ or } 5.32 - 9.86 .$$

Figure 8.23: ANOM for X-Ray Charges by Physician

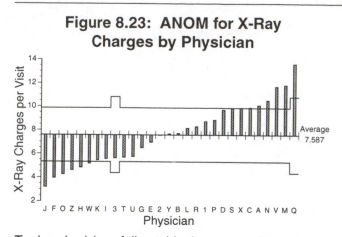

Twelve physicians fall outside the system. Physicians H and S are plotted but not included in the calculation of the average due to their large MRMax values.

Fifteen physicians are "in" the system, 5 are "below" the system, and 7 are "above" the system. Note that there is more variation exhibited in X-Ray behavior than Lab behavior. A discussion similar to that described above for the lab data needs to take place to reduce the inappropriate and unintended variation. Note that one of the new physicians, Physician Q, is one of the "above". If further opportunities for improvement are desired, a separate Pareto analysis for "in," "below," and "above" physicians may be interesting to evaluate where the differences lie and where most of the charges go.

Summary

It is hoped that these examples have demonstrated the enormous versatility of the analysis of means technique, both for percentage data and continuous data. It is amazing how often, through judicious identification of special causes present in systems, an "unpredictable" situation/process/system is suddenly found to be quite predictable. This prediction potential inherent in the use of analytic statistical methods has tremendous implications in terms of:

* budgeting (see the Francis & Gerwels article "Building a Better Budget" in Bibliography)

* forecasting

* measurements of performance relative to goals, and

* subsequent identification of strategies (special cause or common cause) to achieve organizational aims.

Shifting perspective from comparisons of individual units relative to each other allows comparison of these same units relative to the *system* they form and work in. This creates a culture that is truly poised to use the power of "statistical thinking": Only then can the danger of arbitrary numerical goals be fully grasped. Now people can truly work together to understand the organization's current state and plan for a future that will, as Deming has said through his "chain reaction", "create jobs and more jobs."

A Final Word On Tools and Charts

The remainder of the book will now be concerned with synthesizing the material in Chapters 1-8 into an integrated whole. Regarding the tools, techniques, and charts presented in Chapters 6-8, this book is designed for people in the "trenches" who may not have access to a statistician. Nevertheless, they need robust methods that are sound approximations to the statistically accurate ones. Most people do not have the time nor interest to appreciate the subtle differences between I-charts, p-charts, c-charts, u-charts, "X-Bar" charts, R-charts, S-charts, etc. As has been consistently shown in the examples in the text, just plotting one's data over time almost accomplishes 50% of any analysis in and of itself! To quote Ott, when asked about a process for analyzing data: "First, you plot the data. Then, you plot the data. Then, you plot the data. Then, you THINK! Then, you plot the data." In the authors' opinion, very well put!

Lists, grids, and explanations that are intent on "helping" people use the *right* chart in the *right* situation, in the authors' opinion, just cause more confusion and create opportunities to use *more* tools incorrectly. The overall objective is to understand variation! The authors stand behind the "good enough" philosophy of this book and have kept the emphasis on the *thinking* needed to use the analyses correctly. The tools presented in these last two section have tried to "keep it simple" and been designed within a robust context to allow people to go down the correct path in analyzing a situation.

Notes to Chapter Eight

1.   ASQC. *Quality Progress*. March 1996.

2.   Joiner BL. Private communication.

3.   Hacquebord H. Private communication.

4.   Wheeler DJ. *Understanding Variation*.

Chapter Eight Exercises

1. The PTCA Incidence Data

A cardiologist went screaming into a hospital QA director's office because two colleagues were "above average" for the number of incidences in which a patient had to be rushed to the OR during a PTCA procedure. A statistician received a call from the distraught QA director and calmly requested the data. They are presented in the following table:

MD	# Incidences	# PTCA	# Incidences / # PTCAs
1	1	36	.0278
2	4	53	.0755
3	4	79	.0506
4*	2	58	.0345
5	5	110	.0455
Total	16	336	.0476

* Screaming Cardiologist

1a) Use an Analysis of Means via a p-chart to compare the cardiologists' rates. Are the two "above average" culprits truly above average?

1b) Based on the analysis in (a), should a common cause or special cause strategy be used for improvement?

1c) Based on your answer in (b), comment on the current process for improvement:

Each undesirable "incidence" is subjected to a painstaking review. Recommendations are made and implemented.

Does this process sound familiar? Intuitively, this seems like a "common sense" approach to problems of this nature. In this current example, what kind of cause (common or special) does the strategy assume?

In this process's defense, how could one see whether progress was indeed being made using this strategy?

1d) For those who would like a more "rigorous" statistical analysis, instead of using 3 standard deviations as in (a), calculate *three* sets of limits using the following multipliers instead of 3 (taken from Table 8.1):

2.07 (Overall 10% risk), 2.30 (Overall 5% risk), 2.76 (Overall 1% risk)

Did this expose anything we may have missed using the "approximate" nature of 3 standard deviations?

2. The 911 Signing Data

A major medical center was contracted to respond to 911 calls. By law, if a crew arrives on the scene and the person involved refuses treatment, he/she must sign a waiver stating that treatment was refused. High numbers of refused treatments can get rather costly. In reaction to an increase in signings, the medical center instituted a policy that a crew would be fined for every signing that resulted from a dispatch. Apparently, the theory was that the patient's refusal to cooperate resulted from a lack of skill on the part of the crew.

Data were obtained on 40 individual medics as to the total number of calls responded to and the resulting number of signings. They are sorted from smallest to largest percent. For what it's worth, everyone "knew" that Medic #39, who had the highest number of waivers, had poor people skills.

8

Medic	# Waivers Signed	# Patients seen	% Waivers Signed
1	3	41	7.32
2	9	95	9.47
3	2	16	12.50
4	9	71	12.68
5	12	94	12.77
6	26	182	14.29
7	28	187	14.97
8	13	86	15.12
9	28	184	15.22
10	26	170	15.29
11	36	226	15.93
12	11	68	16.18
13	10	58	17.24
14	40	226	17.70
15	28	154	18.18
16	41	224	18.30
17	35	186	18.82
18	7	37	18.92
19	29	153	18.95
20	15	79	18.99
21	11	57	19.30
22	23	118	19.49
23	39	195	20.00
24	4	20	20.00
25	35	173	20.23
26	14	67	20.90
27	14	67	20.90
28	31	142	21.83
29	40	175	22.86
30	40	173	23.12
31	16	66	24.24
32	24	94	25.53
33	33	129	25.58
34	42	164	25.61
35	26	101	25.74
36	39	150	26.00
37	39	149	26.17
38	35	120	29.17
39	42	139	30.22
40	17	56	30.36

2a) Construct a p-chart and do an analysis of means for this data. Feel free to either use a three standard deviation band or 3.18 for a formal 5% risk or even 3.62 for a 1% risk. What do you notice? What should be done about Medic 39?

2b) Is the fining policy a common cause or special cause strategy? From your analysis, is the problem the process or the people?

2c) Is there a low aggressive data strategy that might help to further localize a significant opportunity in this process? How would one know if it worked?

2d) If there is any fining to do, who should *really* be fined?

3. The C-Section Data

For the C-Section data shown in your text, data were collected on the 15 individual physicians who practiced at the hospital. It is shown in the following table:

MD	C-Sections	Deliveries	% C-Sections
1	32	196	16.33
2	59	353	16.71
3	38	309	12.30
4	63	350	18.00
5	41	356	11.52
6	55	309	17.80
7	32	229	13.97
8	34	233	14.59
9	59	356	16.57
10	32	337	9.50
11	30	317	9.46
12	68	350	19.43
13	47	288	16.32
14	70	370	18.92
15	33	215	15.35
Total	693	4568	15.17%

3a) What type of analysis might expose a hidden special cause in the process?

Before you do any analysis, what do you need to know about how the data were collected?

3b) Perform an analysis of means by physician. You can take the approximate route and use 3 standard deviations. Or, you can be more rigorous and use 2.61, 2.83, and/or 3.29 standard deviations (10%, 5%, and 1% risks, respectively).

Is there any hidden opportunity?

3c) The data were presented in blinded fashion to these doctors. For the subsequent seven months, the aggregated C-section rates were 13.53%, 10.85%, 14.5%, 13.12%, 10.94%, 13.85%, and 12.31%. Does this represent improvement? Can you prove it statistically?

3d) Before the data presentation, the system was stable at 15.17% and had 693 c-sections out of 4568 births (aggregation of 2/91-12/93 data). The seven follow-up months seem stable and had 237 c-sections out of 1861 births (aggregation of 1/94-7/94 data). Use analysis of means to test whether the difference is significant.

4. The Dictation Data

The transcription department was trying to get a handle on dictation load from a particular department. She collected a data point every two weeks for approximately two months summarizing each MD's performance as well as the department's performance. She was curious about possible differences between the MDs regarding dictation "style" and chose to look at the average number of lines per dictated report. The data are given below:

Time	MD 1	MD 2	MD 3	MD 4	MD 5	MD 6	MD 7	MD 8
1	32.7	39.2	35.0	37.0	30.7	33.0	32.8	31.7
2	31.7	31.7	18.3	26.4	37.5	23.7	37.9	24.8
3	31.5	37.2	33.1	31.7	38.2	24.3	38.1	34.8
4	43.5	32.5	33.6	24.3	34.1	33.7	32.7	32.6
5	27.2	27.0	35.6	32.6	31.3	20.8	31.3	31.9
6	27.4	36.8	31.7	31.5	32.1	30.0	37.3	28.0
7	35.0	23.3	25.8	33.7	32.3	31.3	37.7	22.9

Summary numbers from the department are:

Time	Total Lines	Total Reports
1	5,098	178
2	3,802	136
3	3,734	121
4	6,046	183
5	6,962	254
6	5,592	178
7	4,487	146
Total	35,721	1,196

4a) Find the median moving range for each MD and combine them to find the median moving range for ALL MDs. Using the (3.865 x MMR) criterion, are there any suspicious data points?

4b) Sketch a control chart for each MD to further check for outliers.

4c) Find the average of each MD's stable process as well as the overall average of the "system." Use analysis of means to calculate the common cause variation for each MD around this system average. Plot each individual MD's result and determine whether each in "in" the system, "above" the system, or "below" the system.

4d) Based on the analysis, is there any hidden opportunity for improvement among the MDs?

4e) What can this department predict, based on this data, for a workload in terms of number of reports for any two-week period? Total lines of transcription?

4f) After assessing the stability of this system, do they have the luxury of reasonably predicting the budget for this department for the entire year? How would they know whether or when to adjust the budget? Where would 90-98% of the workloads for a typical two-week period for this department fall?

8

5. The ER Lytic Data

An ER supervisor was receiving vague anecdotal comments about problems with the process of mixing thrombolytic drugs. He decided to study the process by which patients with a suspected heart attack obtained these crucial drugs. The supervisor collected data on the next 55 patients treated for such a condition (i.e., studied the current process). He recorded the number of minutes it took from the time the patient came through the door until the patient received the drug. These times are given below and are sorted in the order in which the patients were treated. This supervisor had some potential theories in mind regarding the variation in the process. Thus, he recorded which shift was on duty. He listed these as: Shift = 1 (7 AM-3 PM) or Shift = 2 (any other time, i.e., 3 PM-7 AM. He also thought that it was important to know how many RNs were on duty at the time. These additional pieces of information will be considered later in the analysis.

Order	Time	Shift	RN	Order	Time	Shift	RN
1	9	1	2	30	40	1	2
2	20	2	2	31	50	1	2
3	20	1	3	32	30	2	2
4	20	1	2	33	58	1	2
5	37	2	2	34	43	2	2
6	55	1	2	35	20	1	2
7	37	2	2	36	18	2	2
8	20	2	2	37	28	2	2
9	37	2	1	38	16	1	2
10	29	2	2	39	20	1	2
11	33	2	2	40	58	2	2
12	33	2	2	41	32	2	2
13	6	2	2	42	16	2	2
14	100	2	2	43	35	1	2
15	98	1	2	44	40	2	2
16	20	2	2	45	16	1	2
17	73	1	2	46	16	1	2
18	14	2	2	47	18	1	2
19	50	1	1	48	22	2	1
20	25	1	2	49	22	1	2
21	40	1	2	50	55	1	2
22	120	1	2	51	31	1	1
23	18	2	2	52	20	2	2
24	44	2	2	53	15	2	2
25	24	1	1	54	21	2	2
26	10	1	2	55	55	1	1
27	106	2	2				
28	22	1	2				
29	15	2	3				

5a) Do a run chart for these times. Do they seem to represent a stable process?

5b) Do a control chart for these data. How many outliers, if any, do you find? What is the time for the "average" patient (Does the "average" patient even exist?)? A better question is,

What is the range of times experienced by 90-98% of the patients? If "everything that could possibly go wrong" went wrong, how long would it take for a patient to receive the thrombolytic drug? Is this kind of variation acceptable?

5c) Is a common cause or a special cause strategy going to be more useful to improve this process?

5d) The supervisor had a theory that the times on the 7AM-3 PM shift would be shorter. If you feel that it is appropriate, test this theory using the common cause strategy of stratification via a stratified histogram. In other words, do a histogram of the data for Shift 1 data and compare it with a histogram for the data for Shift 2. Be sure to use the same scale. What do you notice?

5e) Can you confirm the results in (d) via analysis of means? What about this theory—do they seem to be different?

5f) The supervisor also had a theory that if more RNs were on duty, the times would be shorter. What plot might help to test that theory? Do a scatter plot of Time vs. #RNs on duty (Should outliers be included or not?). Is there a strong relationship?

5g) Is it necessary to go to the next level of data "aggressiveness", (cutting new windows), or can you think of some other way to study the current process?

6. The DRG Analysis of Means Data (Part 1)

A medical center was given feedback about their performance for a specific DRG regarding lengths of stay (LOS) and total charges. They were told to "do something about it."

They were able to obtain the LOS and total charges for every patient over the last year with that DRG (78 cases). The data are on the following pages in patient admit order, i.e., its "naturally" occurring time order. The moving ranges are also shown. A summary appears at the end. It includes the numbers you need to do a meaningful statistical analysis: median LOS, median Total charges, average LOS, average Total charges, and both median moving ranges.

6a) The run charts are also shown. Do a runs analysis. Do there seem to be any apparent special causes? Has the process improved? Is it any worse? Has it been stable?

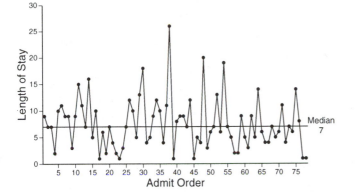

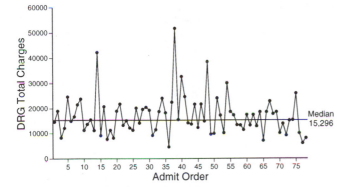

6d) Would there be a way to look at in-house data or to study the current process to localize an opportunity? What kind of a strategy is this? In other words, could "slicing" and "dicing" the data be useful? Any suggestions on how to "slice" and "dice"?

6b) Based on your runs analysis, construct the appropriate control chart. What is the range for the typical LOS (90-98% of the time) for this DRG? Total charges?

For each response, what constitutes a "train wreck"? Are there any?

6c) If one wanted to improve this process, is a common cause or special cause approach necessary?

What if the insurers got "tough" and demanded a special report for any case either having a length of stay greater than 15 days or charges greater than $20000? Would this improve anything? This would be treating what kind of cause (common or special?) as what kind of cause (common or special?)?

How have organizations you are familiar with, including your own, handled similar situations?

Admit Order	LOS	Charges	LOS MR	Charges MR	Admit Order	LOS	Charges	LOS MR	Charges MR
1	9	14736			41	9	24744	1	7956
2	7	19062	2	4326	42	9	14289	0	10455
3	7	8351	0	10711	43	7	13738	2	551
4	2	12207	5	3856	44	12	21684	5	7946
5	10	24756	8	12549	45	1	12390	11	9294
6	11	14991	1	9765	46	5	21765	4	9375
7	9	16791	2	1800	47	4	14961	1	6804
8	9	21589	0	4798	48	20	38654	16	23693
9	3	23842	6	2253	49	3	9641	17	29013
10	9	11330	6	12512	50	6	9971	3	330
11	15	13755	6	2425	51	7	24163	1	14192
12	11	15505	4	1750	52	13	17259	6	6904
13	7	11242	4	4263	53	6	10239	7	7020
14	16	42333	9	31091	54	19	30171	13	19932
15	5	9219	11	33114	55	7	18746	12	11425
16	10	20802	5	11583	56	5	17364	2	1382
17	1	7765	9	13037	57	2	13423	3	3941
18	6	11332	5	3567	58	2	13312	0	111
19	2	8238	4	3094	59	9	11441	7	1871
20	7	18973	5	10735	60	5	17562	4	6121
21	4	21845	3	2872	61	3	13234	2	4328
22	2	13310	2	8535	62	9	17556	6	4322
23	1	15150	1	1840	63	5	12949	4	4607
24	3	12227	2	2923	64	14	18632	9	5683
25	7	11299	4	928	65	6	7170	8	11462
26	12	20172	5	8873	66	4	18617	2	11447
27	10	14230	2	5942	67	4	22868	0	4251
28	5	19697	5	5467	68	7	17846	3	5022
29	13	20519	8	822	69	5	18606	2	760
30	18	19287	5	1232	70	6	10174	1	8432
31	4	9244	14	10043	71	11	13957	5	3783
32	5	11513	1	2269	72	4	9244	7	4713
33	9	18809	4	7296	73	7	15199	3	5955
34	12	24100	3	5291	74	6	15393	1	194
35	10	18299	2	5801	75	14	26043	8	10650
36	4	4691	6	13608	76	8	10117	6	15926
37	11	22511	7	17820	77	1	6109	7	4008
38	26	51830	15	29319	78	1	8174	0	2065
39	1	15594	25	36236	Median	7	$15,296	4	$5942
40	8	32700	7	17106	Average	7.5	$16,939		

7. The DRG Analysis of Means Data (Part 2)

As it turns out, it was quite easy to identify the primary physician involved in the treatment of each case. The next page shows another arrangement of the data. Since the data seem to be from a common cause process, it has been rearranged to be traceable to the physician (input) who oversaw the case. Seventeen physicians had multiple admissions for this DRG. The cases for a particular physician are arranged in their admit date time order. The "train wrecks" identified in Part 1 have been omitted since they represent cases atypical of the process and do not necessarily represent the doctor's usual practice style. They are shown as empty cells.

Since there may be variation among the doctors, a better estimate of the common cause would be desired. To obtain this, one would take the moving range between cases for a particular physician. Then, one could find the overall median moving range when all the physician data estimates are combined (doctors with only one case do not yield a moving range).

You are given the overall averages for both LOS and total charges. You are also given the median moving ranges from which to calculate the standard deviation to be used in your analysis of means. You will probably get a smaller estimate of the standard deviation than your original control chart analysis. This is because the doctor-to-doctor factor has been "removed." In theory, this actually gives you a more discriminating "yardstick."

7a) Calculate the common cause band for each physician (use 3 standard deviations), given the number of cases he or she oversaw. You will need to do this for N=1,2,3,4,5,6,7. (The table on page 189 lists the number of cases by physician.)

7b) Plot each physician's average and draw in the centerline of the overall average. This is also the average taken from your control charts for Part 1—ANOM is "slicing" and "dicing" that average!

Draw the common cause band around the center line. Judge whether each physician is "in" the system, "above" the system, or "below" the system. Have we found any "bad apples"? Did we find any potential opportunity?

7c) Should we use a common cause or special strategy for further analysis of the data? What might you suggest as another "slicing" and "dicing" strategy? Might a Pareto analysis of some sort identify how 20% of the process could address 80% of a potential opportunity?

MD	LOS	Charges	LOS MR	Charges MR
1	11	14991		
1	4	9244	7	5747

MD	LOS	Charges	LOS MR	Charges MR
2	9	11330		
2	7	24163	2	12833

MD	LOS	Charges	LOS MR	Charges MR
3	10	24756		
3	3	23842	7	914
3	6	9971	3	13871
3	1	6109	5	3862

MD	LOS	Charges	LOS MR	Charges MR
4	4	14961	3	
4				
4	7	18746		
4	5	17364	2	1382

MD	LOS	Charges	LOS MR	Charges MR
5	2	8238		
5	5	19697	3	11459
5	10	18299	5	1398
5	1	12390	9	5909
5	5	17562	4	5172
5	5	18606	0	1044

MD	LOS	Charges	LOS MR	Charges MR
6	1	7765		
6	1	15150	0	7385
6	1	15594	0	444
6	2	13312	1	2282
6	3	13234	1	78
6	4	18617	1	5383

MD	LOS	Charges	LOS MR	Charges MR
7	15	13755		
7	8	32700	7	18945

MD	LOS	Charges	LOS MR	Charges MR
8	2	12207		
8	2	13310	0	1103
8	12	24100	10	10790
8	9	24744	3	644

MD	LOS	Charges	LOS MR	Charges MR
9	7	11299		
9	5	11513	2	214
9	6	10239	1	1274
9	9	11441	3	1202
9	9	17556	0	6115

MD	LOS	Charges	LOS MR	Charges MR
10	9	14736		
10	9	16791	0	2055
10	16		7	
10	13	20519	3	
10	9	14289	4	6230
10	6	10174	3	4115

MD	LOS	Charges	LOS MR	Charges MR
11	11	13957		
11	7	15199	4	1242

MD	LOS	Charges	LOS MR	Charges MR
12	7	19062		
12	11	15505	4	3557
12	10	20802	1	5297
12	4	21845	6	1043
12	3	12227	1	9618
12	5	21765	2	9538
12	6	7170	1	14595

MD	LOS	Charges	LOS MR	Charges MR
13	9	21589		
13	4	9244	5	12345
13	4	4691	0	4553
13				
13	6	15393		
13	8	10117	2	5276

MD	LOS	Charges	LOS MR	Charges MR
14	7	8351		
14	12	20172	5	11821

MD	LOS	Charges	LOS MR	Charges MR
15	5	9219		
15	12	21684	7	12465
15	3	9641	9	12043
15		30170		20529
15	2	13423		16747

MD	LOS	Charges	LOS MR	Charges MR
16	10	14230		
16	14	18632	4	4402

MD	LOS	Charges	LOS MR	Charges MR
17	7	11242		
17	13	17259	6	6017
17	4	22868	9	5609
17	14	26043	10	3175

MD	LOS	Charges	LOS MR	Charges MR
18	7	17846		

MD	LOS	Charges	LOS MR	Charges MR
19	1	8174		

MD	LOS	Charges	LOS MR	Charges MR
20	6	11332		

MD	LOS	Charges	LOS MR	Charges MR
21	11	22511		

MD	LOS	Charges	LOS MR	Charges MR
22	7	18973		

MD	LOS	Charges	LOS MR	Charges MR
23	18	19287		

MD	LOS	Charges	LOS MR	Charges MR
24	5	12949		

MD	LOS	Charges	LOS MR	Charges MR
25	9	18809		

MD	LOS	Charges	LOS MR	Charges MR
26	7	13738		

Average of all cases' LOS = 7.0
MMR of LOS = 3

Average of all cases' charges = $15,846
MMR of charges = $5,286.5

MD	Ave. LOS	Ave. Charges	N LOS	N Charges
1	7.5	12117.5	2	2
2	8.0	17746.5	2	2
3	5.0	16169.5	4	4
4	5.3	17023.7	3	3
5	4.6	15798.7	6	6
6	2.0	13945.3	6	6
7	11.5	23227.5	2	2
8	6.2	18590.3	4	4
9	7.2	12409.6	5	5
10	10.3	15301.8	6	5
11	9.0	14578.0	2	2
12	6.5	16910.9	7	7
13	6.2	12206.8	5	5
14	9.5	14261.5	2	2
15	5.5	16827.4	4	5
16	12.0	16431.0	2	2
17	9.5	19353.0	4	4
18	7.0	17846.0	1	1
19	1.0	8174.0	1	1
20	6.0	11332.0	1	1
21	11.0	22511.0	1	1
22	7.0	18973.0	1	1
23	18.0	19287.0	1	1
24	5.0	12949.0	1	1
25	9.0	18809.0	1	1
26	7.0	13738.0	1	1

8

Chapter Nine
Data Skills as a Conduit for Transformation

A New Perspective on Teams, Tools and Data Skills

Before moving on to the realities of training and the case studies, a summary of the ideas presented so far is in order. It is a human tendency to immediately "dive in" to quality improvement. Organizations often attempt to improve simply through "benchmarking," the art of studying current best processes in your industry, and trying to copy examples of successful organizations. Unfortunately this will merely doom you to failure. One cannot even begin to benchmark without knowing what questions to ask the benchmarked organization. It is not as simple as observing someone, being "impressed," and declaring that "We're going to do that, too." *How* are you going to do it? Your organization has its own unique culture. Mere copying will cause the aforementioned "random walk," Brownian motion effect of Chapter 2, and much resulting organizational frustration. More damage than improvement will result. Understand the basic theory of QI and have a plan. Do not underestimate either the possible effects on the psychology of your culture or the unexpected negative backlash.

The reality of designating continuous quality improvement as an organizational goal by itself is necessary, but not sufficient for improvement. This has the effect of causing QI to be perceived as pulling energy away from normal daily tasks which already take up over 100% of everyone's time. The issue is not QI, but **transformation**. Whereas QI can become an energy drain, transformation pulls the energy inward to create an organizational **synergy**. Teams are a necessary part of it, but there are things an organization must do in parallel with the teams' efforts to complement them and create the aforementioned synergy.

It is hoped that the previous chapters as well as the suggested references will help build education as to the *theory* behind quality improvement. The process, variation, and data concepts also allow one to get started immediately without making a typical mistake: creation of too many formal project teams working on issues insignificant to the organization's business strategy and future survival.

The theory is needed by *everyone* in the culture. It helps to create unified work teams with a common language and sense of purpose. These teams can then recognize all work as a measurable process with both internal and external suppliers and customers. This knowledge must become routinely used by front-line teams to be truly effective. An efficient use of data, awareness of variation, and proper reaction to both creates a strong foundation in which project teams are *implicit* in daily work.

Blaming processes instead of people will increase morale and reduce fear. Dysfunctional behavior related to confrontation and blame of lower level workers can be minimized when organizational management sets expectations of *zero* tolerance for this. People will finally be able to recognize that what they previously perceived to be individual, unique problems (special causes of variation) were really the same few problems over and over again in various guises (common causes).

Routine process thinking exposes the true, *hidden* opportunities in the *lack* of daily processes as well as existing hidden time and data "inventories." Part of the hidden opportunity for management is the realization that *special causes* of variation (i.e., "problems") at a *local level* may actually be symptoms of *common causes* of variation at a much *higher level*. Examples of those higher levels include organizational purchasing, technical training, communication skills training, maintenance, promotion, and hiring processes.

Once again, the issue is transformation, not merely improvement. Transforming current managerial behavior through these skills will cause profound improvement of an organization and its culture. However, once the organization is aligned, additional issues and questions (beyond the scope of this book) remain. Consider: Will mere improvement keep you in business five to ten years from now? What processes will help the organization face and deal with unexpected changes in the outside culture? What processes will help you innovate? Do these processes formally exist today? (See the books by Deming, Neave, and Rummler-Brache.)

9

Revisiting Projects and Project Teams

Transitioning to implicit QI work teams can be awkward. Many problems in the transition relate to:

- understanding a situation as an isolated incident rather than a process

- solving "world hunger" problems—inadequate problem definition

- implementing "known" solutions with neither a pilot nor data collection to assess (and hold) the gains

- overuse and improper use of tools

- premature and poorly designed data collection

- lack of consideration of data collection as a process.

These are universal, common problems.

It is also a common error to begin with too many projects working on obvious superficial problems. Once again, beware: The problems that march into your office are not important; the important problems are the ones of which no one is aware.

Obvious problems are usually symptomatic of a much deeper complexity which, if not addressed, will end up even more complex. Knee-jerk reaction usually results in an **additional** layer of complexity which temporarily alleviates the superficial symptom, but causes problems elsewhere.

There are two kinds of projects. The first and most important are those related to the organization's key strategic issues. The team members and facilitators should be mostly top management. Key informal culture leaders must also be involved. These projects can become quite lengthy because they get to the deep root causes of problems which have been merely patched up in the past. In the initial phase of quality improvement, these should be few, high level, and limited in scope.

The other kind of project is what is known as a "task team." These are very limited in scope and are used to get the work force working as a team both within and between departments. In essence, they are pilot projects for learning and testing quality improvement skills while working on significant departmental daily operational problems. They should last no more than two or three months each. An excellent example of a task team is found in the Keene Clinic case study.

To summarize, projects are necessary, but not sufficient. Initially, keep them few and limited. Top management must form a team on a key strategic issue. The work force learns statistical thinking and improvement by improving their daily work through the use of task teams lasting no more than two to three months each.

A comparison of a typical QI approach with that of transformation is contrasted in Table 9.1.

Table 9.1: QI vs. Transformation

QI	Transformation
"One shot" skills training via courses	Routine, continuous education through daily work
(Many) teams of "key" personnel (Focused on daily operational issues)	(Few) top management-led teams (Focused on key strategic issues)
Heavy emphasis on tools	Entire work culture educated in QI theory
(3-15% of opportunity) (Obvious, current problems) 　　Formal problem identification 　　Problem solving tools 　　Management guidance teams 　　Formal team reviews 　　Storyboards 　　QI coordinator and structure	(85-97% of opportunity) (Hidden problems) 　　Appreciation of systems 　　Psychology 　　Variation 　　Use of data to test improvement theories 　　Continuous establishment and documentation of 　　routine processes important to customers
Team facilitators	Change agents
Numerical goals	Understanding variation, Process capability
Management behavior 　　Manage status quo 　　Solve problems 　　Reactive response to variation 　　　　(Treat as unique, special causes) 　　Choose projects, review progress 　　Send people to "courses"	Management behavior 　　Understand/improve processes 　　Facilitates problem-solving 　　Proactive response to variation 　　　　(Asks: common or special cause?) 　　Exhibit QI skills through behavior 　　Teach QI through routine daily work and meetings
Quality "certain percent" of the job and explicit	Quality 100% of the job and implicit

9

Figure 9.1, "The Fundamentals of Variation," represents the basic tenets of process-oriented thinking put into a data framework. They are the principles which the authors have found to be required of everyone in a transforming organization. As deceptively simple as they seem, it takes years to make them a "routine" part of one's organizational culture. Yet, the productive power they will unleash in an organization is enormous.

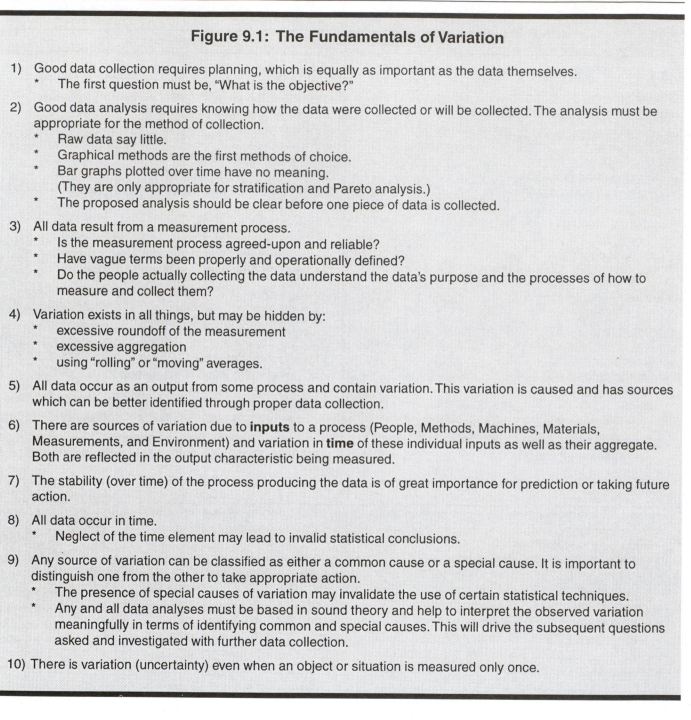

Figure 9.1: The Fundamentals of Variation

1) Good data collection requires planning, which is equally as important as the data themselves.
   * The first question must be, "What is the objective?"

2) Good data analysis requires knowing how the data were collected or will be collected. The analysis must be appropriate for the method of collection.
   * Raw data say little.
   * Graphical methods are the first methods of choice.
   * Bar graphs plotted over time have no meaning.
     (They are only appropriate for stratification and Pareto analysis.)
   * The proposed analysis should be clear before one piece of data is collected.

3) All data result from a measurement process.
   * Is the measurement process agreed-upon and reliable?
   * Have vague terms been properly and operationally defined?
   * Do the people actually collecting the data understand the data's purpose and the processes of how to measure and collect them?

4) Variation exists in all things, but may be hidden by:
   * excessive roundoff of the measurement
   * excessive aggregation
   * using "rolling" or "moving" averages.

5) All data occur as an output from some process and contain variation. This variation is caused and has sources which can be better identified through proper data collection.

6) There are sources of variation due to **inputs** to a process (People, Methods, Machines, Materials, Measurements, and Environment) and variation in **time** of these individual inputs as well as their aggregate. Both are reflected in the output characteristic being measured.

7) The stability (over time) of the process producing the data is of great importance for prediction or taking future action.

8) All data occur in time.
   * Neglect of the time element may lead to invalid statistical conclusions.

9) Any source of variation can be classified as either a common cause or a special cause. It is important to distinguish one from the other to take appropriate action.
   * The presence of special causes of variation may invalidate the use of certain statistical techniques.
   * Any and all data analyses must be based in sound theory and help to interpret the observed variation meaningfully in terms of identifying common and special causes. This will drive the subsequent questions asked and investigated with further data collection.

10) There is variation (uncertainty) even when an object or situation is measured only once.

In integrating these tenets into an organization, several "sacred cows" of data management will be challenged. In addition, inevitable errors will be inherent in a new, initially counter-intuitive method of thinking. This is all part of the learning process.

Organizations tend to exhibit wide gaps in knowledge regarding the proper use, display and collection of data. These result in a natural tendency to either react to anecdotal data or "tamper" due to the current data systems in place. Figure 9.2 summarizes the most common errors in data use, display and collection. It is by no means an exhaustive list, but early recognition may help to keep an organization's efforts on track.

Figure 9.2: Eight Common Statistical "Traps"

Trap 1: *Treating **all** observed variation in a time series data sequence as special cause*
- The most common form of "tampering"—treating common cause as special cause.

  * Frequently seen in traditional monthly reports: month-to-month comparisons; year-over-year plotting and comparisons; variance reporting; comparisons to arbitrary numerical goals.

Trap 2: *Fitting inappropriate "trend" lines to a time series data sequence*
- Another form of "tampering"—attributing a specific type of special cause (linear trend) to a set of data which:
  - contains only common cause.
  - contains a different kind of special cause, usually, a "step" change(s) in the process average.

  * Risk or severity adjustments of data through linear regression is a subtle manifestation of this trap.

Trap 3: *Unnecessary obsession with and incorrect application of the normal distribution*
- Ignoring the time element in a data set and inappropriately applying enumerative techniques based on the normal distribution

  * This can cause misleading estimates and inappropriate predictions of process outputs (aggregated averages, standard deviations, Year-to-Date summaries). This is a case of "reverse" tampering—treating special cause as if it is common cause. **A data summary should not mislead the user into taking any action that the user would not take if the data were presented in a time series**.

- Inappropriate routine testing of all data sets for normality.
- Misapplying normal distribution theory and enumerative calculations to binomial data (percentages based on ratios of occurrences of individual events relative to the number of possible opportunities) or Poisson distributed data (counts of events where the number of possibilities of occurrence are infinite).

Trap 4: *Incorrect calculation of standard deviation and "sigma" limits*
- Grossly overestimating (inflating) the true standard deviation by using the "traditional" calculation.

  * Because of this inflation, people tend to arbitrarily change decision limits to two (or even one!) standard deviations from the average or "standard." The *three* standard deviation criterion with the *correctly* calculated value of sigma gives an *overall* statistical error risk of approximately 0.05.
  * The two best estimates of standard deviation for a given situation are obtained from the time sequence of the data:
    The **Median** Moving Range divided by 0.954, which is *robust to outliers; or
    The **Average** Moving Range divided by 1.128, which is typically taught in control chart texts.
    (This estimate can be influenced by outlying observations and process shifts, but not to the extent of the "traditional" calculation.
    (If there are no special causes in the process, these two estimates, as well as the "traditional" calculation, will yield approximately the same number.)

Trap 5: *Choosing **arbitrary** cutoffs for "above" average and "below" average*
- Ignoring the "dead band" of common cause variation on either side of an average

  * The dead band is determined directly from the data. As a result, approximately half of a set of numbers will naturally be above (or below) average. The potential for tampering appears again—treating common cause as special cause.
  * Incorrect calculation of the standard deviation can inflate the estimate of the common cause variation, and artificially widen the dead band.

* "Robust to outliers" means the analysis is largely unaffected by outliers.

Trap 6:   *Misreading special cause signals on a control chart*
   • Only searching for the special cause at the time period when the control chart gave an out-of-control signal

      *   Just because an observation is outside the calculated three standard deviation limits does not guarantee that the special cause occurred at then. It is extremely useful to do a **runs analysis before** construction of any control chart.

Trap 7:   *Attempting to improve processes through the use of arbitrary numerical goals*
   • Ignoring the natural, inherent capability of the process

      *   Any process output has a within a common cause range. It can perform only at the level at which its inputs will allow it to perform. Whether they are necessary for survival or arbitrary, goals are merely wishes. Data must be collected to assess a process's natural performance relative to a goal.
      *   The most prevalent form of tampering is interpreting common cause over time as special cause, either in a positive or negative sense, for individual deviations of process performance from the goal (Trap 1).
      *   The other prevalent form of tampering results from failure to recognize the dead band of common cause around an average in a data summary (Trap 5). This leads to individual performances judged relative to being above or below an arbitrary goal as opposed to being "inside" or "outside" the process, particularly if the goal falls inside the dead band. This method has no recognition or assessment of capability, and people inside the system (common cause) can be arbitrarily and incorrectly identified as special causes, once again either in a positive or negative sense.

Trap 8:   *Using statistical techniques on a time sequence of "rolling" or "moving" averages*
   • Another, hidden form of "tampering"—attributing special cause to a set of data which could contain only common cause.

      *   The "rolling" average technique can create the appearance of special cause even when the individual data elements exhibit only common cause.

A Change in Managerial Perspective and Behavior

The data skills and customer focus of continuous improvement also have profound implications on the psychology of the work culture. A helpless, powerless feeling among most employees can result from the natural tendencies to:

• blame people

• use arbitrary goals

• judge performance in a system where the odds are at least 85 to 15 against the employee

• work around poorly designed processes

• use "smile or else!" approaches to handle angry customers who are also victims of the same processes

• ignore the reality and presence of demotivators

Dean Spitzer notes, "Too many managers underestimate the importance of what they consider minor irritations, not realizing how large these irritations loom in the subjective experience of the employees. To employees stuck in the middle, these demotivators are not minor at all."[1] Employees are suspicious of empowerment and change because, in their minds, "Here comes another one! Nothing is really going to change. It will just lead to results which don't work, and we'll get blamed... again. It takes enough energy just to get through the day. My job already takes up over 100 percent of my time!"

"Why not let managers and supervisors handle things? They get paid to get blamed...It's part of their job...Let them fix it!" Yes, but in actuality who *truly* has the capability to understand the work and processes as they *really* occur?

For transformation to take root in a culture, all levels of management, supervision, and informal culture leaders should initially become proficient in the skills listed in Figure 9.3 and exhibit their behaviors:

Figure 9.3: Management Behaviors Required for Improvement and Transformation

1) Resist the tendency to treat every problem that walks into one's office as a "special cause" and immediately "solve" it. Facilitate the employees who work in the situation to understand the sources of variation and address root causes. React with *questions*, not necessarily action.

2) Facilitate the conversion of anecdotes about perceived problems into data; design a data collection on work in progress or a **flowchart** to document the process (or lack of a process) within which the anecdote is occurring. Good data (which includes flowcharts to reduce *human* variation) are helpful in stripping the emotion out of a situation and getting a helpful pre-existing measure of the problem's extent.

3) Using various flowcharts (top-down, detailed, deployment, work area) to better understand and improve their own departmental work processes and customer relationships.

4) Take a good, hard assessment of current data collections and reports. Question the objective of each: how it is collected and measured, and whether it adds any value to the organization—(Is it answering the question that it **really** needs to answer?)

5) Avoid overuse of written surveys. There is a tendency to make written surveys amorphous in objectives and overload them with "excess baggage". Instead, substitute routine **talking** to customers, both internal and external, through focus groups and help **clarify perceptions** of troublesome situations. When necessary, this will **focus** the objectives of any subsequent data collection and result in simple, efficient surveys which can be meaningfully analyzed.

6) Do not react to numbers alone, whether presented in tables or individually. Instead, use **graphical displays** (run charts, control charts, analyses of means) to understand and react appropriately to variation. *Insist* that data reports be presented in a similar format.

7) Understand that human resistance to change is natural and will require extreme patience. Have the maturity not to personalize resistance behaviors exhibited by the culture.

8) Exhibit mature behavior in addressing dysfunctional situations of blame. Set the expectation of zero tolerance for such behavior in the future. Routinely blame the process instead of the people.

9) Put quality on a par with finance. Every meeting should include either: videotape, education item, discussion of current data reports & displays, or understanding a departmental process and customer relationships through the use of quality tools.

10) Equip the work culture in crucial non-technical skills such as active listening, conflict resolution, social behavior styles, efficient meeting management.

Routine use of these skills while simultaneously demonstrating their use to the culture creates an atmosphere where transformation has a chance to flourish and succeed. The fact that these are tangible skills to be immediately applied will accelerate comprehension of their subtleties. People must obtain core competency skills to become:

- process-oriented in evaluating a situation

- chart-oriented in displaying and analyzing data and

- non-tampering in response to variation.

A Quick Word About Meetings

Product inventory is a significant hidden cost of waste in manufacturing. A service industry like medicine has its equivalent in time inventories. Poorly run, inefficient meetings are some of the most costly sources of organizational waste. It would be interesting to plot the aggregated number of meetings for an organization. In addition, if one could somehow operationally define a "worthwhile" meeting and have participants agree on a process to classify each meeting as "worthwhile" or "not worthwhile," what would the plot of "percent worthwhile meetings" look like?

Do not underestimate meetings as a source of waste! To quote a sign the authors once saw: "We will continue to have these meetings until we find out why no work is getting done!"

To paraphrase Brian Joiner's comment from Chapter 2, "Vague meetings with vague objectives yield vague results." Has one ever thought of what effect a standardized, operationally defined meeting process would have on an organization? Talk about reducing variation!

There are many good sources on effective meetings. *The TEAM Handbook* is one. Jana Kemp's organization, Meeting and Management Essentials, is devoted strictly to meetings and meeting management. From the authors' experience, several common themes emerge about effective meetings:

1) Every meeting should have a focused, central *objective* around which it is planned.

2) Only personnel relevant to the objective should attend.

3) A *detailed* agenda based on the objective with *times* assigned to individual items should be sent out ahead of time and *reviewed* at the start of a meeting.

4) One member should be formally assigned the role of "facilitator." This role rotates. The facilitator has formal permission to keep track of time, short circuit "tangents," maturely control dysfunctional dynamics, encourage participation, and help the group accomplish its objective. The facilitator does not actively participate in agenda item discussions, and is totally focused on the meeting process.

5) Typically, many conclusions reached in meetings are individually *implied* from discussion. This leads to little effective action. The facilitator needs to make sure that any conclusions are stated *explicitly* in complete sentences agreed upon by all participants.

6) The agenda for any follow-up meeting is "roughed out."

7) Every meeting is evaluated in terms of what went well, what could have gone better, and an explicit improvement for the next meeting.

An example of an effective meeting agenda and summary is found in the coding project examples in Chapter 11. Several useful references are provided in the Bibliography.

Summary

Returning to literal data skills, Figure 9.4 is a bullet summary, expressed in terms of skills. These skills should become routine in any organization.

A more macro perspective of the ideas discussed in this chapter is summarized in a deployment flowchart developed by David Wessner of HealthSystem Minnesota using Rummler-Brache methodology.[2]

Figure 9.4: Summary of Skills to Be Routine in All Organizations

Understand Your Process
- Convert anecdotes
- Understand internal and external customer relationships and their true needs; interconnectedness of processes
- React with questions, not necessarily action
- Flowchart
- Always consider six problems with a process (Figure 3.5)
- Plot data/obtain baseline

Ensure Data Quality
- Eliminate wasteful data (no objectives (PARC), vaguely defined process outputs)
- Avoid unnecessary, vague, written surveys
- Convert anecdotes (define and tabulate occurrences)
- Conduct **simple, efficient** collections at the appropriate level of "aggressiveness"
- Remember the data collection process itself is not trivial (Figure 6.3)
- Use data as a basis for **action**

Localize Problems
- Operationally define "fuzzy" outputs
- Stratify by process input to expose special causes

Assess / Hold Gains
- Use run charts and control charts

Plot "Hot" Numbers, i.e, the Numbers That Make You "Sweat"
- Remember "tampering" losses are incalculable

"When you don't know, you don't know!"
- Ask questions!
- Allow observed variation to drive questions asked

Beware of Arbitrary Numerical Goals
- Ask, "Is the process **capable** of achieving that goal?"

Notes to Chapter Nine

1.   Spitzer DM. *SuperMotivation: A Blueprint for Energizing Your Organization from Top to Bottom.*

2.   Rummler GA and Brache AP. *Improving Performance.*

Chapter Ten
Training and Education: Learning is a Process

Key Ideas

- Learning is a process.

- Training must take into account the needs of adult learners.

- Do not gear training for self-sufficiency in a short time frame.

- One course cannot change behavior. Creative curricula with continuous reinforcements are required.

- Physicians have different immediate needs than administrative personnel, even though many long-term needs are the same.

Many quality improvement education efforts do not have clear goals other than the nebulous "quality training." There is no denying that they are very well-intentioned. People work hard and intuitively do their best. However, truly objective analysis would show that many training programs are not necessarily designed with the "customer," i.e., work force, in mind. Courses typically overwhelm participants with too much conceptual knowledge and jargon in a lecture format and passive participation through unrealistic, rote exercises. The focus tends to be on skills, skills and more skills in a compressed time frame.

The typical mixed audience training session, as administered through a human resource or other department is just not conducive to problem solving. "Here are the dates. Please sign up for a slot" results in more of a mini-university rather than a team atmosphere. Even training courses targeted to specific departments tend to be ineffective due to the overly formal structure and lack of focus on a real problem. Motivation to learn and use tools and skills is lost by bogging down in their minutiae. Many times both the instructors and participants assume an objective of self-sufficiency. Implicit in this assumption is that the participants will be left to decide how and when to apply the methods. As will be discussed, when people have not been shown how to use information properly, they generally misapply it.

Many a disaster has also occurred as a result of "train the trainer" programs. These are programs in which outside resources are used to train a select few, who then train the organization including other trainers. Once again, this is an opportunity (virtually guaranteed) for Deming's Funnel Rule 4 ("random walk," Brownian motion) to add unintended human variation to a situation.

A goal of complete self-sufficiency in methods and skills through a course or series of short courses is unrealistic. Yet, training is delivered as if self-sufficiency were the objective.

The key to successful training is not to teach methods and skills, but to teach people how to use these skills—how to solve their problems. Any conceptual knowledge should support a problem solving process.

In addition, even if the correct knowledge is taught, there is still a process by which people understand and assimilate new information. This process involves the following four phases; only the latter two assume self-sufficiency:
- Awareness
- Breakthrough in Knowledge
- Breakthrough in Thinking
- Breakthrough in Behavior

Each of these four phases is part of the human psychological process. Each has its unique, deliberate pace. All learning launches participants on a journey through these phases. The human change process takes time. Any training that goes beyond an individual's current phase is wasted and could actually be counterproductive by creating unneeded psychological frustration.

Barriers

One of the biggest disappointments in a quality improvement effort occurs when concepts learned in a course do not translate into action. Human nature being what it is, logic is not always persuasive. Formidable barriers are erected by people's natural resistance to change, the link between statistical thinking and methods and "math anxiety", and a job that already takes over one hundred percent of their time. The impact of these barriers is virtually impossible to overestimate.

Unique problems are encountered when teaching adult learners. A partial list includes: participants' perceived lack of immediate applicability, inappropriate material

10

being taught, people's natural resistance to change (even though they acknowledge the need for change), courses quickly getting ahead of what people are capable of realistically absorbing, and, probably most important, the inertia caused by the company's need to stay in business the best way it currently knows how. Thus, the new knowledge is not immediately applied and it is soon forgotten, if indeed it was learned properly in the first place.

In *Firing on All Cylinders*, Clemmer recommends the following as important steps in teaching adults:

- understand why the skill is important

- discuss the specific behaviors involved in the skill

- watch a demonstration of the skill

- practice the skill

- receive constructive feedback

- identify opportunities for using the skill.

Training for training's sake can create some awareness, but little else. This is not necessarily bad, but the awareness created by a course whose objective is self-sufficiency could also have negative repercussions. This is especially true if knowledge and use of the skills is subsequently neither noticed nor rewarded. Further damage occurs when, despite a multitude of classes taught, management discovers the "bottom line" is minimally affected. When management does not participate in training or does not model the appropriate skills, negative consequences also result.

No course or instructor can change people. People must change themselves. Unless the delivery of the education addresses this issue and sparks individual internal motivation, it has no value. Long-held beliefs must be challenged in such a way that people accept the challenge presented and become excited about being led into the future.

Beyond Awareness

Proper education puts training in a perspective. The awareness it creates is seen as the potential beginning of an ultimate journey toward a breakthrough in thinking and behavior, the final phase of understanding and assimilating knowledge. However, there is another phase which must take place before the education can translate into truly

meaningful action. The education/awareness phase must be followed by a necessary but awkward transition phase, a **breakthrough in knowledge.**

This phase is extremely difficult to impose on a culture for reasons discussed previously, and it is naive to believe that one or even a series of short, intense courses geared toward self-sufficiency can change a lifetime of ingrained habits. *A flurry of teaching activity should not be confused with impact.*

It is not realistic to expect an immediate or even a necessarily correct application of material recently learned. In fact, part of the breakthrough in knowledge phase will involve learning from **mis**applications of skills through the filter of old habits. "Thinking statistically" in terms of processes and properly identifying and understanding variation are many times, and especially initially, overwhelming and counter-intuitive.

Breakthrough in knowledge is similar to a comment Steve Allen made when he hosted "The Tonight Show". Allen is a master at interviewing audience members and ad-libbing, and when a woman asked him: "Mr. Allen, do they get your show in Philadelphia?", his reply was, "Well, they see it, but they don't get it."

People are being pushed out of their comfort zones, and they must have time to acclimate as well as see proof that the culture values this change. If management demonstrates the desired behaviors, acts as teachers/coaches, rewards use of the behaviors, and allows people to take pride in their everyday work, the training process will still be deliberate, but it will accelerate and have a chance of succeeding.

A fascinating article on education for purposes of changing behavior is "Measuring training from a new science perspective," by Jim Rough.[1]

A Sample Curriculum

Appendix A contains an eight-session syllabus developed as a seminar by Balestracci for "transforming" HealthSystem Minnesota (HSM) culture. The sessions are spaced one week apart. Each is 2 hours long. At various times throughout the year, "Running Effective Meetings," a 4-hour course developed by Joiner Associates, is offered. It might seem tempting to condense this all into a continuous 2 day "one shot" course; however, the 8-week format has proven quite effective. People need time to truly absorb and assimilate the material. Exercises are designed for them to notice the simple, obvious applications in their everyday work.

Although designed for transformation, the skills can easily be adapted and expanded for more formal project use by a facilitator who truly understands them. It would actually be more effective to educate a team during the natural course of its project. However, it has also been useful for team members to have had an awareness of basic improvement concepts and worked in a department where the supervisor was practicing skills as taught in the seminar.

Much of the time is spent in discussion to address barriers and people's fear of change. As a result, some scheduled material may not be covered, but that really is not a big issue. The education is really an investment in the future. Can it spark people's "wherewithal" to keep learning? The discussion is crucial in addressing people's fear and resistance so they will take a personal stake in transforming the organization. This course can only start them on their journey toward quality improvement.

While not every class member does every assignment, at least one person does each assignment for a given class. All assignments are inevitably discussed in class, which shows the realities, difficulties, and natural mistakes in learning the improvement process. It is helpful to participants and easy for the instructor to be extremely positive and supportive of the class members' efforts. As participants become more convinced of the philosophy, they also begin to notice their department's resulting resistance. This creates some interesting discussion on the psychology of change and strategies for dealing with it.

It is a near certainty that someone will call the day before class and say that lack of time prevented them from completing the assignments and the reading. Should they come to class? The answer is always an unhesitating, "Yes!" During the sixth session of one of the seminars, one such person declared in a tone of confusion, surprise, and anger, "I haven't done any of the assignments and only about one-third of the reading, but, you know, I can't help it...*you've got me thinking differently!*" Exactly.

Thus far at HSM, the participants have been mostly middle management and different levels of supervisors. The approach of short seminars spread over many weeks is usually enough to convince them that their job indeed must become one of understanding and improving processes...but the odds are at least 85 to 15 against them. Who is going to change the systems to better those odds? How can a culture help these people succeed? They leave the seminar with the best of intentions. How can one capitalize on this energy?

Remember from Figure 2.6 that 25-50 percent of management must truly make an effort to change behavior to create the "critical mass" effect. This "critical mass" effect must be kept in mind and be the objective of the initial design of an education program. Attaining it will make the subsequent breakthroughs in cultural knowledge, thinking, and behavior much easier. Concentrate initial education on the people needed for critical mass and make it part of their jobs to teach it to their departments through routine daily work.

From the discussion on "benchmarking" in Chapter 9, consider the curriculum for what it is: an example of a new transformation approach which seems to have a higher success rate than intense "short course" formats. If you find it appealing, try to understand the theory behind its design and adapt it to your organization. It is in a constant state of improvement. One year from now, it may have evolved beyond its current form. Every seminar yields many improvements for the next group.

What About the Physicians?

The typical front-line physician has neither the time, patience, nor interest to sit through such a course. This is especially true if their compensation depends on productivity. Quite frankly, it is a poor short-term strategy to try to convince physicians of the importance of the skills and to teach skills to such an actively resistant culture. Physicians have their own ideas about this "QI stuff." What core knowledge and format would increase the probability of the "critical mass" effect among physicians?

Berwick makes a good case for involving physicians immediately in the process.[2] However, just as the temptation to form too many administrative teams should be resisted, so should the temptation to initially form a parallel, "clinical QI" effort.

10

The authors have great respect for Jack Silversin and his current work on the psychology of physician behavior when faced with change. His work contains six suggestions and considerations to address this major challenge:

- Ask physicians what is means to be part of the group. Do they understand the obligations as well as the privileges?

- Are day-to-day internal issues stemming from lack of both agreement and commitment to the group's goals, i.e., resulting from "me, my, mine"? Is there an absence of passion for a shared commitment?

- Are there skilled and motivated physician-administrators at the unit level, as well as at the top? Are such positions an honor or a chore?

- Do nonphysician staff members view the physicians as advocates of service or as barriers?

- Is there alignment among the leadership? Otherwise, philosophy and mission discussion with front-line physicians is a waste of time.

- Is the atmosphere such that it fosters a healthy ventilation of differences? Can resolution of philosophical difference be linked to the bottom-line business success of the group?

These questions were developed in 1985 (!) and are just as applicable now as then; however, the only reason they may cease to be relevant and applicable is best stated by Silversin himself:

> There is a real danger to postponing action... When "the wolf is at the door" and the competition is growing at your group's expense, it will be too late to achieve an effective response.

Due to increased competition, it is becoming imperative for a group's medical leadership and physicians to create a synergy by aligning behind a common vision with the physicians especially sharing a high level of commitment to a common purpose. Physicians can strive toward personal goals, but they must acknowledge the group and behave in ways that support its mission and objectives.

Due to an unwritten cultural rule of physicians valuing their autonomy and guarding their independence, many groups have intentionally created organizations that allow a number of physicians to practice under one roof while maintaining their autonomy, causing a "me, my,

mine" attitude rather than "ours." Such a lack of alignment slows an organization's decision-making process and jeopardizes the ability to respond rapidly to the pressures of an external environment where the public's expectations are on the rise. Quality *care* is now *assumed*, but service, convenience, and a "high-touch" experience are becoming equally important to consumers.

Task-oriented physicians (the norm) see no such need to explore the philosophical underpinnings of their group practice. They grow impatient with such a process, which quickly becomes extremely political when the true issues are philosophical.

Achieving alignment on philosophical issues is not only worthwhile, but essential. Leadership must recognize the nonalignment is rooted in professional tradition which, although self-serving, has, until now, been successful. However, it would be a mistake to overreact be centralizing power, making decisions without involving others, and tightening the reins — guaranteed to increase frustration and noncompliance. How does one strike a balance between autonomy and account-ability to the group?

OOPS!

Hindsight is 20-20. The experience of HealthSystem Minnesota demonstrates some of the problems with trying to move QI too quickly with physicians. HSM addressed the physician issue in 1990 by forming ten clinical teams on common conditions (asthma, breast mass, chest pain, cholesterol, depression, hypertension, low back pain, menopause, pharyngitis, and urinary tract infection). Informal physician leaders were "volunteered" and given cursory training in the FOCUS-PDCA model of improvement. Needless to say, the variation in perceptions of what the teams were supposed to accomplish was rampant. So were opinions about proper and appropriate treatment of the clinical conditions. Virtually all teams made their scope too wide (solving "world hunger"), did their best but naturally floundered (some folded), and lost track of why they were formed.

The article by Eddy[4] is highly recommended for its discussion of the range of variation that exists in treatment of common diagnoses. Many physicians used the project teams to test strongly held "pet" theories. The frustration and inappropriateness of attempting research in an unstable environment (see Chapter 4) were discovered. Data collections on actual work in progress were hopelessly contaminated. Exposing individual variation practice patterns through the use of flowcharts was fiercely resisted. There was heavy reliance on published literature data. Six teams yielded significant organizational results, but it took over two years!

A Summary of the Initial Clinical Teams and Physician Involvement

The following summarizes the problems encountered by the clinical teams and some reasons they occurred. The lessons were incorporated into a modified approach (to be discussed shortly) which is currently used with physicians.

1) Too ambitious for 1990 state of cultural knowledge

   - Lack of direction (No overall organizational "aim"/focus) and "buy-in" from culture
   - Culture perceived QI as "Thou shalt..."

2) People "doing their best" to facilitate without understanding the theory

   - Acronym (FOCUS-PDCA) without understanding its theory/applications

   - Lack of support materials
   - Reading texts like *The TEAM Handbook* with no knowledge of how to use it

3) Underestimation of complexity of improvement process

   - Difficult clinical topics
   - Learning new process (filtered through "clinical trial paradigm"—no perception of needing a new, entirely different process)
   - Team dynamics and psychology
   - Jobs which already took up over 100% of their time.

4) Clinical trial paradigm

   - Heavy concentration on medical outcomes, not necessarily current processes of delivering care (inadequate consideration of internal "customer-mindedness")
   - Desire to test pre-conceived solutions vs. expose "positive" variation in current care processes (difficulty of collecting data on work-in-progress)
   - Reliance on literature recommendations without parallel studies of existing processes of care in an everyday culture

5) Teams floundered too long—gave QI a bad reputation among physicians ("Two years for this?!")

   - Projects too broad: No overall organizational strategy (Where does the major opportunity exist within this condition? Diagnosis? Access? Treatment? "Improvement in general" should become a sequence of smaller projects on prioritized issues identified through customer needs assessment and data collection within the condition)
   - Lack of understanding of variation in current, existing processes (minimal flowcharts)
   - Lack of understanding of root causes of variation—anecdotal arguments about solutions around "pet theories."

6) Vast underestimation of dynamics of change (solution implementation, cultural resistance to change, holding the gains)

   - Consolidation of lots of good information, but no robust dissemination process
   - Use of written memos and single educational "events": minimal impact

10

- Resistance to studying work in progress to generate a case with data
- Resistance to data collection on whether proposed gains were achieved and held

What was the net result? A lot of good information to disseminate, but, more importantly, invaluable learning about the psychology of transformation and change, both cultural change and human factors of individual change.

Points to ponder:

- Most doctors already deliver excellent care. QI education should not imply otherwise.

- Health care is a **process** which leads to an output...Doctors depend on a series of complex processes to deliver care. They are part of the system and have internal customers.

- *The wasteful variation and unpredictability of these processes represent the major opportunity for improvement.*

Summary: Core Knowledge for Buy-In

After teaching many of the administrative management and nursing supervisors, it finally came to the point where buy-in from "Joe and Jane Front-Line Doc" was crucial. Their lack of knowledge and misperceptions

about QI were presenting a formidable barrier to organizational transformation. The many rapid changes in health care have added to the sense of lost control experienced by many physicians. It is no surprise that one social consequence of QI is resistance. Physicians perceive it as someone else "looking over their shoulder." As Berwick has pointed out, they feel "accused."[5]

With this in mind, self-sufficiency in QI skills is not an objective. The main objective is to overcome misconceptions and make the physicians aware of their place in a system designed for a core process of delivering health care. Presentations of data on routine daily work can provide the convincing that physicians typically need to change behavior. QI is the scientific method applied to the delivery of health care.

At HSM, a four-session seminar was designed with each 90-minute session scheduled one week apart. Arrangements have been made for CME credit. It is hoped that even though some physicians may come to the seminar thinking one thing they will leave thinking another. The hoped-for natural progression is from skeptical to positive. The Syllabus for Educating Change Agents appears in Appendix A, and the Physician QI Seminar in Appendix B.

Notes to Chapter Ten

1.   Rough J. "Measuring Training From a New Science Perspective".

2.   Berwick DM. "The Clinical Process and the Quality Process."

3.   Silversin J. "Get Your People in Sync!".

4.   Eddy DM. "Variations in Physician Practice: The Role of Uncertainty."

5.   Berwick DM. "The Clinical Process and the Quality Process."

Chapter Eleven
Case Study Examples of Quality Improvement from Coding Project Demonstration Sites

The CRAHCA/Medicode QI Coding Project applied QI principles to the coding process in three medical groups. The case studies that follow describe the distinctive experiences of these three groups. The Project Advisory Committee guided unity of purpose and consistency in measurement in all sites. Each group implemented the QI principles and conducted project measures to reflect its own unique practice setting, culture, issues, and resources.

An analysis of key improvement themes and issues common to all three practices during the project follows in Chapter 12. You are encouraged to consider these experiences in light of your own, compare them with other discussions in the literature, and use them to direct your own quality improvement efforts.

Case study: small single specialty practice

ASHEVILLE CARDIOLOGY ASSOCIATES

Asheville Cardiology Associates, P.A. (ACA) is a 16-physician single specialty group which has served the Asheville, North Carolina area since 1971. At the project's beginning in 1991, ACA employed 10 FTE physicians. Six additional cardiologists have joined ACA since then, including two in 1992. A pediatric cardiologist joined ACA in 1994.

Located in a small city surrounded by a rural area with scattered smaller communities, ACA physicians provide services and consultations in two local hospitals. In addition, ACA serves 18 counties in a 65-mile radius. In October 1992, ACA opened its first satellite office in Hendersonville, North Carolina. The opening of this site expanded coverage an additional 30 miles, and added two more hospitals to ACA's inpatient coverage.

Directed towards its patients, ACA's mission statement reads:

> The physicians and staff of Asheville Cardiology Associates are dedicated to providing compassionate and cost-effective cardiac evaluation, treatment, and care of the highest quality to those we serve in Western North Carolina and the surrounding region. We strive to consistently improve our services by emphasizing the continuing education of all our staff members and continual assessment of our results. It is our goal to meet and exceed the expectations of all we serve. We will work to provide an environment within our organization that will provide a respectful, fair, healthy and rewarding employment opportunity for all while maintaining our commitment to our families and our personal and professional growth.

Description of major practice components

Reimbursement issues: The practice serves about 57 percent Medicare patients, with the remainder of their business divided as 30 percent commercial payors; 8 percent Medicaid; 3 percent self-pay and other; and 2 percent managed care. Prior to the project, ACA had begun to recognize the increasing complexity of reimbursement, especially as the Health Care Financing Administration (HCFA) moved Medicare reimbursement to its Resource-Based Relative Value System (RBRVS) and significantly revised its Evaluation and Management codes in January, 1992. Other payors have moved to more rigorous claim filing and documentation requirements as well.

Management style: ACA has been a very traditionally managed medical group, governed by a board of directors composed of twelve cardiologists, nine of whom are stockholders. The board sets group policies, and the administrator has responsibility for implementation of those policies. As in many traditional practices, each doctor has functioned somewhat independently of the others, although each does not have a specific nurse assigned only to him. (A female physician joined the practice in 1994.) Physicians do their own coding. Coding issues are discussed as needed during weekly physician meetings.

In July, 1993, the ACA board voted to ensure that all physicians have a working knowledge of Deming's philosophy. Reorganization of the board occurred in January, 1994 to disband a variety of separate committees. This change created the position of part-time medical director. This position has the authority to release time and resources to further empower the management in its efforts to improve processes and daily operations.

The practice board chairman as well as two physicians on the board who were very interested in QI began moving to a more process-focused management approach several months before the coding project began. The physicians requested the hiring of a Quality Improvement Director to assist the organization in developing a QI program (see the "How They Got Started..." chapter).

While communication between departments could be described as "fairly good" prior to project involvement, procedural change was usually initiated and conducted by the department primarily responsible for the activity, without consistent, organized involvement of other departmental staff. For example, early ACA project minutes noted that "'they' were planning to make changes in the superbill". This implied that possibly not all the key staff involved in using the superbill were involved in the process. The danger existed that the new form under development would still not correct coding process problems.

Staff activities: Eleven of the sixteen physicians practice invasive cardiology and perform heart catheterizations (caths). All caths are performed at one hospital. Several physicians contribute additional procedures including atherectomies, angioplasties, balloon valvuloplasties, electrophysiology studies (EPS), and insertions of pacemakers and implant-able cardioverter devices (ICDs). There are seven physician assistants (PAs) on staff; each is certified by national regulatory agencies and registered with the North Carolina Board of Medical Examiners. The PAs work closely with the cardiologists at the hospitals to assist with initial evaluations, daily hospital rounds, patient discharge, heart catheterizations, and a variety of hospital tests. PAs are responsible for coding their work. Their coding is not reviewed by their supervising physician.

4.5 full-time equivalent (FTE) registered nurses (RNs) assist with office tests and procedures, see patients in the various clinics, and answer telephone calls concerning patient care. In the first project year (10/91-10/92), ACA had 5,665 physician and 1,123 nursing visits, with 10,964 telephone calls taken by the nursing staff.

Four medical assistants are responsible for preparing the patients for examination; drawing blood for lab

work, and escorting patients through the office. Five cardiovascular technicians assist nurses and physicians with treadmills and exercise echocardiograms, connect and scan holter monitors, run EKG tests, and check pacemakers. The practice utilizes four echocardiogram technicians that obtain ultrasounds images for various tests. There are 11 support personnel in the front office that handle scheduling, patient registration and patient check-out. Within the medical records department, there are five clerks and four transcriptionists. The Business Office contains 10 clerks and two persons who also provide computer support. Nearly 40 administrative and support staff assist clinical staff with practice activities.

While practice turnover was approximately less than five percent practice-wide, it still indicated the need for established procedures and processes that could be easily and consistently conveyed to new staff regardless of department or functional level. This would help to ensure processes were consistently applied as employees were added or existing position responsibilities or procedures changed.

ACA's information management needs were becoming increasingly complex due to practice growth and increasingly stringent reimbursement and documentation requirements. During the project, the practice was also involved in a computer conversion. This moved them toward a faster, more efficient system utilizing two major practice management software packages. As in all conversions, there was hope that the new system would really do not only what the practice needed today, but would be flexible enough to meet increasing electronic billing and electronic payor remittances. ACA now believes that the software has provided greatly improved access to both billing and clinical information, with greater flexibility and responsiveness for account research and follow-up.

Processes to be improved: Coding was a process of primary interest to ACA. Coding varied by physician. Some physicians used an extensive list of CPT-4 codes not appearing on the superbill, while others used outdated, "generic", or other incorrect or inexact codes. This was particularly of concern given the evaluation and management codes introduced in 1992.

In addition to coding, some ACA staff perceived that several other processes needed improvement. These included claims follow-up, denials, obtaining records needed to support bills from outside facilities, obtaining current patient data through the registration process, etc. ACA had neither a precertification policy nor a practice-wide system for utilization review updates.

Even though the core number of physicians was relatively small, the number and variety of practice settings and services provided by ACA providers resulted in insurance billing that was very complex. It was a challenge to obtain required supporting documentation completely and consistently in a system with so many different inouts.

When the project began, the billing process allowed claim submission delays of up to six months. This meant a backlog of approximately $20,000 in unbilled accounts. Patients were being billed, and the practice was receiving late reimbursement. No follow-up was conducted on claims that were submitted late, denied or remained unpaid. Incomplete patient information caused a slowdown in claims filing. Some claims were submitted but denied because the time between the date of service and the date allowed by payors such as Medicare was too long. Information received from other providers was not always complete or timely. Finally, ACA had no policy for standard medical record documentation.

Due in large part to unclear billing statements, insurance staff spent 75 percent of their time answering calls and subsequently researching the callers' questions. Patients and payors called because of late and incomplete billings. Claims for some services were not filed at all. An average of 50 calls per day were received after each monthly billing.

In 13 percent of the cases studied at the project's start, physicians who oversaw the performance of certain procedures such as labs and EKGs were not listed as having ordered the procedure. This also created reimbursement delays and denials.

The site was experiencing a number of other issues related to appropriate payment, including overpayments due to secondary insurance filings which occurred at the time of the primary filing; no follow-up or refiling of denied commercial claims; duplicate billing cards sent from hospital to group for same patient/service; and slow filing of out-of-town holter monitor claims.

How they got started with QI

- **Introducing the concepts and project; training.**

ACA became interested in the coding project in August, 1991 after CRAHCA issued a call for demonstration sites. The group saw the need to more fully understand and improve their billing process. They wanted to know which providers accounted for most of ACA billings; which had the slowest turnaround time; and how to improve billing follow-up. Reimbursement had already been identified as a priority issue. ACA believed that the project could assist with its improvement.

Several ACA physicians served as leaders at two hospitals which had already begun QI implementation. They had attended the hospitals' QI education programs, were convinced of QI's potential benefits, and wanted to develop a quality program in their practice. Because ACA physicians are also involved in research, they felt the model was a natural approach to process improvement. Their decision to pursue quality improvement was confirmed when they hired Marilyn Haas as Director of Quality Improvement. Haas was viewed as a natural "quality champion" due to her nursing and administrative background and personal commitment to quality in medicine. During her time at ACA, she has worked to educate all physicians, directors, and staff about quality improvement issues and techniques.

- **Introducing QI to practice customers-board, physicians, other staff**

"We began our QI project by involving those physicians who were already interested in and/or knowledgeable about QI," states Haas. The practice formed a Quality Council made up of ACA's most enthusiastic QI supporters. The Council is made up of three physicians, the administrator, and the Director of Quality Improvement. The three physicians were charged with selecting the quality improvement model (the series of steps to identify and solve process errors) and with overseeing an implementation plan. The Quality Council's major responsibility is to oversee the quality of care delivered throughout the organization. It provides overall direction regarding the issues to be studied and monitored. Staff at all levels can submit ideas to council members for project consideration. In addition, the group conducts periodic surveys to learn more about patient and staff concerns.

11

After practice managers and supervisors were briefed about the benefits of a QI program, ACA established an office QI committee consisting of supervisors and employees who would give input about processes to be improved.

Physicians and staff were surveyed to learn what areas they thought needed improvement. Six physicians responded to a QI Project Suggestion memo. This memo was used to generate suggestions for improvement in processes directly relating to the physicians.

A number of other clinical and administrative issues were identified. The physicians identified categories of need, worked to reach consensus, then voted on the issues. The physicians identified nursing protocols as the greatest area of need, followed closely by issues regarding study/test result turnaround times; responses to referring physicians; and patient escorts. The physicians ranked "nursing protocols" highest because they perceived this as having the greatest impact on patient care. These physicians believed such protocols would allow the nurses to more accurately respond to patient phone questions and would provide for consistent response among the nurses. The physicians felt that protocols would improve in pre-appointment consistency, patient education, nurse response to reported symptoms, and would reduce the time it took to respond to patient inquiries.

Next, the Quality Council reviewed the surveys and decided which processes would be tackled by the quality teams. Decisions about which processes to study were based on the processes identified by the largest number of physicians and staff as critical to patient care and practice operations. To promote the continuing interest of physicians and employees at this early stage, the council proposed process improvements to benefit both of those customer groups. Because ACA physician assistants work full-time at the hospital, they were not included in office process teams.

The Council reappraises the overall quality improvement program annually to identify program components to be added, altered, or deleted. As an example showing an application of the PDCA concept, Figure 11.1 shows ACA's interpretation of steps in the PDCA process. They outlined their telephone patient management improvement activities. While the work of that team was beyond the scope of the coding project, it shows an effort to implement a step-by-step, process-oriented approach.

**Figure 11.1a: An Interpretation of the 10-Step Process/PDCA Method
Asheville Cardiology Associates**

STEP 1: Assign Responsibility
Establish QI Focus Team. Team responsible for active participation in monitoring and evaluation of telephone triage and protocol implementation.

STEP 2: Delineate Scope of Care
Establish an inventory of the area's clinical activities. Telephone logs reviewed to develop telephone symptom protocols.

STEP 3: Identify Important Aspects of Care
Identify aspects that are high-risk, high-volume, and/or problem-prone.

STEP 4: Identify Indicators
Indicators selected were measurable variables related to the structure, process, or outcome of care.

STEP 5: Establish Thresholds for Evaluation
Establish thresholds of the acceptance levels based on clinical/quality assurance literature and/or experience of the organization.

STEP 6: Collect and Organize Data
Collect data and organize them for comparison (fishbone cause-and-effect diagram).

STEP 7: Evaluate Care
Evaluate identified causes, trends, and patterns in processes which are being considered for improvement (flowchart).

STEP 8: Take Actions to Solve Problems
Develop and enact action plans to improve care. In-service education to all parties involved.

STEP 9: Assess Actions and Document Improvements
Assess and document effectiveness of improvement actions (refer to histogram, scattergrams, and pie diagrams).

STEP 10: Communicate Relevant Information to the Organization QI Program
Document and report findings/conclusions through all channels, including physician QI Council and Board.

11

Figure 11b: Flowchart of PDCA Interpretation
Asheville Cardiology Associates

PROCESS OF QUALITY IMPROVEMENT

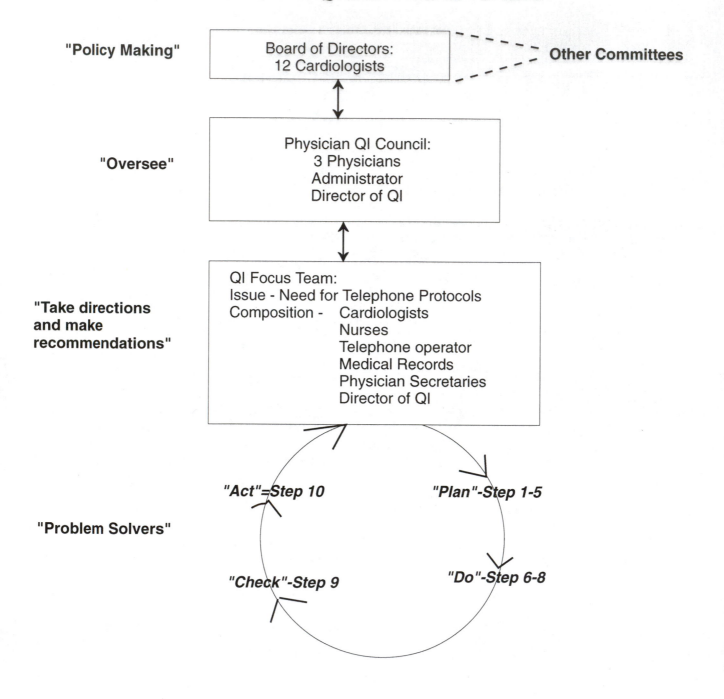

After Haas received training through courses then led by Deming, the site's quality improvement efforts began. "We jumped right in," she says, "and I taught process thinking as we went along." Much was learned by staff as they served on the teams. Formal training for all supervisors and employees occurred in July and November, 1993. The first course was a two-hour introduction attended by all staff; the second program lasted 16 hours, and was offered to all supervisors and some key staff positions. ACA physicians are now required to attend formal training through the Deming-method courses.

ACA received minimal additional training specific to this project. A Medicode consultant spent a day with ACA staff to discuss and review effective medical record audit procedures. These procedures were used in assessing the quality of medical record documentation related to coding.

ACA chose to establish two teams and to work on several issues simultaneously to promote buy-in to the concept by both physicians and staff. One QI team was formed to work on the physicians' concerns, and another was formed to address staff concerns. The first physician team was formed to address the need for nursing telephone protocols as identified by physicians. The second team formed to investigate "better preparation of patients for their office visits". An operational definition of "better preparation" included such issues as arrival time, appropriate dress for test to be conducted, and information needed for examination and processing (history, medications, etc.). With input from medical records and the billing department. the third QI team looked into coding and reimbursement.

The ACA teams determined the frequency with which they met. All teams are multidisciplinary in structure, involving at least one representative from each area involved in the process under study. The Director of Quality Improvement served as facilitator and recorder at the team meetings when the teams were getting started. The QI Director reported team progress during Quality Council meetings. As the teams gained experience, department supervisors moved into these roles.

- **Team development**

A physician interested in the project (who happened to <u>not</u> be on the Quality Council) served as the liaison between the other physicians and the coding project team. Proposed changes as developed by the coding team were communicated to the other physicians, and their responses were collected through his participation in weekly physician meetings. Many written documents were circulated to keep everyone informed. These included proposed changes and opportunity for comment and revision. Physicians were advised by the Director of Medical Records about changes during weekly meetings. She attended at least two meetings with the group physicians to discuss changes and gather input. Root causes of process problems were identified by the project committee. The team used flowcharts and pie charts to communicate their findings and process improvement suggestion as well as written and oral communications.

ACA created a flowchart that represented the current process. Next, billing, coding, and medical records staff along with cardiac and echocardiograph technicians brainstormed and discussed system improvement ideas. Based on these discussions, the team felt the problems were so obvious that additional data were not required before work on improvement could begin. The fishbone diagram (Figure 11.2) identifies some of the obstacles and flowcharts (Figures 11.3 and 11.4) illustrate the improved processes.

11

**Figure 11.2: Ishikawa Analysis (Fishbone Diagram):
Out-of-Town Holter Tests-Asheville Cardiology Associates**

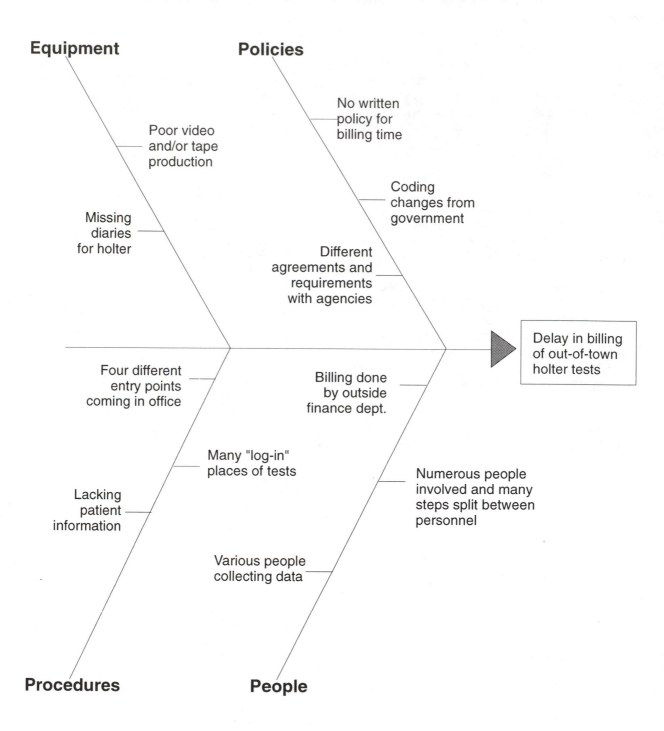

Figure 11.3: Echo Test Coding Process - Asheville Cardiology Associates

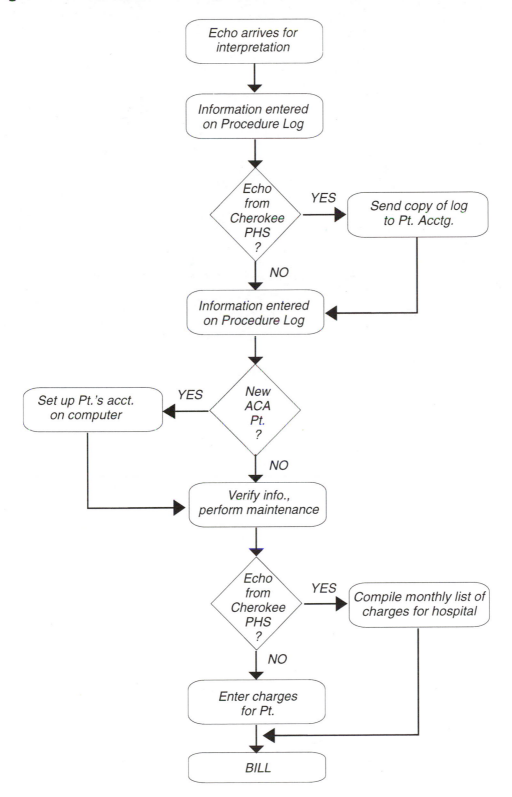

11

Figure 11.4: Billing for Inpatient Admission - Asheville Cardiology Associates

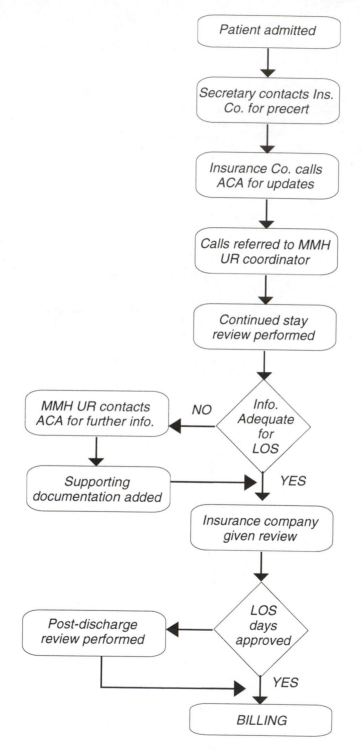

Coding project data collection and analysis

Each demonstration site was asked to conduct both baseline and final measures on four macro issues:

- turnaround time from date of service to claim submission
- medical record audit
- claim denial/resubmission rates
- claims edit review

ACA's baseline measurements were taken in March, 1992. 10 medical records were reviewed for each of 10 physicians, equalling 100 records. Final measurements were conducted in January, 1993. 10 medical records were reviewed for each of 12 physicians (including two physicians added March/July 1992), totalling 120 records. Figure 11.5 represents a data collection checklist used by ACA for this project.

Figure 11.5 Asheville Data Collection Checklist

Full Name	Plate Stamped	ADM Date	DC Date	DX Given	DX ADEQ to Code	Receive Promptly	M.D. Initials	Correct Codes	All Proc. Listed
1									
2									
3									
4									
5									
6									
7									
8									
9									
10									
11									
12									
13									
14									
15									
16									
17									
18									
19									
20									

11

Table 11.1 summarizes the site's information regarding its project measures. The table shows the percentage of occurrence for each category for both baseline and final measures.

TABLE 11.1
Summary of Baseline and Final Measurements: Project Macro Measures
Asheville Cardiology Associates

Measure	Baseline	Final
1. Turnaround (days): Service to Claim Submission		
a. Incorrect information on patient registration forms	64%	40% *estimate: not re-audited
b. Incomplete hospital cards	58%	32% *estimate: not re-audited
c. Turnaround-hospital services to billing date	21 days	1 day
d. Unbilled from 1/1/91-4/91	$20,000	$0 unbilled at 12/92 measurement
2. Supportable Coding Documentation		
a. Goal at baseline: 100% of claims will have coding supported by appropriate documentation	no written policy or procedure	See 2.b.
b. Supporting documentation attached to claims submitted	62%	100% A new software program adding during the project produces hard copy whenever documentation is needed. This assumes correct coding.
c. Services documented but not coded	13%	6%
d. Services coded but not documented	4%	1%
e. Number of missing in-office patient signatures	64%	42% (The difference between baseline and final is believed to have been about 22% but not formally measured)
3. Denied/Resubmitted Claims Ratios		
a. Medicare claims denied (goal at baseline: less than 10% denial rate)	25%	8%
b. Services (fluro, lab, supplies) not charged on superbill	13%	5.7%
4. Claims Edit Review (Medicode Claims Edit Manager)		
a. Goal at baseline: 95% of hospital/office charge tickets accurately reflect which physician performed the services rendered	Prior to project, 13% not attributed accurately to physician who oversaw/ ordered care	100%
b. Goal at baseline: 100% appropriate use of E/M codes as mandated by HCFA	No statistic	73.4% of superbills in office 87.3% of charts from hospital

The operational definition of "appropriate" was "coded so the bill was not denied".

As part of the measure for Macro Measure 3, "Denied/ Resubmitted Claims Ratio", 13,000 claims with dates of service between September 1991 and January 1992 were reviewed. A computerized claims audit system developed by Medicode-Claims Manager-was used to conduct this measure. According to the Medicare regulations as programmed into Claims Manager, 522 claims (4 percent) were candidates for denial. After this review, ACA had several questions.

The edit identified some claims as "would be denied by Medicare". However, since this was a retrospective review, the practice knew it had not received denials for these same claims. This indicated that the edit on the Medicode system was more rigorous than the way in which ACA's Medicare carrier was implementing denials. However, it was valuable for ACA to see these potential denials, since policy is ever-changing and rules can be redefined and readministered depending on a variety of factors.

According to the claims edit, the place of service was also seen as important to accurate coding For example, a procedure normally done as an inpatient that is coded as outpatient is a prime target for denial. In addition, the system indicated some claims were deniable because they were for telephone consults, not on-site office or hospital visits.

The site found the claims edit to be useful in raising their awareness of precise payor requirements as compared with their actual denial experience, and potential areas for improvement should payors begin more stringent enforcement of coding requirements.

What they learned and what improved

ACA further stratified its baseline and final measures by physician to identify trends. The information was shared with physicians on an individual basis by the Director of Medical Records. After the data were shared, the Director noted "considerable improvement in this process." However, data to define "considerable" were not collected. Physician response to the information was generally positive. Many commented that they believed a process improved through such data would improve efficiencies and reduce their "hassle factor."

By far the greatest problem related to inpatient billing (Table 11.1, item 1.b.) was that physicians were not following the procedure of stamping the inpatient billing card. Stamping gives ACA support staff important information needed for billing, including patient demographic data, admission date, admitting

physician, and Medicare status. Sometimes the stamp was not available, but unstamped cards were usually the result of a physician who simply did not do the stamping. Physicians viewed stamping as an unimportant clerical task that took extra time from their clinical work.

Due to staff time and availability constraints, final measures of macro measures "percent complete hospital cards" and "percent incorrect patient registration forms" were not obtained. Despite the fact that data were not available on these measures, the perception of the Director of Medical Records was that these process elements had drastically improved thanks to a combination of front desk and clinical staff efforts.

In addition to the quantitative macro measurements, site staff involved with the project found additional benefits in using QI to address coding problems. Perhaps most important of these was an increased awareness of the complete coding process, especially among physicians, which resulted in changed behavior. Following their involvement with the project, the physicians more consistently stamped the billing card.

Through the efforts of the project team, the ACA encounter form was significantly revised to include more complete coding options and correct codes for the most frequently performed procedures. THe physicians and other staff felt the form was more user friendly, as it more accurately reflected the needs of all its users.

Issues related to supportable coding were improved not only through the project team's direct efforts, but also through improvements gained by installation of the new computer system and its options for custom report programming.

As a result of the project, new employees with coding or business office responsibilities as well as those who are retrained into those positions are given flowcharts of how relevant processes work.

Site self-evaluation: tools, project measures and experience

At the end of the project, each demonstration site was asked to evaluate its experience with application of QI concepts and tools to improvement of its coding process. ACA gave the following responses in this evaluation:

11

- **Which QI tools and techniques were most useful?**

ACA used the following QI tools and techniques during the coding project:

- brainstorming

- flowcharts

- cause and effect "fishbone" diagrams

- team meetings, with meeting minutes taken and distributed for comment

- pie charts

Because the team's sophistication level was still developing, quantitative analysis tools like histograms were not used at ACA for this project. Later teams at ACA have used these tools. An example of an scattergram used (beyond the scope of the coding project) by the ACA protocols team appears as Figure 11.6.

- **Which measurements and/or analyses were of the most value to the coding quality improvement effort?**

ACA found the medical record documentation audit and study of their claims follow-up system to be very useful. The flowcharts allowed the teams to quickly see the key process issues. The fishbone diagrams organized their thoughts and helped them focus on the root problems.

According to ACA's Director of Patient Accounting, "The end result of our involvement is that we've identified where many of our problems lie. The project made ACA staff aware of the problems and has changed their attitude about many activities related to coding. Most staff are really trying to 'do it right the first time' by seeing that complete and accurate coding information appears on the claim form before submission and/or transmission."

A number of site-specific issues were also identified through the project by each site. At ACA, these micro-level improvements included study of the precertification process. The team identified a need for precertification data to appear in the computerized cath scheduler, as well as a need for payor information and authorization numbers to be part of the claims filing system.

Difficulties and how they were overcome

Says Haas, "In retrospect, we believe that one of our biggest barriers to successful, lasting improvements has been that we did not educate all our physicians from the beginning. We had to 'backtrack' to educate all the physicians including those who were not particularly interested or knowledgeable, as their lack of involvement has created some slowdowns to improvement efforts. A core of physicians were initially involved, but we later found that the 'uneducated' physicians were tampering with the process."

The ACA physicians who were enthusiastic from the outset believed increased demands for quality, cost-effective service at all levels were leading toward continued change. They viewed implementation of a quality program as critical to survival. Some delay in training of all physicians was due in part to difficulties in getting all the physicians in one place at one time.

Haas believes that the staff were motivated by the QI approach, and no significant barriers to change were encountered from them—they felt empowered and enjoyed participating in the improvements. Some of the coding problems were found to be the result of problems with getting accurate billing information. Haas believes that getting secretarial input upfront in the improvement process will reduce these problems.

ACA now has a full-time employee physically located at each of its two major hospitals. To maximize their productivity, these staff are cross-trained to manage other critical activities in addition to coding. For example, one person manages inpatient coding for ACA patients half-time, with the other half devoted to catheterization scheduling. At the other hospital, the ACA staff person spends 50 percent of her time on payroll issues and the other 50 percent on inpatient coding. As a result, the rate of completed inpatient coding information has significantly increased, with corresponding improvement in billing turnaround times and reduced denials related to late billing.

ACA has developed monthly "insurance outstanding" reports with enough information to allow insurance staff to efficiently follow up on outstanding claims. As for documentation, certain procedures which require medical notes are filed via hard copy instead of via electronic medical claim filing, and are flagged on the form itself with the notation, "requires medical notes." Also, by now having an ACA staff member working on-site at each hospital, the delay between date of service and posting date of hospital charges has been dramatically reduced.

ACA experienced the following benefits from its application of QI to the coding process.

- Savings were realized. Claims filed with supporting documentation; coding supported by documentation; and correct coding resulted in more full and timely payment. ACA identified other issues that were areas of potential savings, which led to the review of the claims denial process that began after the project. Elimination of rework with its associated staff costs was seen as very important.

- Communications with staff in facilities outside the practice were improved. ACA worked with hospital staff regarding precertifications, using the fax and approval monitoring. The actual project team was expanded to include those outside the practice like the hospital utilization review staff.

- Studying the process assisted in a proactive way by preparing the practice for Medicare's comparative performance reviews. The skills gained in applying QI to the coding process will be used as ACA addresses other ongoing practice issues like patient registration. Continuing QI efforts have continued beyond the technical end of the CRAHCA/Medicode project, including a team working to achieve 100 percent accuracy on patient registration forms.

An update: two years' post-project

Two years after the original coding project, ACA is still committed to quality improvement. The original teams are still in place. They are currently assessing what new improvements can be made. A number of new monitors, including expanded patient surveys, are in place. ACA notes that it remains more difficult on one hand to conduct improvement work through teams, however, it is better than alternatively making poor decisions in isolation. In addition, Haas has gone on to obtain additional advanced nursing training and a PhD.

Figure 11.6: Scattergram of Response Time to Chest Pain Telephone Calls

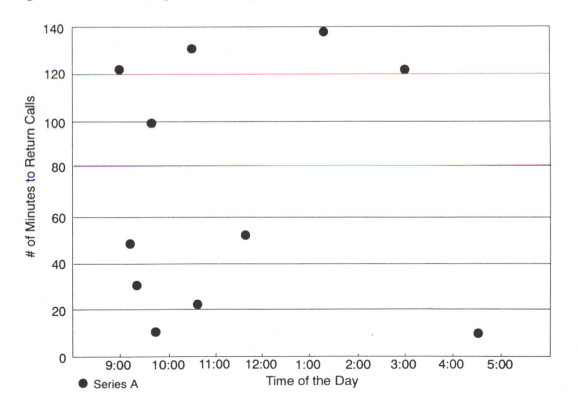

11

Case study: mid-sized multispecialty practice

THE HITCHCOCK CLINIC,
KEENE DIVISION

The Hitchcock Clinic Keene Division (Keene) is a 50-physician multispecialty group which has served in Keene, New Hampshire since 1948. On December 1, 1993, Keene officially became known as the Keene Division of The Hitchcock Clinic. The Hitchcock Clinic is in turn the Lebanon, New Hampshire component of the Dartmouth-Hitchcock Medical Center.

Like ACA, Keene is located in a small city surrounded by a rural area with scattered smaller communities. Keene physicians provide services and consultations to the Cheshire county area and serve on the medical staff of the Cheshire Medical Center (CMC), located literally next door to the group. Keene has had a particularly close relationship with CMC.

Guiding the practice at the time of the project was the Keene Clinic Mission Statement, which read:

> The physicians and staff of Keene Clinic are committed to caring for the community by providing professionally excellent medical services within the framework of multispecialty group practice.
>
> We are committed...
>
>> to patient satisfaction by providing care that is compassionate, cost effective, readily available, courteous and personal, while maintaining the patient's autonomy, dignity and confidentiality.
>
>> to the development of a group culture which fosters quality performance, loyalty, collegiality, and fairness in all its endeavors. The organization will provide all employees with a competitive compensation and benefits program which will attract, retain, and motivate talented people.
>
>> to maintaining a leadership position as the primary provider of physician services to patients in Southwestern New Hampshire and the neighboring Connecticut River Valley area. The scope of the Clinic's services shall be determined by the needs and demands of the communities it serves as well as its ability to provide such services.

> to a mutually supportive relationship with The Cheshire Medical Center. The Clinic will also work to develop strong relationships with academic centers for tertiary care, research and teaching.

> to governance which can support the mission and goals of the Clinic, and which preserves physician ownership and direction of the organization. To ensure survival of the organization, the Clinic will function within the dictates of sound financial management.

Description of major practice components

Reimbursement issues: The practice serves about 75 percent fee-for-service and 25 percent managed care patients. As did ACA, Keene had begun to recognize increasing reimbursement complexities. Keene anticipated that other payors will move to more rigorous claim filing and documentation requirements as well. Their work with the coding project was particularly affected by HCFA's new evaluation and management codes, as one of their two project teams was focused on family practice.

Management style: During the time of the project, Keene operated with a traditional, physician-led medical group management style, which it had held for over 40 years. Stockholder physicians held a voting stake in the major decisions affecting the practice. In 1989, efforts to address some practice issues using QI principles began (see how they got started with QI). The practice had structured physician/nurse relationships to include direct physician-nurse support or team nursing support of the physician dependent upon the department.

While practice communication between departments could be described as "fairly good" prior to project involvement, Keene physicians were not generally knowledgeable about the reimbursement and procedural implications of their coding practices. Communication with physicians and staff were often "hit or miss", with memos regarding a variety of practice issues not received or read. In addition to standard memos, physicians and others received updates on coding criteria changes via departmental and operations committee meetings. However, as coding was viewed largely as clerical and less important to practice success, it had been difficult to improve coding behavior in a consistent, comprehensive way.

Staff activities: Keene Clinic staff includes physicians, mid-level providers and other staff providing a broad spectrum of services, including primary care, internal medicine and surgical subspecialties, and mental health. The size of the physician panel has remained relatively constant for several years.

Positive morale and economic conditions have kept the number of employees who voluntarily leave the practice low. With Keene's diverse array of services, policies and procedures that are consistent and effective across functional areas became particularly important, and such efforts became a challenge for the practice.

Processes to be improved: Many of the departmental areas at Keene had different coding procedures, priorities, and communication strategies. As the practice worked to make processes more effective and efficient, coding became a natural focus for improvement efforts.

How they got started with QI

- **Introducing the concepts and project; training.**

When the project began, Keene already had 10 active QI teams, with six staff persons trained as team facilitators. The site received minimal additional training specific to this project. A Medicode consultant spent a day with the Business Office Manager, the Physician Business Services Supervisor, and the Manager of Patient Care Services reviewing effective medical record audit procedures. These procedures were used in assessing the quality of medical record documentation related to coding.

- **Introducing QI/project-board, physicians, other staff.**

Keene physicians were educated about coding issues by Business Office personnel through a series of department meetings which included lunch.

The Medical Director and administrator were charged with selection of the quality improvement model and approach that the teams would use, and with developing an implementation plan for the team's work. The Chair of the Practice/Procedures Committee, which later evolved into the Quality Improvement Committee, was involved in the planning process.

A 1989 survey of employees and physicians indicated a desire for increased involvement of employees and physicians in decisions affecting daily operations and a more focused sense of ownership.

Four clinical and four non-clinical staff were represented in the project through the Family Practice team, with five clinical and two non-clinical staff represented on the General Surgery/ Orthopaedics Team.

The initial Charge Submission Team developed the macro and micro measures that the two department specific teams used to gauge their progress. The initial project data were collected by this team. Both General Surgery/Orthopaedics and Family Practice decided to study coding improvement, but with different focuses. Family Practice selected office-based coding and General Surgery/Orthopaedics selected hospital-based coding.

As with the other demonstration sites, the practice did not go through a mass QI "roll-out". Instead, the practice used a project-specific approach. Prior to the project various teams were organized to look at important processes, most notably patient registration. Other Keene QI teams have looked at medical records, patients with portable catheterizations, chemotherapy, billing, and payroll processing.

The practice's previous QI experience was an important consideration in choosing Keene as a project demonstration site. Kathleen Iannacchino, RN had served as Keene's Quality Improvement Coordinator since the position was created in 1989. The administrator had made the decision that this position was needed after studying the role of quality in the practice. His ideas were supported by what he heard at a conference disseminating the results of the National Demonstration Project in Boston that year. The Board agreed that in order to be both effective and efficient, practice-wide efforts needed to be coordinated through one area. A job description of the Quality Improvement Coordinator appears as Figure 11.7.

The Quality Improvement Coordinator's role has been to "spread the wealth" of QI techniques by involving as many different people as possible on teams, providing both on-the-job and external training.

11

In 1989, Keene had organized its Quality Improvement Committee to serve as the advisory team for oversight and coordination of all quality improvement projects. Some team members had QI training through personal reading, attending seminars, etc. Training was coordinated through the Quality Improvement Coordinator and Administrator, and was provided to all physicians and staff who were on project teams.

The QI Committee was comprised of physicians, an administrator and assistant administrator, the director of nursing, the clinic medical director, the laboratory manager, a patient representative, and the managed care medical director. The QI Committee commissions teams to work on issues, and is the body to whom teams report results and recommendations. The Keene Board of Directors approved the work of the coding project teams before they began their work.

Figure 11.7: Keene Clinic Job Description: Quality Improvement Coordinator

TITLE: Quality Improvement Coordinator
DEPARTMENT: Administration
REPORTS TO: Administrator
JOB CLASSIFICATION: -----
EMPLOYEES DIRECTLY SUPERVISED: Administrative Secretary and Patient Representative

QUALIFICATIONS: Must possess tact and poise in dealing with people, both individually and in groups. A Bachelor's degree in either Business Administration or Health Administration is required. Additional training as a nurse, medical technologist, or physician assistant preferred.

SUMMARY: Performs a variety of duties related to the Clinic's efforts in continuous quality improvement through participative management, group dynamics and data accumulation and analysis. Serves as the organization's expert on the theory and practice of continuous quality improvement.

GENERAL RESPONSIBILITIES:

1.   Meets or exceeds standards of performance as established for employment at Keene Clinic.

2.   Assists in the identification and prioritization of problems to be assigned to project teams.

3.   Assists in the identification of participants for quality improvement project teams.

4.   Serves as project team facilitator, assisting the teams in their efforts by being an instructor, a coach, and a staff resource to the team.

5.   Performs and teaches others the process and tools of quality improvement, including data collection and analysis.

6.   Serves as staff to the Quality Improvement Committee.

7.   Stays current with continuous quality improvement theory and practice through self-instruction, attendance at approved workshops and seminars and networking with businesses and other healthcare providers.

8.   Submits reports and makes presentations as requested.

9.   Complies with all departmental and Keene Clinic policies and procedures.

10. Performs other duties and participates in special projects as appropriate or assigned.

• **Team development**

Keene began the project by organizing its teams. The team specialty areas for project focus were chosen by the Charge Submission Team, which provided oversight to project team activities. Potential team members were invited to participate by the QI Chairman and QI Coordinator. The Keene Oversight Committee, which had previously been examining the charge submission process, was comprised of the following staff:

Keene Oversight Committee

Purpose: To develop a consistent, timely charge submission process

Orthopedic Surgeon-Team Leader-H.R. Hansen, MD
Quality Improvement Coordinator/Facilitator-Kathleen Iannacchino, RN
Manager, Business Office-Jill Bond
Associate Administrator-Mike Chelstowski
CEO/Administrator-David Cooke, CPA
Supervisor, Data Processing-Christine Cunningham
LPN Supervisor-Pediatrics-Dale Randall
Supervisor-Physicians' Business Services-Sylvia Willard

The Oversight Committee developed the two coding project teams including the following staff:

Family Practice Charge Submission Team

Purpose: To examine the process of office-based charge submission

Physician-Team Leader-Don Mazanowski, MD
Ophthalmology Supervisor-Facilitator-Laura Judge
Receptionist-Andrea Adgie
Associate Administrator-Mike Chelstowski
Physician-Family Practice-Mark Newberry, MD
Physician's Assistant-David Segal, PA
Staff Nurse-Linda Thayer, LPN

General Surgery/Orthopaedics Charge Submission Team

Purpose: To examine the process of hospital-based charge submission

Orthopedic Surgeon-Team Leader-H.R. Hansen, MD
Supervisor, OB/GYN-Facilitator-Maria Powers, RN
Manager, Business Office-Jill Bond
General Surgeon-William V. Chase, MD
Staff Nurse-Surgery-Jeanine Key, RN

Supervisor, Orthopaedics-Barbara Taft, RN
Business Office-Mary Miller

Data collected by the team was reviewed at department meetings with both physicians and nursing staff. The physicians on the team solicited input and feedback from their colleagues, then brought that information back to the team. The QI Coordinator served as a liaison between the two teams and facilitated their meetings. She assisted with data collection and analysis so that improvement could be measured.

The Family Practice Team developed excellent ground rules for team meeting management. These rules helped to minimize power and authority issues among team members, and to focus the team on finding and improving root problem causes through data-driven teamwork. Their ground rules were:

1) Attendance is necessary.
2) Promptness is important—please try to be on time for the meetings.
3) Everyone participates in discussion and problem-solving.
4) Effective listening is important. Let a person finish what they're saying.
5) Talk one at a time.
6) The agenda for the following meeting will be discussed before ending each meeting.
7) Minutes will be taken and distributed to all team members.
8) Team meetings will be evaluated by participants.
9) Meetings will finish on time.

Coding project data collection and analysis

Keene followed a step-by-step approach to defining its coding process, studying the process, and implementing and monitoring improvements.

During Step 1, the process focus—coding—was identified by the Charge Submission Team. The team decided to subdivide study of the coding process into the two practice areas. They outlined the problem statement and related goals. The statement and goals were subsequently approved by the board. They identified the coding process customers: payors, whether third-party or patients. The team noted that coding requirements varied by payor, e.g., Medicare carrier.

11

The team defined its objectives for coding as:

1) Charges for services will be submitted within two business days of the date of service or hospital discharge date.

2) Medical records will be received in the departments with the appropriate charge documents attached, with 100 percent compliance expected.

The Family Practice team began by looking at process of office-based charge submission. After improvements in timeliness were demonstrated, the team shifted its focus to a more micro level. They began to study the timely submission of charges for ancillary tests. The team had identified this as an important area for potential savings and prevention of lost revenue.

Keene's baseline measurements were taken in March, 1992. 10 medical records were reviewed for each of four family practice physicians, equalling 40 records. Follow-up measures of the medical chart audit were not conducted, because the team did not find documentation to be a problem during its baseline measures. Keene team members decided to combine the goals of efficient and accurate coding under one heading. Project team efforts were focused upon Macro Measures 1, "Turnaround Days from Service to Billing."

Tables 11.2 and 11.3 outline the project findings of both Keene's family practice and general surgery/orthopaedics teams.

TABLE 11.2
Summary of Baseline and Final Measurements
Project Macro Measures — Keene Clinic: Family Practice

Measure	Baseline	Final
1. Turnaround (days): Service to Billing		
a. Unbilled ancillary charges	a. $14,000 in 3-week period	a. $4,000. 94% of charges submitted within two days using improved Encounter Form
b. Completeness of charge card (related to timely claims submission)	b. 42% returned incomplete	b. 16% returned incomplete
2. Supportable Coding Documentation	No problem (Dec. 1992)	Still no problem (Feb., 1994)
3. Denied/Resubmitted Claims Ratios Have established and maintained a less-than 5% return rate over an entire year.		
a. Ancillary charge cards returned	42%	16% Stat orders had a 0% return rate
4. Claims Edit Review (Medicode Claims Edit Manager)	Baseline not available	Measure not conducted-level of claims data analysis needed not as sophisticated as that provided.

TABLE 11.3
Summary of Baseline and Final Measurements
Project Macro Measures — Keene Clinic: General Surgery/Orthopaedics

Measure	Baseline	Final
1. Turnaround (days): Service to Billing	0-100%; average=50%	Orthopaedics: Submitted within 2 days=68% within 7 days=90% Surgery: Submitted within 2 days=25% within 7 days=43%
2. Supportable Coding Documentation	Baseline and final measures not taken.	
3. Denied/Resubmitted Claims Ratios	Baseline and final measures not taken.	
4. Claims Edit Review (Medicode Claims Edit Manager)	Baseline and final measures not taken.	

Some areas for possible further study were identified, but Keene's project efforts were concentrated on encounter form issues rather than the specifics of claim review.

Figure 11.8: Percentage of Keene Family Practice Ancillary Charges

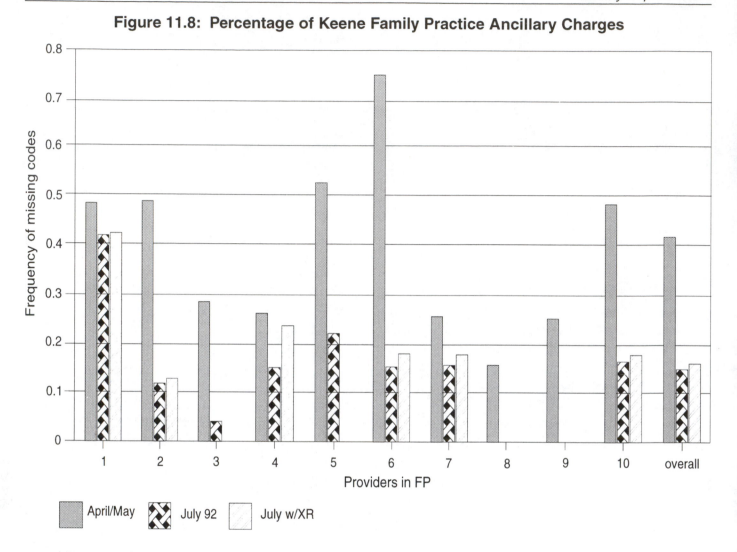

Keene's Step 2 was the process of team development, as described earlier in this chapter.

In Step 3, the team focused on the "diagnosis" of process problems. The Family Practice department staff felt that they were doing a better job with routine charge submission since they began using the encounter form as revised through the project team. The data they collected to check how the improved process was going indicated they were right—they had achieved a 94% compliance rate. The team believed that ancillary charges (lab and x-ray) were being returned for incomplete data. They wanted to examine and improve that process.

Data revealed that the range of ancillary charges returned went from a high of 78% to 18%, with an overall department return rate of 42 percent. Figure 11.8 shows data for April/May, June, July, and August 1992 illustrating the percentage of ancillary charges

with missing diagnosis codes. The approximate cost was $14,000 for unbilled charges in a three-week period. This figure does not include the direct and indirect costs of rework, decreased patient satisfaction, or the delayed billing- reimbursement cycle.

The team asked several key questions during this process:

- What are the root causes of the problems?

- Do STAT orders have missing diagnosis codes?

- Do phone orders include all necessary data?

Step 4 included the actual improvement implementation and monitoring of progress. Information was discussed at a department meeting and followed-up with a memo from the team leader to the other physicians and staff. The knowledge gained had a significant impact on the rate of error. This was evidenced by the decrease in ancillary charges returned. More importantly, behavior changes by providers such as supplying necessary information *at the time of patient scheduling* allowed the work to be done "the right way the first time."

The teams then reviewed the data collected to answer their Step 3 questions. They used graphs and charts to visually analyze the percentages of occurrence for each root problem cause.

In Step 5, the team checked results. They found that most providers had a dramatic decrease in the number of returned ancillary charges and their return rate.

What they learned and what improved

Keene believed that the system problems related to future ancillary service orders (and their accompanying reimbursement) would not have been discovered without the work of the QI teams on the coding process.

Work done by the Charge Submission Team resulted in the development and implementation of the encounter form to replace the charge card. The revised billing/encounter form more accurately reflected the functional needs of all coding process "customers"—physicians, billing clerks, medical records, etc.

As previously noted, the site received financial benefit from the improvement project, as they identified $14,000 in ancillary services not coded for only a three-week period. The project accelerated identification of other savings that could be realized through process improvement, such as services consistently filed with correct codes and appropriate supporting documentation. The project was a first step in further study of the claims denial process, to ensure that rework is eliminated.

After the technical end of the project, Keene has continued its QI efforts to monitor improvements it has implemented and to apply the techniques to new improvement challenges. The teams demonstrated that by simply examining the process and discussing variation, process improvement can be significant. In August, 1992, plans for continued team work included development of a code list for "call-in" lab work. One possible improvement solution that would be explored might be the training of the receptionists maintain such a list and to query any providers who order tests without diagnosis codes.

As with the Asheville site, some final reviews were viewed as less critical by the team, and were shifted in importance during meetings as other items took precedence.

Keene believes that improvement structured through the QI approach provides increased understanding of customer/supplier internal relationships and an appreciation for process complexity. For example, the complex links between the clinical departments and the business office were not clear to many staff before the project. Nursing provides an important link between administrative and clinical services, and is critical to the success of most teams.

The benefits of many different points of view were illustrated in the project teams. Often those without ownership in a process can ask more objective questions about the "whys" and "hows" of a process, which can lead to better improvements. This benefit can be gained by using the brainstorming process in the early part of a project, so that ideas can be freely generated without being prematurely evaluated.

Keene found the medical record audit aspect of the project to be especially useful. The audit pointed out variation within the Family Practice Department regarding levels of coding. In addition, it gave specific feedback to physicians about their coding and provided data that were useful in revising the encounter form.

Keene found that involving those who are not traditionally part of business office form development, but who have to use the form on a daily basis, was an important benefit. As issues about using a process were identified by those who used it (physicians coding on the form, for example), corrective response to those issues could be considered upfront in the design practice. Participants learned how to better work together as a team, providing improved morale with fewer barriers between departments. The resulting continued improvement in this area demonstrates this concept.

As with many practices, Keene found a significant need to increase physician awareness of coding's effect upon reimbursement and other major issues. General Surgery has maintained a timely submission rate of 80 percent and have discussed its project approach and findings with key individuals in all surgical subspecialties. While the Family Practice Department has undergone a number of staff and system changes since the project's end, data gathered through periodic spot checks and anecdotal information to confirm the gains have been held.

11

Some General Surgery (GS) practices adopted the charge process used in Orthopaedics. Department-specific data has been distributed to all of GS and is under discussion at their department meetings.

One reason for the improvement is greater physician awareness of the importance of correct and timely completion of the charge card. Another is that the team made the encounter form into a more efficient tool by including the most commonly used codes on the back of it.

Site self-evaluation: tools, project measures and experience

Which QI tools and techniques were most useful?

The QI tools and techniques used by Keene during the project included:

- brainstorming

- flowcharts

- cause and effect "fishbone" diagrams

- team meetings (meeting minutes)

- project storyboard

Examples of Keene's flowcharts, fishbone diagrams, and team meeting minutes appear as Figures 11.9, 11.10, and 11.11.

Figure 11.9: Lab Charge Process Flow in Family Practice - Keene Clinic

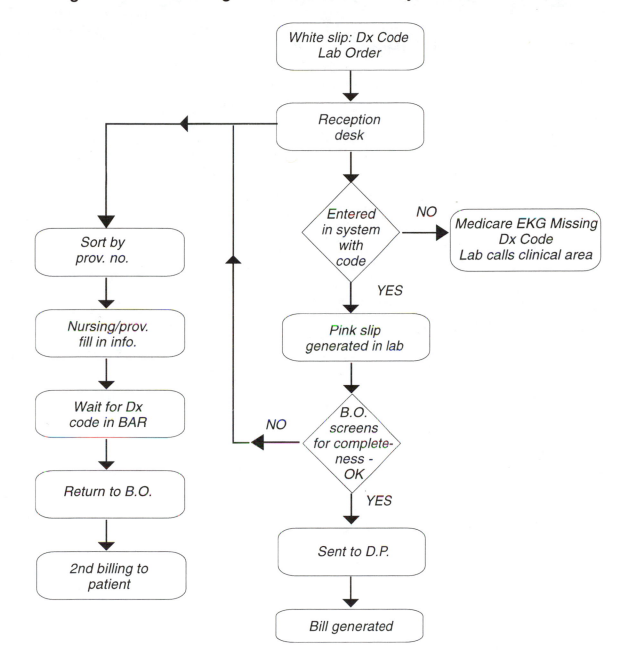

Figure 11.10: Fishbone Analysis of Delay in Charge Card Submission - Keene Clinic

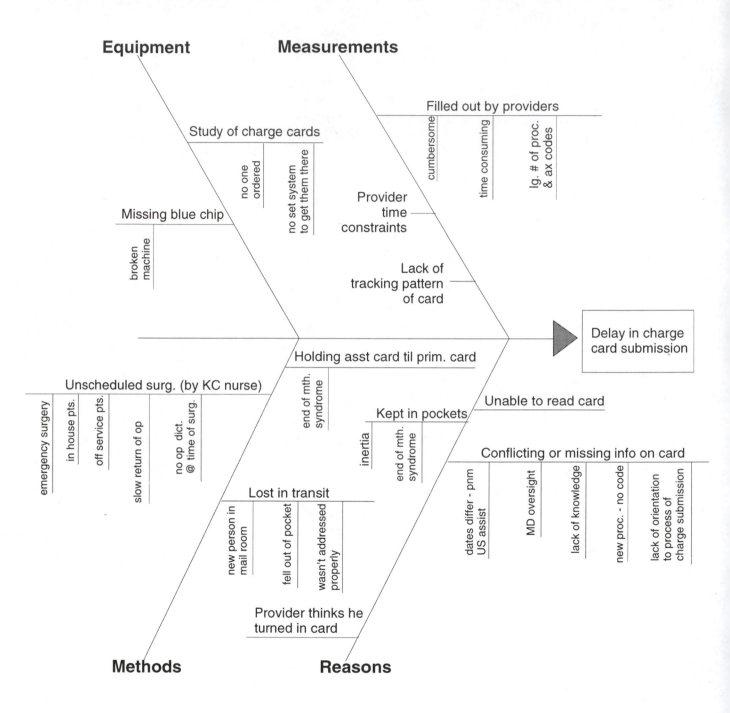

Figure 11.11: Meeting Minutes
Family Practice Charge Submission Team
FRIDAY, APRIL 10, 1992

The meeting began at 12:30 p.m.

1. Previous notes were reviewed.

2. Discussed difficulty of having the minutes typed. (_____) to discuss with ____ about having these minutes typed up by different secretaries.

3. Timeframe of project team reviewed. It was felt that six months was an adequate estimate of how long this project would take.

4. It was felt that the project team should develop data on making efficient changes to the present system. "Not just a bandaid."

5. Problem statement. It was felt the problem statement should be to establish a process that allows for the submission of all office charges (encounter forms) within two business days of the date of service with a target of 95% of these being accurate and complete.

6. The issue of lab and x-ray charge slips being returned was discussed. It was felt that this was part of the whole charge submission.

7. Flow Chart on Charge Submissions.

    1. Appointments are made and put in the computer.

    2. The charge is generated. A sticker is made at that time.

    3. The sticker is placed on the encounter form by the nurse or medical assistant.

    4. The patient is seen by the physician or provider. A note is dictated. Could also be seen as a nursing visit.

    5. Physician or provider fills out the encounter form.

    6. Nurses place on medication, extra medications or supply stickers.

    7. Encounter forms are collected by receptionist that evening or the next morning.

    8. Receptionist screens encounter form.

    9. Brings encounter forms back to provider, if changes or corrections need to be made.

    10. Receptionist sorts encounter forms in provider order and separates out Mathew Thornton Health Plan.

    11. Encounter forms are put in mail basket for pickup.

    12. They are sent to the Business Office.

8. ____ to look at charges within the Family Practice Department to determine how many charge submissions are late, how many mistakes there are.

9. Business Office to track the time differential between the date of service and when they actually get the charge submission. _____ to bring back data on this.

10. The next Charge Submission Committee Meeting will be on May 8th at 12:30 p.m.

Respectfully submitted:

Team recorder

(Copies to committee members)

The teams felt that producing the flowcharts clearly communicated the complexity of the process to those who may have initially thought coding was a simple clerical task. In addition, the flowchart helped to clearly identify areas of rework. Keene was the only demonstration site that used the storyboard format to capsulize their project experiences. They found the storyboard, with its brief text and graphic illustrations of improvement, to be an excellent tool for communicating progress with staff at all levels. The storyboard format that Keene used appears as Figure 11.12.

Pareto charts, histograms, and run charts were not used during the project. The teams and facilitators felt they were not necessary for data display in this case because the teams and facilitators were still in their early learning stages, and an effort was being made not to overwhelm them with statistical tools.

The Claims Manager system provided by Medicode was viewed by the site as an exceptionally powerful tool for looking at data. However, the level of claims analysis required by the project was not as sophisticated as the tool. Keene felt that until a project team has worked together on process improvement for a significant length of time, the amount and structure of the data provided by Claims Manager might be a little overwhelming.

Notes Iannacchino, "Tools are just **tools**—they do not give you magic answers. Information collection should be for the purpose of gathering information, not an end in itself, and must be kept manageable."

The site found that looking at the charge submission side of their practice allowed them to address several processes involved in appropriately documenting and billing for services rendered.

Difficulties and how they were overcome

While staff turnover was not historically a problem for Keene, systems are in place to ensure that new physicians and staff are educated both about the QI process approach as well as the specific processes in which they are involved. Keene uses employee orientation and direct team involvement to educate new staff and continue the learning of those who have worked with QI for some time. As payor and other coding requirements change, physicians and staff are informed through department chairs and department meetings. Teams may be reconvened as necessary if new requirements would alter the improved process.

Physician leadership was found to really accelerate the pace at which improvement can move. Keene found it very helpful to have a physician on the team who was proactive in communicating the team's goals to his peers, and soliciting input from them. The gains in awareness of the interlocked nature of all activities, whether clinical or administrative, need a physician to bridge the gap effectively with increasingly busy clinicians.

The 9-step system displayed in Figure 11.12 was used by Keene project teams as they worked to improve a work process. The Problem-Solving Process is used to guide the team through logical steps of analyzing and improving a work process. It also gives a method to display the progress and activities of the project team.

Figure 11.12: The StoryBoard Tool As Used by Keene Clinic
The 9-Step Problem-Solving Process
(The Storyboard)

STEP 1: DEFINE CUSTOMER REQUIREMENTS
  • *Survey*   • *Flowchart*   • *IPO Model*

STEP 2: COLLECT, ORGANIZE, AND DISPLAY DATA
  • *Survey*   • *Flowchart*   • *IPO Model*
  • *Run Chart* • *Histogram*

STEP 3: LIST AND PRIORITIZE IMPROVEMENT OPPORTUNITIES
  • *Improvement Opportunities Matrix*

STEP 4: DEFINE IMPROVEMENT OBJECTIVES
  • *Objective Statement*

STEP 5: ANALYZE AND SELECT THE ROOT CAUSE
  • *Fishbone Diagram* • *Pareto Chart*

STEP 6: GENERATE POTENTIAL SOLUTIONS
  • *Force Field Analysis*

STEP 7: SELECT THE BEST SOLUTION
  • *Solution Selection Matrix*

STEP 8: IMPLEMENT THE SOLUTION
  • *Implementation Plan Matrix*

STEP 9: TRACK EFFECTIVENESS
  • *Survey*   • *Checklist*   • *Log*

Story Board

DEPARTMENT _____ **NAME(S)** _____

Requirements	Measurement		
Define Requirements	Collect and Organize Data		
Action			
List and Prioritize Improvement Opportunities	Define Improvement Objective	Analyze and Select Most Significant Root Cause	Generate Potential Solutions
Select Best Solution	Implement Solution		Track Effectiveness

Case study: large academic practice

NORTHWESTERN MEDICAL FACULTY FOUNDATION, INC.

The Northwestern Medical Faculty Foundation, Inc. (the Foundation) is a large multispecialty academic group practice comprised of over 400 physicians and health care professionals who are faculty members of the Northwestern University Medical School in Chicago, Illinois. Through providers from 36 different medical and surgical specialties, the Foundation provides tertiary through primary care through a network of 35 clinical practice offices, a residency program and hospital care at Northwestern Memorial Hospital (including Prentice Women's Hospital and Maternity Center), Children's Memorial Hospital, the Rehabilitation Institute of Chicago as well as other associated institutions in the Chicago area.

The practice's mission statement reads as follows:

> It is the Foundation's mission to support the teaching and research functions of the Northwestern University Medical School through a commitment to the Medical School goals and objectives.

> Further, it is our mission to create a health care delivery system in which innovation in the provision of patient care services, use of sound practice management techniques, and responsible allocation of resources are used to create an environment in which health care professionals are educated and prepared to respond to a changing health care environment and future societal medical needs.

> Within this environment, it is our mission to support and facilitate the evolution of scientific endeavors from laboratory to direct delivery of care to our patients.

Description of major practice components

Reimbursement issues: The practice's reimbursement mix is currently about 13 percent self-pay; 22 percent commercial; 25 percent Medicare; nine percent public aid; and 31 percent managed care. During the project, the practice began to look more closely at its traditionally small involvement with managed care. It became evident that coordinating processes across departmental and functional lines, as well as the ability to retrieve and analyze utilization and reimbursement data, would be critical in a managed care environment.

Management style: Foundation departments are governed and managed by its Board of Directors which has ultimate decision and policy-making authority. Members of the Board include the Dean of the Medical School; the chairman of each clinical department in the Medical School that is represented in the Foundation; one section chief from the department of medicine and one from the department of surgery; six Foundation members-at-large; and two or more outside persons who are not health care professionals.

The Foundation is under the day-to-day direction of its President (who is the Dean of the Medical School) and its Senior Vice President/Medical Director. The executive management team is responsible for implementing Board-directed programs as well as for managing certain day-to-day practice activities.

In conjunction with physicians, the Director of Practice Operations and other department leaders, administrators at the specialty department level make decisions about how coding and other administrative functions will be managed. All Foundation departments use the same integrated practice management system for registration, billing, appointment scheduling, and managed care information. Monthly practice activity reports—financial and receivables management reports including various service, income, collection, reimbursement analysis and appointment scheduling information—are distributed by department. Executive management reviews various summary reports of activity across departments.

Staff activities: In addition to its full-time faculty, the Foundation employs over 700 FTE nurses with an RN degree or above, 14 LPNs, and 400 administrative and clerical support staff. Practice management at the department level is decentralized. Of the 36 practice specialties, three clinical areas (obstetrics/gynecology, surgery, and orthopedic surgery) were involved in the coding project. In some areas, coding is handled directly by the physicians, while in others, dedicated coding staff are responsible for coding. In addition, a central administrative department (Professional Fee Support Services) provides coding and reimbursement support.

Processes to be improved: Coding analysis is done in conjunction with information downloaded from the main system and information obtained by audits performed by the Quality Assurance (QA) area of the Professional Fee Support Services department.

Monthly reports provide data regarding certain performance indicators that are shared between departments. However, at the outset of the project, coding process data was not routinely shared nor was such sharing formally approved by upper management. The practice felt that this departmentalized approach might be hiding some opportunities to more effectively and efficiently manage coding. At the beginning of the project, the practice had monitors in place to determine how long after the date of service that charges are posted and claims actually prepared, but were not able to track how long it took before the claims were actually filed after preparation.

When the project began, it typically took 60 days from the date of service before claims for surgical care were submitted. This was because these claims were frequently held for manual processing while operative room reports were found and attached to them. As these were typically high-dollar claims, this delay contributed significantly to accounts receivable. There was no procedure for processing anesthesia claims requiring similar attachments.

How they got started with QI

*   **Introducing the concepts and project; training.**

Prior to the project, some staff members had basic knowledge of QI concepts through basic courses or personal reading. The Foundation did not use the roll-out approach to QI training. The absence of a common QI language or experience made the team's work in defining its purpose and actively involving its members in improvement a very lengthy process (see Difficulties and How They Were Overcome later in this chapter).

Like other demonstration sites, the Foundation received a one-day briefing by Medicode on extracting information from medical records for quantitative assessment purposes. The team used this training in its review of medical records in support of Macro Goal #2 (supportable coding).

Team development. An interdepartmental team was formed to guide project coding process improvement. The team was comprised of:

*   Director, Professional Support Services-Richard Nagengast

*   Manager of Information Systems-Andrew Capron

*   Department Administrator, Surgery-Chris Durovich

*   Department Administrator, Orthopedic Surgery-John Galleazzi

*   Department Administrator, Obstetrics/Gynecology-Connie Wolf

*   Director, Ambulatory Care Services-Nancy Koch

*   Director, Professional Billing-Ann Riordan

*   Project Manager, Ambulatory Care Administration-Anita Majerowicz

*   Manager, Professional Fee Support Services-Debra Gaskin

*   Manager, Medical Records-Carol Matusewick.

Clinical staff were not initially involved on the project team. The Project Manager, Ambulatory Care Administration initially served as facilitator, leader and recorder. Due to personnel changes, responsibility for the project shifted to Richard Nagengast, the Foundation's Director of Professional Support Services in August, 1992. The team was organized in March, 1992 and held its first meeting on April 5, 1992.

11

As the team worked to prioritize its data collection goals and improvement strategies, it was suggested that the use of a smaller taskforce within the team might be effective. The subgroup would work on activities such as process diagrams and flowcharts. Team members with more availability participated in the subgroup.

The team also sought advice about improvement possibilities from practice staff outside the project. They asked a previously established workgroup— the Front-End Systems Team—to exchange data and improvement ideas. This workgroup was initially established as an accounts receivable improvement task force. However, its original focus had expanded to include work on overall practice operations. It had already served for two years as a forum for suggesting broader improvement. The Front-End Team had previously used QI brainstorming in their efforts. The project team felt it natural to present project findings to the Front-End Team and to solicit their feedback. Subsequently, several of the first recommendations for process improvement came from the Front-End Systems team.

Coding project root cause identification, data collection and analysis: The site conducted baseline and final measures on the four project macro issues. A previous arrangement between the Foundation and Medicode had already determined that Medicode's Claims Manager system would be used to analyze potential claims denial issues for the practice. This arrangement extended beyond the limited specialties included in the project.

The project team chose to study the practice's 10 most frequently performed inpatient procedures. Each diagnosis code was represented by at least 10 records. Because of limited staff, it was believed that any additional record review would not allow the review to occur in a timely manner. Records were identified for review through a data search of the practice's billing and accounts receivable system. Table 11.4 lists these codes.

Table 11.4 Codes selected for
CRAHCA/Medicode QI CODING PROJECT
1992 CPT-4 Code Descriptions
Northwestern Medical Faculty Foundation

CPT-4 Procedure Code Number	Procedure Name	Other Descriptors
27130	Arthroplasty	Acetabular and proximal femoral prosthetic replacement (total hip replacement), with or without autograft or allograft
27447	Arthroplasty, knee, condyle and plateau	Medial AND lateral compartments with or without patella resurfacing ("total knee replacement")
30520	Septoplasty or submucous resection	With or without cartilage scoring, contouring or replacement with graft
33512	Coronary artery bypass	Autogenous graft, (e.g.,, saphenous vein or internal mammary artery); three coronary grafts
35301	Thromboendarterectomy	With or without patch graft; carotid, vertebral, subclavian, by neck incision
47605	Cholecystectomy	With cholangiography
58150	Total abdominal hysterectomy	(Corpus and cervix), with or without removal of tubes(s), with or without removal or ovary (s).
59400	Vaginal delivery	Vaginal delivery only (with or without episiotomy and/or forceps) including postpartum care
61712	Microdissection	Intracranial or spinal procedure (list separately in addition to code for primary procedure)
66984	Cataract removal	Extracapsular cataract removal with insertion of intraocular lens prothesis (one stage procedure), manual or mechanical technique (e.g., irrigation and aspiration)

The Foundation's baseline measurements were taken in April, 1992. Medical records were reviewed for each of 49 physicians in the three project specialties, for a total of 165 records reviewed. Final measurements taken in March, 1993 included 69 records for 27 physicians.

Table 11.5 summarizes the site's project measurement information. Since it was thought that the information from the Claims Manager review might provide additional information for the audit process, the medical record audit was conducted after the Claims Manager edit. The team included supporting documentation from outside the medical record in its study, such as invoices, explanations of benefits (EOBs) sheets, and accounts receivable information. By doing this, the site combined measurements for Macro Goal #2 (supportable documentation) and Macro Goal #3 (denied claims ratio).

The Director of Support Services coordinated the baseline data collection. The Professional Fee Support Services QA staff performed the audit and review for the three project departments. The site also did additional data searches through specific practice management systems on the central computer. The Foundation's process to determine coding accuracy for the project diagnoses was:

1) Each inpatient record was abstracted.

A. The post-operative diagnosis and procedure listed on the operative report, pathology report, discharge summary and diagnoses coded on the hospital facesheet were abstracted. The post-operative diagnosis on the operative report was used even though this might not have been the principal admitting diagnosis. However, the team decided this was appropriate since the abstractor reviewed the inpatient medical record documentation to determine the appropriate diagnoses for billing that particular surgical procedure, not the principle condition for the patient's hospital admission.

B. Medicare guidelines published in the *Federal Register* were used in abstracting.

2) This information was then compared to the diagnosis and procedure codes submitted for billing on the invoice.

TABLE 11.5
SUMMARY OF BASELINE AND FINAL MEASUREMENTS PROJECT MACRO MEASURES
Northwestern Medical Faculty Foundation, Inc.

Measure	Base April 1992	Final March 1993
1. Turnaround (days): Service to Claim Submission		
a. Surgical claims	60 days	
b. OB/GYN	No data provided	Both surgical and OB/GYN claims submitted within practice time limits for claim submission
2. Supportable Coding Documentation and 3. Denied/Resubmitted Claims Ratios		
	165 records/49 physicians	64 records/27 physicians
a. Documented but not coded	a. $10,000 potential revenue	
b. Denied claims	b.$110,00(all denial types)	
4. Claims Edit Review (Medicode Claims Manager)		
	No baseline	60,478 total claims reviewed (surg., ortho., OB/GYN)

Data from the Claims Manager edit included an indication that office visits were being billed as minor surgical services which included variable preoperative and postoperative services. Because of the indefinite pre- and postoperative services related to the surgical procedures, the usual "package" concept for surgical procedures could not be applied to them. Other procedures did follow the "package" concept and were not usually billed with an office visit.

In addition, the Claims Manager edit indicated possible unbundling across the three departments. The team decided that further research into these data were needed before any department-level action was taken. As at ACA, subsequent research into these data found that the software's screens for potential Medicare denials were more rigorous than what the practice was actually encountering. This was specifically noted regarding unbundling of lab tests. However, the record audit findings generally supported the findings of the Claims Manager edit.

The team's analysis of "documented but not coded" services showed that while the frequency of such services was low (spanning 13 occurrences and five different codes), the potential lost revenue equalled nearly $10,000.

After locating these improvement opportunities, the team discussed possible improvement solutions. Subsequently, procedures were implemented for processing anesthesia claims requiring attachments.

Due to the variance in how the coding process was carried out in each department, the project was actually measuring a multiple number of coding processes rather than one. Information was collected by the team and for each procedure a graph was used to illustrate the percentage of codes that:

- had supportable documentation

- followed Medicare's rules for global surgery coding

- were upcoded, downcoded, or unbilled

- were invalid or incomplete codes

- were not documented

- had been assessed a late charge

- claim was rejected by the payor.

A sample graph for the procedure "total knee replacements" appears as Figure 11.8.

By comparing the procedure-code specific graphs, the team saw a difference in the types of coding problems by department. Related to the item "had been assessed a late charge", the Foundation had established specific targets for timely submission of claims: a late charge indicated the target was not met. The reasons for delay again varied by department, with delay often associated with obtaining supporting documentation. Other comparisons can be made, but the major point in comparing these measures across departments is to identify opportunities for improvement while indicating who may have already developed a "best practice" in coding.

The project team was very concerned with data collection issues. They were concerned with choosing a sample size that was truly representative. They wanted to weight the importance of different inputs to the process by their problem-causing significance. Sample size was minimized by availability resources of staff, but was at least a starting point for asking further questions about the process. The team discussed at length data stratifications (billing area, department, specialty) that would be most meaningful to them.

Once the team received its initial data, some members wanted to follow the natural inclination to "go fix" the items identified in the baseline measures. However, the facilitator cautioned them that a process overview across departments was still needed, and that action based on one set of measures might be premature.

The OB/GYN department began further study of the extent and possible causes of the unbundling issue as identified through the claims edit. This work led to proposed revisions of the gynecology inpatient voucher as suggested by a team based in the OB/GYN department. This team decided to ask its physicians about coding issues to learn more about what sort of forms, education, etc. would best meet their process needs. The OB/GYN team also identified other coding reference resources that were not currently utilized, and raised awareness about the coding process complexity of the department. The OB/GYN Department used a cause and effect approach and flowcharting to analyzing the problem of unbundling.

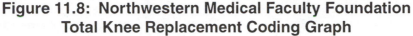

Figure 11.8: Northwestern Medical Faculty Foundation Total Knee Replacement Coding Graph

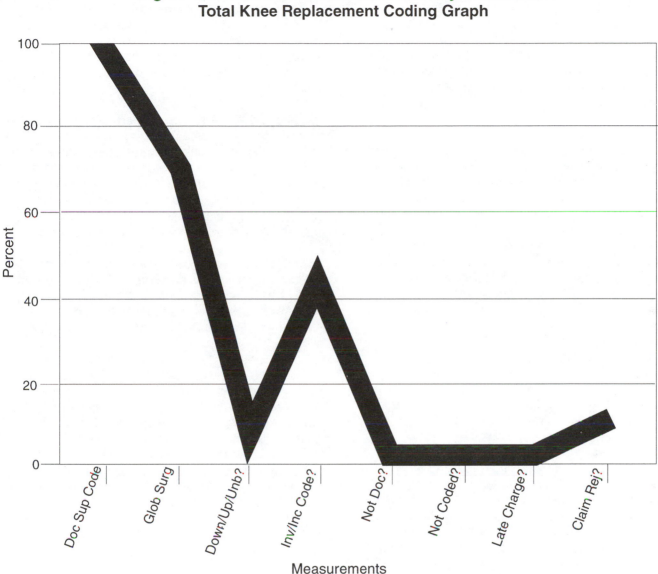

After several months of work, the team made a report to the Foundation's Finance Committee in May 1993 about the project and its findings. The committee endorsed continued efforts to improve coding using the QI approach.

What they learned and what improved

The site notes that it learned a great deal about data collection and sharing simply from the process of analyzing the baseline measures. Through this experience, team members learned that data reporting must be very concise and focused if it is to be understood and used by team participants.

The Foundation believes that project involvement helped to raise awareness among site staff and prepare them for increasing cost and utilization controls from managed care, government, etc. and other players. These external pressures demand that practices really understand their critical processes.

One improvement implemented to address the problem with delayed attachments was a revision of the billing system's procedure code dictionary. Selection criteria were identified to assure that procedures requiring operative reports and/or other payor-specific attachments were flagged to "drop to paper," as opposed to electronic transmission of the claim. A procedure was implemented to procure the attachments within specific timeframes to expedite timely claims submission. After the project, the site planned to work with specific carriers that process claims electronically. They planned to pursue electronic acceptance of claims requiring attachments and to develop a mechanism to transmit additional information in this same manner.

The site plans to build on the credibility of its existing QA structure and the Front-End Systems team for continuing QI activities. At the project's end, it was thought that the Front-End team might break into "task groups" for specific initiatives. The newly established position of director of management engineering will be an integral team member.

Two significant programs have been implemented which were direct outgrowths of the QI project experience and other Foundation quality improvement activity. A new "Audit Assessment" program has been implemented by the Quality Assurance area, using the QI approach to develop recommendations for improvement. Areas of focus include lost charges, levels of service and coding inaccuracies. This represents the restructuring of a function and its reporting relationship. This restructuring is to improve the quality and efficacy of the front-end charge capture process. Both these programs utilize many of the same quality measures used in the QI project.

The site found the medical record/invoice audit to be helpful. It confirmed where coding was being done effectively while highlighting specific documentation issues that really needed attention. In addition, while its data analysis was at a level that was somewhat advanced for the team's functional level during the project, the Foundation found the Claims Manager edit to be helpful because helped to point out potential problems.

Several team members found flowcharting to be a valuable way to quickly see "traffic patterns" in the coding process.

Difficulties and how they were overcome

The site approached the coding project with the support of the Director of Ambulatory Services. While upper management supported the group's involvement, they were not in a leadership role in the project nor represented on the team. Therefore, the perceived importance of the coding improvement effort relative to other organizational priorities was lessened. Some members viewed the project as another "administrative" project and did not see it as a priority for staff and time resources.

In addition, because some felt that project information would not affect physician behavior, they were not convinced of its value. The team leader worked to develop the team's understanding of the value of process improvement, so that concerns about team goals and priorities could be addressed openly and effectively.

The team worked to reduce concerns about data-sharing. Sharing of data regarding error rates and particular process problems was a new experience for some team members. Since little precedent had been set in the culture for sharing between departments, it took some time to develop a comfort level regarding the goals and purposes of data collection and analysis. Over time, some data-sharing did occur.

Another issue arose related to standardization of data collection. Some team members were not comfortable with comparing their data with that of other areas, since their processes varied widely from each other. For example, the OB/GYN department's coding was based on physician communication with the coders, but in the General Surgery area the coders had little physician interaction. Meanwhile, in Orthopaedics, the physicians coded directly without using a coder. The team began data collection soon after forming. However, once the medical record audit began, it became clear that the team members wished to know more about the criteria by which their department's records would be judged. Some members were ready to share data, and encouraged the rest of the team to do so through further discussion. The team members were given information about the criteria for supporting documentation review, as well as the training received from Medicode. Over time, the team discussed the data, and was able to move on.

Perhaps related to practice cultural issues about data-sharing and/or the project's potential usefulness, the team took additional time to take initial steps like flowcharting the current process. They "could not move forward without data." In addition to the time it takes to design an effective data collection system for a complex process, the team also spent some time in working with Medicode to get claims analysis information into a format that more precisely met their needs.

Chapter Twelve
Case Study Analysis

The experiences of the case study demonstration sites were similar in many ways and unique to their practice setting in others. In the following analyses, major improvement issues are discussed by specific topic. Examples from the case studies which most clearly illustrate those issues are included. To assist in understanding your own practice issues and experiences, it is suggested that these evaluations be used in conjunction with the material in Chapters 1 through 10.

Data Collection, Display and Analysis

In ACA's description, we find the statement "Based on these discussions, the team felt the problems were so obvious that additional data were not required before work on improvement could begin." ACA ultimately experienced a positive result from action without data. Since the practice had a very minimal coding and claims follow-up system prior to the coding project, perhaps any work done to establish a process was of value. However, this positive result is more the exception than the rule. How would a team know that it was designing the process with the maximum capability? How would they know if the process was being designed most efficiently, or which process steps might contain the greatest potential for variation? What kind of variation might they contain?

Data overkill ("analysis paralysis") is a real and present danger. At some point, all project sites used a tool that provided process information that was either too detailed or had a focus that didn't match the objective for data collection. The team should clarify which data collection tools and data display formats most closely meet their objectives *before* tools are developed and used. Refer again to Chapter 6 to consider the four strategies of data aggressiveness.

Figure 10.5 is an excellent example of an ACA tool used to disaggregate data and "cut new windows". It was developed with minimal resources and did not require extensive training or tools. However, remember that clear operational definitions must be developed in advance of using such a checksheet to collect data. Even though column headings may seem self-explanatory, don't assume that everyone will interpret them in the same way!

The ACA coding team originally focused on the coding process. Their foray into the related billing system was

a natural part of their learning process. However, each significant, lasting improvement requires clear, specific objectives and related data collection and analysis. Groups commonly have difficulty in narrowing down the processes to study. "Solving world hunger" diffuses energy and makes focus on specific root causes difficult. While the processes are certainly interrelated, a continued, focused data collection and study localizes the problem and keeps the improvement on track.

Using only two data points to make assumptions is a common error in early data collection and analysis. Because resources of time and staff are increasingly tight, it is tempting to delay or even forgo ongoing measurements. In all project sites, some data were measured once at baseline but not remeasured to confirm the results of the implemented improvement. The Foundation project team struggled to balance the knowledge that one data collection alone (the baseline) could not provide sufficient improvement information, but yet there was the need to start somewhere on improvement. Valid samples and the time required to remeasure must be balanced with the realities of other demands on staff time. As described in Chapter 7, two-point measures often mask or distort the root questions that should be asked about a process, and should be avoided.

Used by all project sites, pie charts and similar graphs are a variation on the problem with bar charts. Data is overly aggregated and trends can be assumed where none exist. Pareto charts, histograms and scattergrams are the preferred graphical displays because they fully portray variation. For example, Keene might have used Pareto charts to look at the reasons for charge card returns, and histograms to display submission times.

While improvement efforts without data can provide staff with a sense that "something is being accomplished" or that "things are getting better", valid data measured at routine interval are critical. These data help immensely to ensure that changes made really significant result in process improvement. If the team skips the step of identifying true root causes and moves directly to solutions, major potential for inappropriate action exists. Avoiding data collection often results in a group of people without a unified language to accurately describe and assess the problem.

Goal-Setting and Process Capability

In each project site, there were instances in which goals were set at less than 100 percent. This is sometimes done in an attempt to make improvement seem manageable and/or more possible. A team may feel it creates too much pressure on those doing the work to be "perfect", i.e., to commit to 100 percent. However, this misses the correct focus: is the process as currently designed truly capable of reaching 100 percent?

An ACA example was the goal "100 percent of patient registration forms will be completely and accurately filled in and will be sent to the business office in a timely manner". Will the current process for collecting information on the forms ever allow this goal to be achieved? What steps in the process limit its capability? What if the process doesn't include a step in which the patient is asked for any insurance coverage changes? Without that step, it is very unlikely that the process will *ever* allow the information to be complete *and* accurate *and* forwarded in a timely manner.

It seems the real intent is to provide the business office with patient registration information they need in a timely, complete, and accurate manner. Does this statement of the goal bring to mind more possibilities for improvement than just better form-completion? Perhaps the business office doesn't need the forms at all—perhaps the information can be provided through another, better avenue. If so, effort focused on insistence that no mistakes are made without reconsidering the process might be misplaced.

Another example comes from Keene. As a problem statement, the Family Practice Project Team wrote, "to establish a process that allows for the submission of all office charges (encounter forms) within two business days of the date of service with a target of 95 percent of these being accurate and complete." Notice the use of "all office charges", "95 percent", "within two business days".

Does this problem statement help to define current process capability or to localize a major opportunity? The statement's major elements seem to assume that what is needed is for the process to produce more accurate items within a shorter timeframe. Is the current process capable of doing this? How was 95 percent chosen? By examining these questions, a more focused approach can be taken, which should result in more effective use of energies.

All project sites noted a determination to "do it right the first time". However, would the process allow that to happen?

Process capability is the important issue. If the process is improved, e.g., more efficient, less complex, etc., then it may be capable of meeting 100 percent of a goal. Processes should be redesigned with 100 percent as the goal. If the process is not capable of reaching the 100 percent, the goal may frustrate more than motivate. Such a problem lies with the process not the goal. The reader is referred to Chapter 7, "A Word About Goals".

Reducing Variation=Key to Improvement

The process variations found in ACA's coding and broader billing processes made those processes prime candidates for improvement. This is illustrated in Figure 10.2, in the points "four different entry points coming in office", "various people collecting data" and "different agreements and requirements with agencies". The Foundation included numerous departments that represented several different coding processes. ACA found that by standardizing the inputs and processes to the greatest extent possible, variation was reduced and improvement occurred. Standardization of all processes, particularly complex ones, reduces variation. This should increase efficiencies and thus higher quality process results.

Again, to correctly study variation, we must know if a process is stable. Figure 10.8 displays the frequency of missing diagnosis codes by Keene provider, as a percentage of ancillary charges. Some questions that could be asked about this figure are:

- Was this a stable process during the two data collection points of study? (April/May 1992 and July 1992)

- Was there special cause variation related to Provider #6? (Provider 6 accounted for the only incidence of missing codes that was greater than 50 percent, in the April/May 1992 data collection)

- Was special cause variation the source of the significant decrease in the percentage of missing codes between the April/May and July collections?

Another potentially helpful question might be: what codes accounted for 80 percent of the missing codes? A stratification by codes might indicate a code that is particularly troublesome to use, e.g., poorly defined or a newer code whose use is not well-understood by providers.

Sometimes "natural relationships" can provide a clue toward improvement opportunity definition. For example, the Foundation might conduct further improvement work focused on departments in which physicians directly did the coding, rather than trying to improve all coding processes (including those departments which utilized coders) from the beginning. Or, processes common to several specialty areas, e.g., pediatric immunization follow-up, might include pediatrics and OB/GYN.

Both Keene and ACA teams found that revision of the encounter form to more closely fit user needs was important in reducing variation.

Selection, Suggestions and Solutions

"Suggestions" for areas needing improvement within a practice are often actually proposed solutions. The statement "need for nursing protocols" identified by ACA's physicians is one example. This skips the step of identifying what is being observed that needs improvement. An example of stating an observable occurrence that would lead to process improvement might be "patient care is variable, resulting in miscommunication, repeated tests, etc." Rather than being the actual process to be improved, nursing protocols would be only one possible solution to improving the patient care process. This ACA team may have been more effectively focused on answering the question, "What are you observing due to a lack of nursing protocols?" Again refer to the set of questions posed by Berwick in Chapter 2, regarding "does this ever happen to you?"

Project selection based on anecdote and opinions creates problems with identifying the most important processes to study and finding root causes of process variation. Especially in a Pareto format, data can assist in effective project selection by stripping excess emotion from the selection process.

External pressures upon the practice—payors, consumers, regulators, media—are numerous and constant. Often these external pressures are the catalysts for the practice's consideration of QI. Each of the demonstration sites noted that their interest in QI was stimulated by rapid, continuing changes in their environment. However, it is recommended that QI is chosen proactively, not because it is mandated or perceived as a "quick fix", but because it provides the logical path to sound decision-making.

Whether administrative or clinical, our training often supports a crisis-oriented approach to problem-solving. This can disrupt efforts to manage process improvement from a data-driven approach. For example, a team member may feel they "know all the answers" or want the problem "fixed right away". They may experience frustration when asked to take what is sometimes perceived as a slower path to improvement. When the Keene team experienced this, they used periodic, demonstrated progress to highlight the benefits of the QI approach to those ready to leap ahead without data. While it may not be possible to convince everyone of the value of QI, its use by a majority does result in better decisions and actions.

Upper Management Support of Improvement Efforts

Substantial learning can occur when practices use a project-specific approach to QI implementation. However, the coding project research underscores that demonstrated upper management support for the implementation of even a single team is essential to significant improvement.

At ACA, the Quality Council directed the choice of QI and the Deming method as well as the QI implementation plan. At Keene, the project work was guided by the Charge Submission Team. In both cases, management had established a mechanism to coordinate and evaluate the work of specific project teams.

At Keene, the board approved the goals and approach of the team before their work began. However, such approvals were granted on a project-specific basis. At the Foundation, project activities slowed because several team members did not perceive that the QI approach was valued by upper management. After the technical end of the project, QI received more management sanction through establishment of a standing team. After that, resistance to data-sharing and collection among the Foundation's project team members was further reduced. Since ACA had support for their teams through an established mechanism (the Quality Council), they did not experience these same problems.

Whether project-specific or organization-wide, approval from upper management for QI activities and timelines is important. Even on a project basis, the changes in thinking required to use the QI approach are significant. They represent change not only for those on teams but for everyone, especially upper management. Significant problems can occur if a board learns of "employee empowerment" in vague, potentially threatening terms rather than through an educational process that includes their modelling of QI behavior.

It is up to organizational leadership whether QI learning occurs through major training simultaneously at all levels, or whether the learning and change is more incremental (the project approach). Demonstration site experiences support the premise that the potential level of improvement is directly related to demonstrated management commitment to the QI approach.

Physicians, Patients and Other Customers: What Does the Customer Want?

When looking at the coding process, one of the first questions asked by Keene's Family Practice Project Team was, "what do the insurance companies want?". If a major function of coding is to communicate "services rendered" to payors, payor formats and definitions are important to consider in process improvement. Both external customers (patients, payors, regulators) and internal customers (physicians, nurses, billing office, etc.) were considered in project process improvement.

Physician involvement was shown in all three project sites to be critical to improvement efforts. Physicians are major customers and/or suppliers in virtually every process in the medical practice. For effective process change, they should be included in process improvement from the beginning. When physicians and other clinical leaders are not involved in improvement efforts *at the outset*, they often view the efforts as unimportant to their daily lives, or as another administrative roadblock that reduces their time with patients.

Keene believed that consistent physician participation on their Family Practice Project Team was a major factor in the teams' improvement success. They noted that lack of physician participation on the General Surgery/ Orthopaedics team impeded its progress. At the Foundation, some team members perceived that the coding project was an administrative effort not supported by clinicians. This perception was perhaps supported by the lack of physician representation on the initial team. This lessened the credibility of the data and project among the team members.

There are a variety of ways to involve and interest physicians in improvement efforts. Most people's curiosity is raised when confronted with a question like: "Would you like to be involved in reducing the time you spend doing *x* (looking for medical records, finding exam room supplies, calling for consult information, resubmitting claims denied, etc.)?"

The Foundation's OB/GYN department asked its physician customers what education, forms, etc. would be most useful to them to accomplish coding tasks. ACA surveyed physicians and staff about the issues that they felt were most important to improve.

Direct compensation for work on improvement teams is one strategy to involve clinicians in improvement efforts. However, in a cost-containment era, appealing to quality of work life may be a more viable option for most organizations. Any conditions for involvement (e.g., time to participate in team meetings and data collection, compensation for productivity lost, etc.) must be made clear and applied fairly across physicians.

Clinician involvement should not be limited only to physicians. All relevant clinical customers and suppliers—nurses, assistants, technicians, therapists—should be included when assessing a process for improvement. Nursing and other clinicians played key roles in the project teams at all sites.

In discussions about the many customers in our complex healthcare processes, we often return to focus on the person traditionally called "patient". The patient was included as customer of the coding process both as a potential payor and as someone who could encounter difficulties resulting from ineffective coding process. This was seen in ACA's case study; patient calls to the business office regarding denied bills or delayed payment created significant work and extra steps for patients and staff. Keene included the patient as a potential payor in its initial problem statement.

When considering process improvement, always consider the process' effect on the patient, even if the process is "non-clinical". Inclusion of patients in redesign of those processes most critical to them-patient flow, medical record access, scheduling and registration-is especially important. Whether the person is called "patient", "member", "client" or by another name, process improvement must consider whom the process has really been designed to serve. The patient focus is combined with the view of the other process suppliers and customers to gain true perspective on the current process.

To Team or Not to Team

Some believe that too many teams working on too many issues at once is ineffective. They believe this focuses energy on less-than-significant issues, not on systemic root problems. Division of improvement work into "too many teams" can create its own set of problems, including administrative time for coordination among teams, false divisions between administrative and clinical issues, etc.

ACA found three teams to be an appropriate number with which to begin their improvement efforts. In a larger practice, just three teams might find it difficult to identify and implement significant improvements for the whole practice. Again, the focus should be on those processes that can provide significant improvement—transformation.

Sometimes an ineffective proliferation of teams is the result of over-separation between "administrative" and "clinical" teams. ACA believed that by establishing a team focused on primarily clinical processes and other teams focused on primarily administrative work, they strengthened QI buy-in for both segments. They felt this assisted with education about and experience with the QI model and tools. But because both physicians and administrators were essential process customers and suppliers for the coding process, ACA included both on the coding team..

Most practice processes include elements of clinical and administrative tasks, e.g., medical records management. Developing a clinical team may seem the best route to directly involve clinical staff. However, integration of each type of staff on each team provides the broader perspective needed for significant change. Processes should be selected for improvement primarily for the significance of their improvement potential.

The people who fill various team roles like facilitator and recorder are not required to have supervisory authority over the process. They may not even be supervisors at all. The person who can be the most effective team facilitator sometimes comes from outside the process. By placing persons who are not usually in authority in these team roles, lower-level staff enthusiasm for tackling complex tasks like data analysis and change can be heightened and maintained at a higher level. Group management skills, including conflict resolution, are very important to the facilitator role. The role of recorder requires accuracy and the ability to communicate by effective summaries of conversations and key points.

Such a person can sometimes be perceived by other team members as more fair or less threatening than a formal authority figure. Keene found that just the presence of higher-level administrators on the team sometimes constrained the team as they tried to brainstorm. While management must be informed about team activities and use their findings to make better management decisions, this does not mean they must be a member of every process improvement team.

While lunch may seem to be a trivial issue to some, Keene in particular found food to be a gracious acknowledgement of additional time spent to improve practice operations. Meals provided a social equalizer as well as an icebreaker to smooth the more difficult aspects of the team's work!

Training and Staff Involvement

ACA found that their approach to physician QI training—training some physicians but not all at the same time—slowed down their ability to implement improvement. Since the project, ACA has revised their approach by creating additional opportunities for exposure to QI concepts and quantitative thinking for both physicians and staff (see Chapter 10). In a larger practice, there may be additional pressures to train only certain staff at different intervals. In those cases, the objectives of the organization's improvement efforts guide who gets what training when. The Physician Quality Improvement Seminar (Appendix B) is an excellent way to expose many clinicians to QI concepts before they become involved on a specific team.

The Foundation encountered a barrier to staff involvement common in practices of all sizes—fear of data-sharing. It can be difficult to share data across departmental and functional lines, particularly in complex academic environments. In these settings, departments have often traditionally had great administrative autonomy. The language needed to discuss data and to remove the fear that it "won't be used against me" is time-consuming to learn. No one wants their department to be "the worst".

Resource prioritization and political agendas are other aspects of this barrier. Setting goals and moving ahead with improvement in the face of this barrier takes time, data and persistent energy. For example, the Foundation project team took several months to get comfortable with why data would be shared, what data would be shared, and what the consequences of open problem identification would be. In addition, environmental factors play a role in how improvement can proceed. For example, the medical record audit as conducted at the Foundation would be very different if the coder did not have direct access to the inpatient medical record. Overcoming concerns about QI can be greatly accelerated by clear direction about the whys and hows of a project team. These messages begin with training and awareness-building, and continue through consistent, positive reinforcement from management.

Over time, with consistent management support of the project and the QI approach, the Foundation reduced this barrier. Leadership and acceptance among organizational leaders, especially clinical leaders, was again shown to be related to the success of improvement efforts.

The realities of just how busy people are in their work lives makes upfront planning for concise, effective meetings *critical* to the success of QI efforts. This is evidenced by support such as allowing for reimbursement, time off in trade, etc. Sometimes people can be motivated by a chance for improved "quality of worklife": reducing the "hassle factor", reducing interdepartmental barriers, etc.

Finding a champion for process improvement can take time! At the Foundation, the OB/GYN department administrator emerged as someone who felt comfortable with the QI data-sharing approach. That person served as a leader in data sharing and process improvement. The fact is that not everyone will be excited by a model that can be threatening to some degree. Some people have a greater need for "information" before they make changes. Refer again to Chapter 5.

All three project sites requested additional training in how to accurately obtain and relate medical records information to coding information. In many practice settings, the functions of the medical record or even patient registration, i.e., demographic information have not been effectively integrated with more administrative (particularly billing) data. Until the majority of practices move to a fully integrated automated system with exam-room data entry directly in the patient record, extracting and combining these data in a meaningful way will require additional work.

Practices will no doubt be interested in learning more about how to combine these previously distinct documentation areas.

Summary

It is easy to revert to old priorities while making improvements, but the odds are against lasting positive change with the old approaches. Optimally, data collection and analysis are routine parts of everyone's job, not viewed as special projects that can be conveniently rescheduled. Change requires time. Data collection and improvement monitoring are good uses of the time needed for significant change. The experiences of the demonstration site medical practices in the CRAHCA QI Coding Project support the following key principles:

- Data should be displayed in a non-aggregated form to correctly assess trends.

- Process capability is an important focus of improvement. A focus on goals can distract from real process issues.

- Correct identification of root problem causes and variation within a process is essential to significant, lasting improvement.

- Ongoing involvement of all levels of staff, upper management as well as physicians and other clinicians, is essential to the improvement of healthcare processes.

- Management actions must be supported by data collection and analysis appropriate to the process improvement.

- The needs of the process customer should be primary forces in process improvement.

- Teams are an important way to involve the correct people in process improvement, but significant improvement opportunities, not teams, drives successful improvement.

- When supported by both administrative and clinical management, a common QI training and language, can accelerate improvement efforts.

Bibliography

American Society of Quality Control. "QA/QC Software Directory". *Quality Progress*. April 1996; 29(4).

Andell JL. "Confessions of a Shot Messenger". *Journal for Quality and Participation*. January/February 1996.

Bender AD and Krasnick C. *Quality Practice Management: How to Apply the Principles of Total Quality Management To a Medical Practice*. Swarthmore, PA: Thayer Press, 1993.

Bennett, R et al. *Gaining Control*. Salt Lake City, UT: Franklin Quest Co., 1987.
(can be purchased with a video in a package titled: Gaining Control: The Franklin Reality Model)

Berwick DM. "Improving the Appropriateness of Care". *Quality Connection*. Winter 1994; 3(1).

Berwick DM et al. *Curing Health Care: New Strategies for Quality Improvement*. San Francisco, CA: Jossey-Bass, 1990.

Berwick DM. "Can Quality Management Really Work in Health Care?" *Quality Progress*. April 1992.

*Berwick DM. "Controlling Variation in Health Care: A Consultation From Walter Shewhart". *Medical Care*. 1991; 23(12).

*Berwick DM. "Run to Space" (video of closing keynote address to the Seventh Annual National Forum on Quality Improvement in Health Care). Boston, MA: Institute for Healthcare Improvement, (call 1-617-754-4800 for purchase information).

*Berwick DM. "Seeking Systemness". *Healthcare Forum Journal*. March/April 1992.

*Berwick DM. "Sounding Board: Continuous Improvement as an Ideal in Health Care". *New England Journal of Medicine*. 1989; 320(1).

*Berwick DM. "The Clinical Process and the Quality Process". *Quality Management in Health Care*. 1992; 1(1).

*Berwick DM. "Peer Review and Quality Management: Are They Compatible?" *Quality Review Bulletin*. July 1990.

*Brown MG. "Is Your Measurement System Well Balanced?" *Journal for Quality and Participation*. October/November 1994.

Brown MG. "Why Does Total Quality Fail in Two Out of Three Tries?" *Journal of Quality and Participation*. March 1993.

*CC-M Productions. "The Prophet of Quality". Silver Spring, MD.
Also resource for Deming library including QI successes at Renton (VA) Hospital. 301-588-4095; email: ccm@nmaa.org

Better Management for a Changing World - Featuring Dr. Russell Ackoff (video series). Chicago, IL: Films Incorporated, 1995.
Part 1: "The New World View"
Part 2: "The Big Picture
Part 3: "The New Leadership
Part 4: "Doing the Right Thing Right

Center for Life Cycle Sciences, "Organizational Transformation Newsletter". Port Orchard, WA. (Call 1-360-876-2399 to subscribe. If you want "cutting edge" stuff, this is it!)

*Clemmer J. *Firing On All Cylinders: The Service/ Quality System for High-Powered Corporate Performance*. Homewood, IL: Richard D. Irwin, Inc., 1992.

Clemmer J. *Pathways to Performance*. Rocklin, CA: Prima Publishing, 1995.

Deming WE. *The New Economics*. Cambridge, MA: Massachusetts Institute of Technology, 1993.

Deming WE. "What Happened in Japan?" *Industrial Quality Control*. August 1967.

Bib.

* Highly recommended

*Eddy DM. 'Variations in Physician Practice: the Role of Uncertainty". *Health Affairs*. 1984; 3(74).

Executive Learning Inc. Brentwood, TN: (1-800-929-7890 for preview & purchasing information about the video training modules listed below).
    Series #1 (Healthcare Version)
        "The Flowchart: Picture of a Process."
        "The Cause & Effect Diagram: Understanding the 'Why's'."
        "Team Meeting Skills."
        "Idea Generating Tools"
        "Consensus Decision Making Tools."
    Series #2 (Healthcare Version)
        "Pareto Analysis"
        "Planning for Data Collection"
        "Data Collection Methods"
    Series #3 (Healthcare Version)
        "Variation: The Foundation for Run Charts and Control Charts."
        "Control Charts: Construction & Interpretation."
        "Control Charts: Application."
    *The Practice of Medicine: Regaining the Professional High Ground
        "The Daily Application of Science."
        "Stewardship and Systems Thinking."
        "Telling the Truth."
    *(Outstanding resource for front-line physicians.)

Ferrini-Mundy et al. "How Quality is Taught Can Be as Important as What is Taught". *Quality Progress*. January 1990.

*Frances AE and Gerwels JM. "Building a Better Budget". *Quality Progress*. October 1989.

*Franklin International Institute, Inc. *Gaining Control "The Franklin Reality Model"* (video). Salt Lake City, UT: Franklin International Institute, Inc., 1990. (call 1-800-654-1776 - can be purchased in a package with book *Gaining Control*, by Bennett.)

Fuller FT. "Eliminating Complexity from Work: Improving Productivity by Enhancing Quality". *National Productivity Review*. Autumn 1985.

Gaudard M et al. "Accelerating Improvement". *Quality Progress*. October 1991.

*Glasser, W. *The Control Theory Manager.* New York, NY: Harper Business, 1994. (Good approach for dealing with physicians)

Grinnell JR. "Optimize the Human System". *Quality Progress*. November 1994.

Hacquebord H. "Health Care From the Perspective of a Patient: Theories for Improvement". *Quality Management in Health Care*. 1994, 2(2).

Hare LB et al. "The Role of Statistical Thinking in Management". *Quality Progress*. February 1995.

*Harper A and Harper B. *Team Barriers*. New York, NY: MW Corporation, 1994.
    (Excellent resource containing assessments, check lists, and exercises designed to transform organizational culture. Useful for <u>all</u> levels.)

Holland D and Williams J. "Sharpening Your Executive Competencies". *Healthcare Executive*. July/August 1994.

Huge EC. *Total Quality: An Executive's Guide for the 1990's*. Homewood, IL: Richard D. Irwin, Inc., 1990.

Huyler Productivity Associates, Inc. *MEET Guide to Better Meetings*. Buffalo, NY: Huyler Productivity Associates, Inc., 1992.
    (Call Meeting & Management Essentials 1-800-701-9447 to order.)

*James J. *Survival Skills for the Future* (video). Cambridge, MA: Enterprise Media, Inc., 1993.
    (call Enterprise Media, Inc. 1-800-423-6021 to order.)

*James J. *Thinking in the Future Tense*. New York, NY: Simon & Schuster, 1996.

*James J. *Windows of Change* (video). Cambridge, MA: Enterprise Media, Inc., 1993.
    (call Enterprise Media, Inc. 1-800-423-6021 to order.)

Jeffrey JR. "Preparing the Front Line". *Quality Progress*. February 1995.

*Joiner Associates, Inc. *Fundamentals of Fourth Generation Management* (video series). Madison, WI: Joiner Associates Inc., 1992. Free preview cassette available.
> Call 1-800-669-TEAM to get on mailing list. Excellent resources.
> Module 1: "Fourth Generation Management"
> Module 2: "Voice of the Customer"
> Module 3: "Process and System Thinking"
> Module 4: "Voice of the Process"
> Module 5: "The Language of Variation"
> Module 6: "Using Data to Learn and Improve"
> Module 7: "All One Team"
> Module 8: "Leaders Making Progress"

*Joiner B. *Fourth Generation Management: The New Business Consciousness*. New York, NY: McGraw-Hill, Inc., 1994.

Joiner B and Gaudard M. "Variation, Management and W. Edwards Deming". *Quality Progress*. December 1990.

Juran, JM. *Managerial Breakthrough: A New Concept of the Manager's Job.* New York, NY: McGraw-Hill, Inc., 1964.

Juran Institute. "The Tools of Quality, Part V: Check Sheets". *Quality Progress*. October 1990.

*Kemp JM. *Moving Meetings*. Burr Ridge, IL: Richard D. Irwin, Inc., 1994.
> (Call Meeting & Management Essentials 1-800-701-9447 to order.)

*Massey M. *Just Get It!* (video). Boulder, CO: Morris Massey Associates, Inc.
> (call 1-800-346-9010 for preview and purchase information).

McCoy R. *The Best of Deming*. Knoxville, TN: SPC Press, Inc., 1994.

Meeting & Management Essentials. *Better Meetings for Everyone* Quarterly Newsletter. Boise, ID. (call 1-800-701-9447 for subscription).

Mills JL. "Sounding Board: Data Torturing". *New England Journal of Medicine*. 1994; 329(16).

Migliori, RJ. "Continuous Quality Improvement in Clinical Medicine: The Experience of the Breast Mass CQI Team". *The Bulletin*, 1992; 36(2).

*Mowery N et al. *Customer Focused Quality*. Knoxville, TN: SPC Press, Inc., 1994.

*Neave HR. *The Deming Dimension*. Knoxville, TN: SPC Press, Inc., 1990.

*Nelson EC. "Measuring for Improvement: Why, What, When, How, For Whom?" *Quality Connection*. Spring 1995, 4(2).

Nelson LS. "The Deceptiveness of Moving Averages". *Journal of Quality Technology*. April 1983.

Nolan TW. "Integrating Quality Improvement and Cost Reduction". *The Quality Letter for Healthcare Leaders*. October 1994.

*Nolan TW and Provost LP. "Understanding Variation". *Quality Progress*. May 1990.

Ott ER. *Process Quality Control*. New York, NY: McGraw-Hill, 1975.
> This book has a manufacturing bias, but is well-written and contains a lot of wisdom. It is the best reference on analysis of means.

*Ralston, F. *Hidden Dynamics*. New York, NY: AMACOM, 1995.

*Rough J. "Measuring Training From a New Science Perspective". *Journal for Quality and Participation*. October/November 1994.

*Rummler GA and Brache AP. *Improving Performance: How to Manage the White Space on the Organizational Chart, Second Edition*. San Francisco, CA: Jossey-Bass, Inc., 1995.

Sandberg J. "Strategies for Making Things Happen". Denver, CO: Mountain States Employers Council, Inc., 1992.

Sandberg J. "Why People Resist Change". Denver, CO: Mountain States Employers Council, Inc., 1992.

Scholtes H. "Beginning the Quality Transformation, Part I". *Quality Progress*. July 1988.

Scholtes H. "Six Strategies for Beginning the Quality Transformation, Part II". *Quality Progress*. August 1988.

*Scholtes PR. *The TEAM Handbook: How to Use Teams to Improve Quality*. Madison, WI: Joiner Associates, Inc., 1988.

Bib.

Scholtes PR. *The 7 Step Method for Improvement.* Madison, WI: Joiner Associates, Inc., 1989.

Silva, K. *Meetings that Work.* Burr Ridge, IL: Richard D. Irwin, Inc., 1994.
(Call Meeting & Management Essentials 1-800-701-9447 to order.)

Silversin J and Kornacki MJ. "Building Your Medical Group's Learning Capability". *Group Practice Journal.* July/August 1993.

Silversin J and Kornacki MJ. "Get Your People In Sync!" *Group Practice Journal.* September/October 1985.

SPC Press, Knoxville, TN, 1-800-545-8602. Great source for a variety of materials.

Silversin J and Kornacki MJ. "Shaping Your Group's Mentality". *Group Practice Journal.* September/October 1987.

Spitzer DR. *SuperMotivation: A Blueprint for Energizing Your Organization From Top to Bottom.* New York, NY: AMACOM, 1995.

*Turner D. "Redesigning the Service Organization". *Journal for Quality and Participation.* July/August 1994.

Wheeler DJ. *Advanced Topics in Statistical Process Control.* Knoxville, TN: SPC Press, Inc., 1995.

*Wheeler DJ. *Understanding Variation: The Key to Managing Chaos.* Knoxville, TN: SPC Press, Inc., 1993.

Wheeler DJ and Chambers DS. *Understanding Statistical Process Control.* Knoxville, TN: SPC Press, Inc., 1986.

Education for Integrating Quality
Syllabus for Educating Change Agents

Session 1: Establishing the Mindset

Pre-reading: *(mailed before first session)*
    Berwick: "Continuous Improvement as an Ideal in Health Care"
    TEAM Handbook:Chapter 1
    Neave: Chapter 3

Warm-up: "What do you expect from this series of sessions?"
    Share one thought from the Berwick article.

Joiner Tape #1: "Fourth Generation Management"

CQI vs. Transformation

Joiner Triangle

Ackoff Tape #1: "The New World View"

Evaluation

Assignment:
    1) Complete the work sheet from page 2-17 of the TEAM Handbook
    2) a. Pre-reading for Meeting 2
          b. After finishing the reading, identify a process that has been the "bane" of yourexistence.

Session 2: Some "Basics"/The Importance of Process-Oriented Thinking

---

Pre-reading:
    Philosophy: Joiner: pp. 1-24
    Core Knowledge: TEAM Handbook: pp. 2-1 to 2-16

Warm-up: "If this seems like 'common sense,' what's keeping it from happening in our organization?"

Discuss: "Key concepts" material

Everything is a process

Joiner Tape #3: "Process and System Thinking"

Vital concept: 6 Problems with a Process

Discussion of "bane" processes

Video: "The Flowchart"

Manager/Supervisor's job: To understand/improve processes and customer relationships

Evaluation

Assignment:
    1) Flowcharts are a key department process (Make copies for participants)
    2) Be ready to discuss what you learned from doing this
    3) Pre-reading for Meeting 3

App. A

Session 3: Documenting Key Processes

Pre-reading:
  Joiner: Chapter 3, Chapter 4
  Neave: Chapter 8 "Processes and Systems"
  Berwick: "Seeking Systemness"

Warm-up: "How does looking at our organization as a system change your concept of your job?"

Discussion: Neave's Chapter 8 and Berwick article

Presentation of individual flow charts: "What did you learn when you did your flowchart?"

Ackoff Tape #2: "The Big Picture"

Alignment: How does your process/team fit into the organizational whole?

Data: "philosophy" and collection of data

Data skills as a conduit to transformation

Putting it all together: A "process" for documenting key processes.

Evaluation

Assignment:
  1) Start collecting all reports containing data that you routinely receive.
  2) Pre-reading for Session 4

NOTE: 1) will form part of the agenda for Session 5

Session 4: Introduction to Variation

Pre-reading:
  Joiner: pp. 103-133
  Nolan/Provost: "Understanding Variation"
  Berwick: "Controlling Variation in Health Care: A Consultation from Walter Shewhart"

Warm-up: Share one significant insight from either the "Understanding Variation" or Berwick article.

Transforming from "Statistics" to "Statistical Thinking"

Common Cause vs. Special Cause I: The Medication Error Problem

Data "Aggressiveness"

Common Cause vs. Special Cause II: Introduction to Run Charts

The ten "Fundamentals of Variation"

Review of 6 problems with a process

Evaluation

Assignment:
  1) Find a daily, weekly, or monthly number that makes you "sweat" and do a run chart (Minimum of 15 data points).
  2) Continue collecting routine reports.
  3) Review and catch up on previously assigned reading
  4) Use the "process" template to understand more deeply one of your key processes.
  5) Review "Understanding Variation"

Session 5: Becoming Proactive in Response to Variation

Pre-reading:
        Joiner: pp. 59-77, Chapter 9
        Article: "Building a Better Budget"

Warm-up: Comment on how you observe data being used in any aspect of our organization as to
                appropriateness of collection/analysis/display/action.

Presentation of data reports:
     1)   What data currently being collected is either totally of no value to you or of no value to you in its current form?
     2)   What data would you like to receive **routinely** in graphical, run chart form?

Determining the common cause of a process: How to convert a run chart into a control chart.

Strategies for reducing variation.

Watch out for percentages!

Ackoff Tape #3: "The New Leadership"

Evaluation

Assignment:
        Pre-reading for Session 6

Session 6 A Process for Self-Managed Teams: Introduction to the 7-Step Process

Pre-reading:
        Kume: "What are Pareto Diagrams?"
        Article: "Accelerating Improvement"
        Joiner: Chapters 10-12

Warm-up: Give an example this past week of "management reactions to variation."

Six Common Statistical Traps

Joiner Tape #6: "Using Data to Learn and Improve"

A discussion/summary of the "7 Step Method for Improvement"

Evaluation

Assignment:
        Catch up on reading and review

App. A

Session 7: Putting It All Together

Pre-reading:
        Article: "The Role of Statistical Thinking in Management"

Warm-Up: What scenario presented in the article fits our organization?

Joiner Tape #8: "Leaders Making Progress"

Evaluation

Assignment:
        Pre-reading for Session 8

Session 8: Resistance to Change

Pre-reading:
        Joiner: Chapters 13 & 14
        "Resistance to Change"
        Article: "Why TQM Fails in Two Out of Three Tries"

Warm-Up: Share one "A-hah!" from the reading.

Jennifer James Video: "Windows of Change"

Donald Berwick, M.D. Video: "Run to Space"

Discuss things learned over the course of the seminar

Plan for the future:
        1)   How do we keep the momentum going?
        2)   What kind of support is needed?

* See CC-M Productions in the Bibliography to find the Ackoff videos.

Appendix B
Physician Quality Improvement Seminar

Essential Knowledge for a Changing Health Care Environment

Learning Objectives:

1. Distinguish between traditional quality assurance and continuous improvement
2. Apply concepts of "Process", "Customer", and "Variation" to everyday work
3. Construct run charts and control charts to understand and improve their work processes
4. Understand the danger of sub-optimizing a process at the expense of the whole system

All Sessions are 90 Minutes

Session 1: Basic Concepts

Pre-reading:

Berwick:	"Continuous Improvement as an Ideal in Health Care"
Berwick:	"The Clinical Process and the Quality Process"
Berwick:	"Making Real Change: Improving the Appropriateness of Care"
Eddy:	"Variations in Physician Practice: The Role of Uncertainty"

Materials:

Joiner Video 1:	"Fourth Generation Management"
Joiner:	"Key Quality Improvement Concepts"
Huge:	Unifying Principles and Four Stages of Transformation

Agenda:

20 min.	Warm-up: Individual Expectations
30 min.	Video
15 min.	Discussion of Video
	Joiner Triangle
	Process/Customers/Variation
	Other unifying principles
15 min.	QA vs. QI
	Discussion of two Berwick articles
10 min.	Evaluation

Session 2: Process and Variation

Pre-reading:

Nolan & Provost:	"Understanding Variation"
Berwick:	"Controlling Variation in Health Care: A Consultation from Walter Shewhart"

Agenda:

20 min.	Warm-up: Share one insight from the reading

15 min.	Process-oriented thinking
	What is a process?
	Six sources of problems with a process
10 min.	Continuous improvement vs. clinical research
10 min.	Expose unintended and inappropriate causes of variation
	Common vs. Special causes of variation
25 min.	Video: "Stewardship and Systems Thinking"
10 min.	Evaluation

Session 3:   Optimizing the Whole

Pre-reading:

| Neave: | Chapter 8, "Process and Systems" |
| Berwick: | "Seeking Systemness" |

Agenda:

20 min.	Warm-up: Share one insight from the reading
45 min.	Video: "Run to Space"
15 min.	Discussion: How does the concept of "systemness" change the physician's concept of his/her job?
10 min.	Evaluation

Session 4:   A Proactive Approach to Variation

Pre-reading:

| Hacquebord: | "Health Care From the Perspective of a Patient: Theories for Improvement" |
| | Run Chart/Control Chart Handout |

Agenda:

10 min.	Warm-up: Share one insight from the reading
10 min.	Construction and interpretation of run charts
15 min.	Construction of control charts
30 min.	Common vs. special causes
	Understanding and interpreting variation via control charts
	Understanding common cause variation via stratification and other relevant data
	Discussion of examples created from their data and other relevant data
15 min.	Discussion: "What are you going to do differently?"
10 min.	Evaluation

Solutions to Chapter Exercises

Chapter Seven Exercises

1. Aggregated Medication Error Data

1a) Begin by constructing a run chart (Figure 7.20):

Plot the data in time sequence. *Do not plot December 1994 since the month is not yet complete.* (It is interesting though, that even though the month is half-complete, the number of errors does not approach half of a typical month. Does this give you any ideas for future data collection?)

Check for **trends.** Since there are more than 20 data points, a trend is a sequence of seven or more consecutive points all increasing or all decreasing. (Had there been fewer than 20 points, six consecutive points all increasing or all decreasing would be sufficient.) The longest trend is six points from August 1993 through January 1994. No signs of a special cause.

Check for **alternation.** There is no series of 14 or more points alternating up and down. The longest sequence of alternating points is 6, from December 1993 through May 1994. No special causes yet.

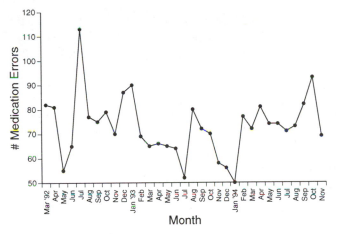

Next, find the median. Sort the data from smallest to largest, then count the total number of data points, N. In this case N = 33. Since N is odd, the median is the $\frac{33+1}{2}$ = 17th smallest number, or 72. Note that this is also the 17th largest number.

Month	Sorted Medication Errors	Sorted Order		Month	Sorted Medication Errors	Sorted Order
1/94	50	1st		8/94	73	18th
7/93	52	2nd		5/95	74	19th
5/92	55	3rd		6/94	74	20th
12/93	56	4th		9/92	75	21st
11/93	58	5th		2/94	77	22nd
6/93	64	6th		8/92	77	23rd
3/93	65	7th		10/92	79	24th
5/93	65	8th		8/93	80	25th
6/92	65	9th		4/92	81	26th
4/93	66	10th		4/94	81	27th
2/93	69	11th		3/92	82	28th
11/94	69	12th		9/94	82	29th
10/93	70	13th		12/92	87	30th
11/92	70	14th		1/93	90	31st
7/94	71	15th		10/94	93	32nd
3/94	72	16th		7/92	113	33rd
9/93	72	17th				

Next, draw the median line on the plot and circle the runs:

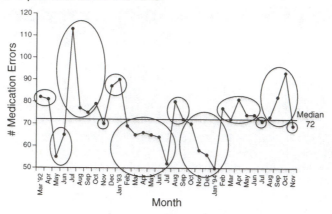

Note that September 1993 and March 1994 had results exactly on the median. When identifying runs, these points do not break a run. A run is broken only when the line *crosses to the other side* of the median.

The next step is to check for **long runs**, i.e., length eight or greater. In this plot, the longest run is length 6, from February 1993 through July 1993. This is not enough to declare a special cause.

Finally, count the **number of runs**. This plot contains 12 runs. Since there are two points exactly on the median, they are subtracted from the total number of data points for the purposes of counting runs and using Table 7.3. Thus we have 33 - 2 = 31 data points. Table 7.3 indicates we should expect between 11 and 21 runs, again indicating no evidence of a special cause.

To summarize:

Test	Criterion	Result	Special Cause?
Trend	With more than 20 points, 7 consecutive increases or decreases	Longest was 6	No
Alternation	14 consecutive alternating up or down	Longest was 6	No
Long runs	8 consecutive on same side of median	Longest was 6	No
Number of runs	With 33-2=31 points, we expect 11-21	12 runs	No

There were no special causes. In other words, the process has been running consistently and predictably during the entire 33-month period. The average has not changed. If the "20% improvement" from 1992 to 1993 received lots of attention, it indicates incorrect application of a special cause strategy. People may have been rewarded for events beyond their control.

A better strategy would be a common cause approach. A first step might be to take the entire data set and stratify the errors by process inputs. Some possible areas of stratification include type of error, physician, type of medication, pharmacist, transcriber, time of day, day of the month, etc. A brainstorming session could be helpful in generating other inputs for stratification.

1b) Table 7.11 describes the method for converting a run chart into a control chart. Since we've already done the runs analysis and found no special causes, we can begin with step 4, and compute the moving ranges.

Recall that the moving ranges are the absolute value of the difference between each point and the previous point. In other words, from each data point, subtract the previous value. (Note that the first data point has no associated moving range because there is no previous point.) If the difference is negative, drop the minus sign so that the difference becomes positive.

The calculation is shown for the first seven moving ranges:

Month	Medication Errors	Moving Range Calculation		Moving Range
		Difference	Absolute Value	*
3/92	82			
4/92	81	81-82= -1	1	1
5/92	55	55-8= -26	26	26
6/92	65	65-55= 10	10	10
7/92	113	113-65= 48	48	48
8/92	77	77-113= -36	36	36
9/92	75	75-77= -2	2	2
10/92	79	79-75= 4	4	4
11/92	70		9	
12/92	87		17	
1/93	90		3	
2/93	69		21	
3/93	65		4	
4/93	66		1	
5/93	65		1	
6/93	64		1	
7/93	52		12	
8/93	80		28	
9/93	72		8	
10/93	70		2	
11/93	58		12	
12/93	56		2	
1/94	50		6	
2/94	77		27	
3/94	72		5	
4/94	81		9	
5/94	74		7	
6/94	74		0	
7/94	71		3	
8/94	73		2	
9/94	82		9	
10/94	93		11	
11/94	69		24	

Sort the moving ranges and calculate their median:

Moving Range	Sorted Order	Moving Range	Sorted Order	Moving Range	Sorted Order
0	1st	4	12th	12	23rd
1	2nd	4	13th	12	24th
1	3rd	5	14th	17	25th
1	4th	6	15th	21	26th
1	5th	7	16th	24	27th
2	6th	8	17th	26	28th
2	7th	9	18th	27	29th
2	8th	9	19th	28	30th
2	9th	9	20th	36	31st
3	10th	10	21st	48	32nd
3	11th	11	22nd		

To find the median, count the total number of data points, N. In this case N = 32. Recall that the number of moving ranges is one less than the total number of data points. Since N is even, the median is the average of the $\frac{32}{2}$ = 16th smallest number and the next largest. These values are 7 and 8, respectively, making the MMR 7.5. Note that they are also the 16th and 17th largest numbers.

Next, calculate MRMax, the maximum difference between two consecutive months that would be expected from a common cause system. The calculation is MRMax = 3.865 x MMR = 3.865x7.5 = 29.0. Thus if any two consecutive months differ by more than 29 errors, it is evidence of a special cause.

In this case, there are two points exceeding MRMax - the moving ranges associated with 7/92 and 8/92. A closer look reveals that they are the two moving ranges that include July 1992. The number of errors in July 1992 was 113, which appears to be an outlier (an unusually high number of errors).

To calculate the common cause limits, use the following equations:

    Upper Control Limit (UCL) = Average + (3.14 x MMR)

    Lower Control Limit (LCL) = Average - (3.14 x MMR)

The average of all the data is 72.9, so the limits are:

    UCL = 72.9 + (3.14 x 7.5) = 72.9 + 23.6 = 96.5

    LCL = 72.9 - (3.14 x 7.5) = 72.9 - 23.6 = 49.3

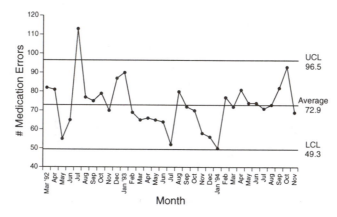

As expected, July 1992 exceeds the upper control limit, but all the other months are within the common cause band of variation. We can conclude:

• A typical month has 73 errors.

• Any one month could range from 49 to 97 errors and still be from a common cause system.

• July 1992 was an outlier. The appropriate strategy for that month would be to look for events or changes in process inputs specific to July 1992 (if the information is still available).
• In general, the process is a common cause system. To improve the system, a good strategy would be to aggregate all the data *except July 1992*, and stratify by process inputs.

Note that the average could have been recalculated with the outlier deleted. However, it only drops the average to 71.7, not an appreciable difference. Had the difference been more substantial, it would make sense to replot the data using the new average.

As suggested with the runs analysis, a common cause strategy would be the best approach. This in-house data set operated at the first level of data aggressiveness. The next step is to study the current process. If the original data can be traced to the appropriate process inputs, stratification would continue to be at the first level of data aggressiveness. If they cannot be traced, stratification would then move to the next aggressiveness level. Regardless of traceability, the current data set has established a baseline for process monitoring and can be used to evaluate future improvement efforts. If the process improves, we would expect to see an indication of a special cause (with the average number of errors decreasing).

2. The Adverse Drug Event Data

2a) Begin by constructing a run chart (Figure 7.20):

Plot the data in time sequence.

Check for **trends.** Since there are more than 20 data points, a trend is a sequence of seven or more consecutive points all increasing or all decreasing. (Had there been fewer than 20 points, six consecutive points all increasing or all decreasing would have been sufficient.) The longest trend is 5 points, which occurs from March 23 - 27. (Note that the trend from March 3 - 7 covers five days but only counts as a trend of four - since the value on March 6 was a direct repeat of the previous value, it does not count as part of the trend.) No signs of a special cause.

Check for **alternation.** There is no series of 14 or more points alternating up and down. The longest sequence of alternating points is 8, from March 26 through April 2. No special causes yet.

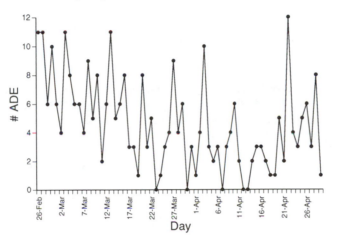

Next, find the median. Sort the data from smallest to largest, then count the total number of data points, N. In this case N = 64. Since N is even, the median is the average of the $\frac{64}{2}$ = 32nd smallest number and the next largest.

These values are both 4. Their average and thus the median is 4. Note that these are also the 32nd and 33rd largest numbers.

Day	Sorted ADE	Sorted Order	Day	Sorted ADE	Sorted Order	Day	Sorted ADE	Sorted Order
3/23	0	1st	4/4	3	23rd	3/5	6	44th
3/30	0	2nd	4/6	3	24th	3/6	6	45th
4/7	0	3rd	4/8	3	25th	3/12	6	46th
4/12	0	4th	4/15	3	26th	3/15	6	47th
4/13	0	5th	4/16	3	27th	3/29	6	48th
3/19	1	6th	4/24	3	28th	4/10	6	49th
3/24	1	7th	4/27	3	29th	4/26	6	50th
4/1	1	8th	3/2	4	30th	3/4	8	51st
4/18	1	9th	3/7	4	31st	3/10	8	52nd
4/19	1	10th	3/26	4	32nd	3/16	8	53rd
4/29	1	11th	3/28	4	33rd	3/20	8	54th
3/11	2	12th	4/2	4	34th	4/28	8	55th
4/5	2	13th	4/9	4	35th	3/8	9	56th
4/11	2	14th	4/23	4	36th	3/27	9	57th
4/14	2	15th	3/9	5	37th	2/29	10	58th
4/17	2	16th	3/14	5	38th	4/3	10	59th
4/21	2	17th	3/22	5	39th	2/26	11	60th
3/17	3	18th	4/20	5	40th	2/27	11	61st
3/18	3	19th	4/25	5	41st	3/3	11	62nd
3/21	3	20th	2/28	6	42nd	3/13	11	63rd
3/25	3	21st	3/1	6	43rd	4/22	12	64th
3/31	3	22nd						

Next, draw the median line on the plot and circle the runs:

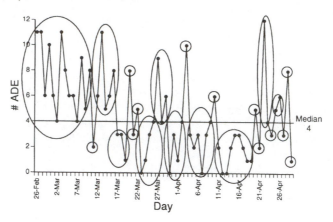

Note that several months had results exactly on the median. When identifying runs, these points do not break a run. A run is broken only when the line *crosses to the other side* of the median.

The next step is to check for **long runs**, i.e., length eight or greater. In this plot, the longest run is length 12, from February 26 through March 10. Even though this covers 14 days, two of them had values of 4, i.e., the median. They are not included in the count of the run length. This is evidence of a special cause. Note that there is another long run (length 9) from April 11 through April 19.

Finally, count the **number of runs**. This plot contains 22 runs. Since there are seven points exactly on the median, they are subtracted from the total number of data points for the purposes of counting runs and using Table 7.3. Thus we have 64 - 7 = 57 data points. Interpolating from Table 7.3 indicates we should expect between 23 and 35 runs. This is further evidence of a special cause.

To summarize:

Test	Criterion	Result	Special Cause?
Trend	With more than 20 points, 7 consecutive increases or decreases	Longest was 5	No
Alternation	14 consecutive alternating up or down	Longest was 8	No
Long runs	8 consecutive on same side of median	Longest was 12	Yes
Number of runs	With 64-7=57 points, we expect 23-35	22 runs	Yes

There is evidence of a special cause of variation. The process average decreased. This could either indicate an improved process with fewer errors, or a backslide into underreporting. A good question to ask might be, What system was in place to hold the gains?

Let's look at the recent stable system, which appears to begin March 17. The Runs analysis follows:

Begin by constructing a run chart (Figure 7.20):

Plot the data in time sequence.

The longest **trends** and sequences of **alternation** are the same as in the plot for all the data. No special causes were detected with these tests.

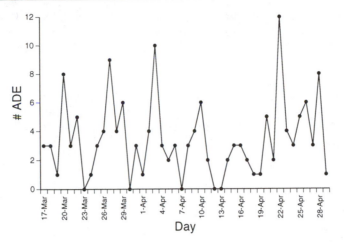

Next, find the median. Sort the data from largest to smallest, then count the total number of data points, N. Now N = 44. Since N is even, the median is the average of the $\frac{44}{2}$ = 22nd smallest number and the next largest. These values are both 3, so their average and thus the median is 3. Note that these are also the 22nd and 23rd largest numbers.

Day	Sorted ADE	Sorted Order	Day	Sorted ADE	Sorted Order	Day	Sorted ADE	Sorted Order
3/23	0	1st	4/21	2	16th	4/2	4	31st
3/30	0	2nd	3/17	3	17th	4/9	4	32nd
4/7	0	3rd	3/18	3	18th	4/23	4	33rd
4/12	0	4th	3/21	3	19th	3/22	5	34th
4/13	0	5th	3/25	3	20th	4/20	5	35th
3/19	1	6th	3/31	3	21st	4/25	5	36th
3/24	1	7th	4/4	3	22nd	3/29	6	37th
4/1	1	8th	4/6	3	23rd	4/10	6	38th
4/18	1	9th	4/8	3	24th	4/26	6	39th
4/19	1	10th	4/15	3	25th	3/20	8	40th
4/29	1	11th	4/16	3	26th	4/28	8	41st
4/5	2	12th	4/24	3	27th	3/27	9	42nd
4/11	2	13th	4/27	3	28th	4/3	10	43rd
4/14	2	14th	3/26	4	29th	4/22	12	44th
4/17	2	15th	3/28	4	30th			

Next, draw the median line on the plot and circle the runs:

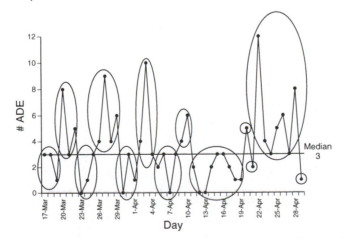

Note that several months had results exactly on the median. When identifying runs, these points do not break a run. A run is broken only when the line *crosses to the other side* of the median.

The next step is to check for **long runs**, i.e., length eight or greater. In this plot, the longest run is length 7, from April 11 through April 19. Even though this covers 9 days, two of them had values of 3, i.e., the median. They are not included in the count of the run length. (The same is true for a run covering April 22 through April 28 - there are only 5 non-median values, so the run is of length 5, not 7.) This is not enough to declare a special cause.

Finally, count the **number of runs**. This plot contains 13 runs. Since there are twelve points exactly on the median, they are subtracted from the total number of data points for the purposes of counting runs and the Table 7.3. Thus we have 44 - 12 = 32 data points. Table 7.3 indicates we should expect between 11 and 22 runs. There is no evidence of a special cause.

To summarize:

Test	Criterion	Result	Special Cause?
Trend	With more than 20 points, 7 consecutive increases or decreases	Longest was 5	No
Alternation	14 consecutive alternating up or down	Longest was 8	No
Long runs	8 consecutive on same side of median	Longest was 7	No
Number of runs	With 44-12=32 points, we expect 11-22	13 runs	No

There is no evidence of any special cause of variation. It appears that this is a stable time period with 3 error reports on a typical day. Note the high value of 12 on April 22. This was due to a new fax machine that was set to the wrong paper size. It resulted in an atypically large number of errors.

2b) The effect of the new education can be evaluated by performing a runs analysis of the stable system together with the newly collected data.

Begin by constructing a run chart (Figure 7.20):

Plot the data in time sequence.

As before, the longest **trends** and sequences of **alternation** are the same as in the plot for all the data. No special causes were detected with these tests.

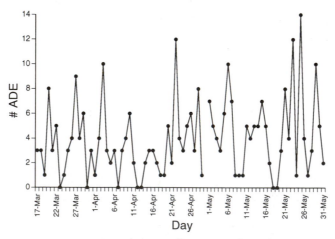

Next, find the median. Sort the data from smallest to largest, then count the total number of data points, N. Now N = 75, since the value for April 30 is missing. N is now odd, so the median is the $\frac{75 + 1}{2}$ = 38th smallest number, 3. Note that this is also the 38th largest number.

Day	Sorted ADE	SortedOrder	Day	Sorted ADE	Sorted Order	Day	Sorted ADE	Sorted Order
4/30	*		3/17	3	26th	4/20	5	51st
3/23	0	1st	3/18	3	27th	4/25	5	52nd
3/30	0	2nd	3/21	3	28th	5/2	5	53rd
4/7	0	3rd	3/25	3	29th	5/11	5	54th
4/12	0	4th	3/31	3	30th	5/13	5	55th
4/13	0	5th	4/4	3	31st	5/14	5	56th
5/18	0	6th	4/6	3	32nd	5/16	5	57th
5/19	0	7th	4/8	3	33rd	5/30	5	58th
3/19	1	8th	4/15	3	34th	3/29	6	59th
3/24	1	9th	4/16	3	35th	4/10	6	60th
4/1	1	10th	4/24	3	36th	4/26	6	61st
4/18	1	11th	4/27	3	37th	5/5	6	62nd
4/19	1	12th	5/4	3	38th	5/1	7	63rd
4/29	1	13th	5/20	3	39th	5/7	7	64th
5/8	1	14th	5/28	3	40th	5/15	7	65th
5/9	1	15th	3/26	4	41st	3/20	8	66th
5/10	1	16th	3/28	4	42nd	4/28	8	67th
5/24	1	17th	4/2	4	43rd	5/21	8	68th
5/27	1	18th	4/9	4	44th	3/27	9	69th
4/5	2	19th	4/23	4	45th	4/3	10	70th
4/11	2	20th	5/3	4	46th	5/6	10	71st
4/14	2	21st	5/12	4	47th	5/29	10	72nd
4/17	2	22nd	5/22	4	48th	4/22	12	73rd
4/21	2	23rd	5/26	4	49th	5/23	12	74th
5/17	2	24th	3/22	5	50th	5/25	14	75th
5/31	2	25th						

Next, draw the median line on the plot and circle the runs:

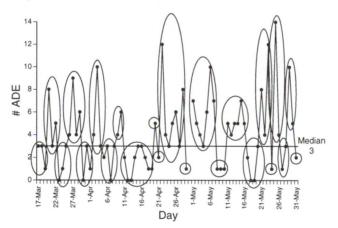

Note that several months had results exactly on the median. When identifying runs, these points do not break a run. A run is broken only when the line *crosses to the other side* of the median.

The next step is to check for **long runs**, i.e., length eight or greater. In this plot, the longest run is length 7, from April 11 through April 19. Even though this covers 9 days, two of them had values of 3, i.e., the median. They are not included in the count of the run length. (The same is true for a run covering April 22 through April 28 - there are only 5 non-median values, so the run is of length 5, not 7.) This is not enough to declare a special cause.

Finally, count the **number of runs**. This plot contains 23 runs. Since there are fifteen points exactly on the median, they are subtracted from the total number of data points (76 - 1 = 75 because of the missing 4/30 value) for the purposes of counting runs and using Table 7.3. Thus we have 75 - 15 = 60 data points. Table 7.3 indicates we should expect between 24 and 37 runs. There is evidence of a special cause.

To summarize:

Test	Criterion	Result	Special Cause?
Trend	With more than 20 points, 7 consecutive increases or decreases	Longest was 5	No
Alternation	14 consecutive alternating up or down	Longest was 8	No
Long runs	8 consecutive on same side of median	Longest was 7	No
Number of runs	With 75-1-15=60 points, we expect 24-37	23 runs	Yes

It seems that the education has had some effect. The question, again, is whether the effect can be maintained. Note that it is still not back to the level that resulted from the initial education. Although, could this possibly be because definitions of errors are clearer and people are being more careful only due to the attention being given Adverse Drug Events?

3. The Newspaper Bar Graph Problem

3a) The display is not very clear and has several problems:

1. The bars are drawn up and down from 0. This is essentially an arbitrary goal. It is not good for evaluating the stability of the process, i.e., whether there have been any significant changes.

2. The wage and benefit graph suffers from the same problems as the bar graph in Figure 7.1. If there were trends in the data, it would be nearly impossible to follow them because the two indices get in the way of each other.

3. There is no way to assess whether the data are from a common cause system.

It would be appropriate to ask questions about the stability and the long term trends in the data.

3b) Begin by constructing a run chart (Figure 7.20):

Plot the data in time sequence, then check for **trends** and **alternation.** Note that there are less than 20 data points. Therefore, a trend is a sequence of six or more consecutive points all increasing or all decreasing. (Had there been more than 20 points, seven consecutive points all increasing or all decreasing would have been required.)

Productivity

The longest trend is 4 points, from 1989 through 1992. The longest series of alternation is also 4 points, which occurs twice. No signs of a special cause.

Wages

The longest trend is three points, which occurs four times throughout the period. The longest sequence of alternating points is five, which occurs twice. No special causes yet in wages.

Benefits

The longest trend is four points, from 1980 through 1983. The longest alternating sequence is six points, from 1984-1989. Thus far, there are no special causes in any of the indices.

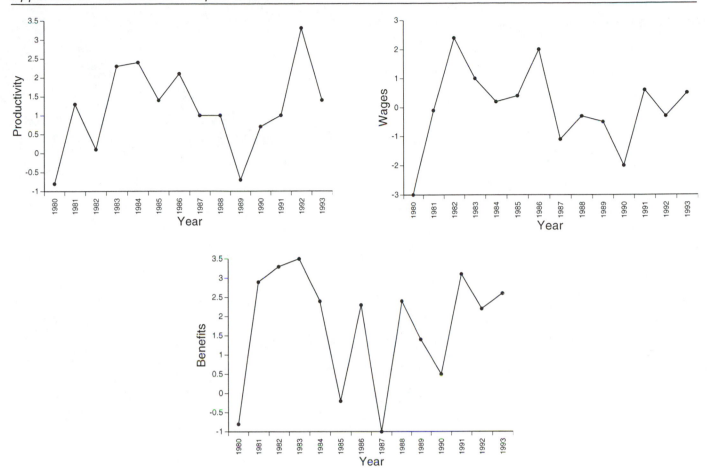

Next, find the median. Sort the data from largest to smallest, then count the total number of data points, N. In this case N = 14. Since N is even, the median is the average of the $\frac{14}{2}$ = 7th smallest number, and the next largest. The medians for productivity, wages, and benefits are 1.15, 0.05, and 2.35, respectively.

Year	Sorted Productivity	Year	Sorted Wages	Year	Sorted Benefits	Sorted Order
1980	-0.8	1980	-3.0	1987	-1.0	1st
1989	-0.7	1990	-2.0	1980	-0.8	2nd
1982	0.1	1987	-1.1	1985	-0.2	3rd
1990	0.7	1989	-0.5	1990	0.5	4th
1987	1.0	1992	-0.3	1989	1.4	5th
1988	1.0	1988	-0.3	1992	2.2	6th
1991	1.0	1981	-0.1	1986	2.3	7th
1981	1.3	1984	0.2	1988	2.4	8th
1985	1.4	1985	0.4	1984	2.4	9th
1993	1.4	1993	0.5	1993	2.6	10th
1986	2.1	1991	0.6	1981	2.9	11th
1983	2.3	1983	1.0	1991	3.1	12th
1984	2.4	1986	2.0	1982	3.3	13th
1992	3.3	1982	2.4	1983	3.5	14th

App. C

Next, draw the median line on the plot and circle the runs:

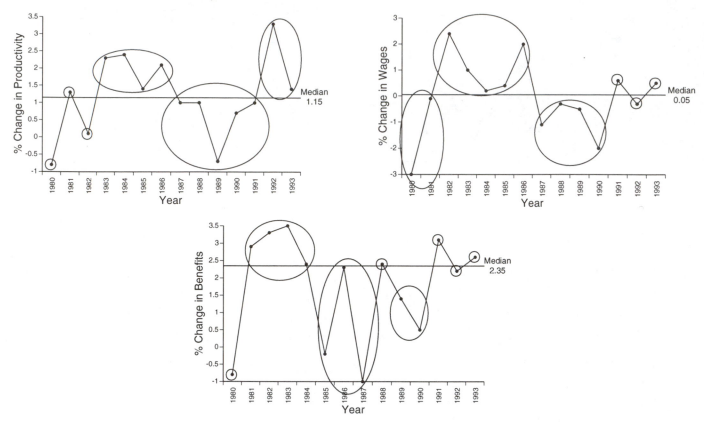

The next steps are to check for **long runs**, i.e., length eight or greater, and to count the **number of runs**. Since there are 14 data, table 7.3 indicates we should expect between 4 and 11 runs.

Productivity: The longest run is length 5, from 1987-1991, and the plot contains 6 runs.

Wages: The longest run is 5 points and there are 6 runs

Benefits: The longest run is 4 points and there are 8 runs.

To summarize, none of the runs tests showed special causes for any of the tests. From a runs perspective, it appears that all three are operating in a common cause mode.

3c) Table 7.11 describes the method for converting a run chart into a control chart. Since we've already done the runs analysis and found no special causes, we can begin with step 4, and compute the moving ranges.

Recall that the moving ranges are the absolute value of the difference between each point and the previous point. In other words, from each data point, subtract the previous value. (Note that the first data point has no associated moving range because there is no previous point.) If the difference is negative, drop the minus sign so that the difference becomes positive.

Year	Productivity	MR	Wages	MR	Benefits	MR
1980	-0.8	*	-3.0	*	-0.8	*
1981	1.3	2.1	-0.1	2.9	2.9	3.7
1982	0.1	1.2	2.4	2.5	3.3	0.4
1983	2.3	2.2	1.0	1.4	3.5	0.2
1984	2.4	0.1	0.2	0.8	2.4	1.1
1985	1.4	1.0	0.4	0.2	-0.2	2.6
1986	2.1	0.7	2.0	1.6	2.3	2.5
1987	1.0	1.1	-1.1	3.1	-1.0	3.3
1988	1.0	0.0	-0.3	0.8	2.4	3.4
1989	-0.7	1.7	-0.5	0.2	1.4	1.0
1990	0.7	1.4	-2.0	1.5	0.5	0.9
1991	1.0	0.3	0.6	2.6	3.1	2.6
1992	3.3	2.3	-0.3	0.9	2.2	0.9
1993	1.4	1.9	0.5	0.8	2.6	0.4

Sorted Prod. MR	Sorted Wage MR	Sorted Ben. MR	Sorted Order
0.0	0.2	0.2	1st
0.1	0.2	0.4	2nd
0.3	0.8	0.4	3rd
0.7	0.8	0.9	4th
1.0	0.8	0.9	5th
1.1	0.9	1.0	6th
1.2	1.4	1.1	7th
1.4	1.5	2.5	8th
1.7	1.6	2.6	9th
1.9	2.5	2.6	10th
2.1	2.6	3.3	11th
2.2	2.9	3.4	12th
2.3	3.1	3.7	13th

To find the median, count the total number of data points, N. In this case N = 13. Recall that the number of moving ranges is one less than the total number of data points. Since N is odd, the median is the the $\frac{13+1}{2}$ = 7th smallest number. The values of MMR are 1.2, 1.4, and 1.1 for productivity, wages, and benefits, respectively. Note that they are also the 7th largest numbers.

Next, calculate MRMax, the maximum difference between two consecutive years that would be expected from a common cause system. The calculations are:

Productivity: MRMax = 3.865 x MMR = 3.865 x 1.2 = 4.6

Wages: MRMax = 3.865 x MMR = 3.865 x 1.4 = 5.4

Benefits: MRMax = 3.865 x MMR = 3.865 x 1.1 = 4.2

Thus if any two consecutive years differ by more than 4.6 percent in productivity, 5.4 percent in wages, or 4.2 percent in benefits, it is evidence of a special cause. None of the moving ranges exceed MRMax.

3d) To calculate the common cause limits, use the following equations:

Upper Control Limit (UCL) = Average + (3.14 x MMR)
+2 sigma limit = Average + (2.1 x MMR)
-2 sigma limit = Average - (2.1 x MMR
Lower Control Limit (LCL) = Average - (3.14 x MMR)

The limits are:

Productivity

UCL = 1.18 + (3.14 x 1.2) = 1.18 + 3.77 = 4.95
+2 sigma limit = 1.18 + (2.1 x 1.2) = 1.18 + 2.52 = 3.70
- 2 sigma limit = 1.18 - (2.1 x 1.2) = 1.18 - 2.52 = -1.34
LCL = 1.18 - (3.14 x 1.2) = 1.18 - 3.77 = -2.59

Wages

UCL = -0.01 + (3.14 x 1.4) = -0.01 + 4.40 = 4.39
+2 sigma limit = -0.01 + (2.1 x 1.4) = -0.01 + 2.94 = 2.93
-2 sigma limit = -0.01 - (2.1 x 1.4) = -0.01 - 2.94 = -2.95
LCL = -0.01 - (3.14 x 1.4) = -0.01 - 4.40 = -4.41

App. C

Benefits

UCL = 1.76 + (3.14 x 1.1) = 1.76 + 3.45 = 5.21
+2 sigma limit = 1.76 + (2.1 x 1.1) = 1.76 + 2.31 = 4.07
-2 sigma limit = 1.76 - (2.1 x 1.1) = 1.76 - 2.31 = -0.55
LCL = 1.76 - (3.14 x 1.1) = 1.76 - 3.45 = -1.69

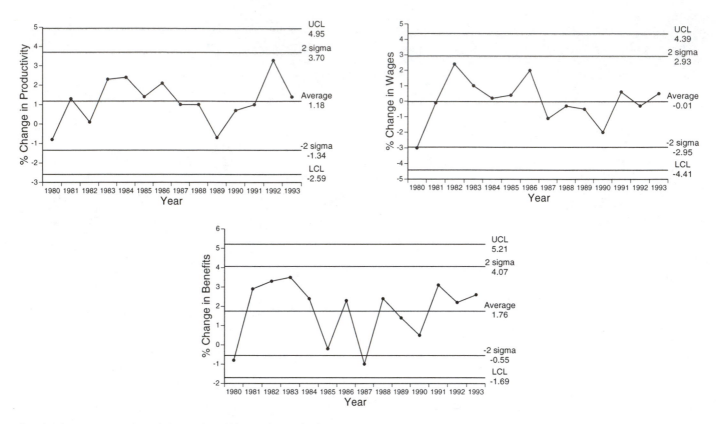

Again there are no special causes. We can conclude:

• Productivity is steadily increasing at 1.18% per year; benefits are steadily increasing at 1.76% per year; and wages are essentially stagnant after adjustment for inflation. They are all common cause systems.

• While the total variation is wide, about 90-98% of the time the results will fall between the +2 sigma and -2 sigma limits.

• Even with the stable, steadily increasing productivity and benefits, it is possible to have individual years where productivity and/or benefits decrease. This is not necessarily an indication of the economy suddenly changing. It is most likely common cause variation. It just means that, at the end of the year, a calculation is performed and the resulting number ends up being less than the previous year. It could still be indicative of the process's positive average. (Think of the coin flips.)

4. The Patient Satisfaction Survey Data

4a) The data collection process suffers from a serious lack of planning. The people who fill out the cards do not necessarily represent "typical" patients; most likely they are the very happy or the very angry. As a result, their opinions are likely to be contradictory, and any decisions based on them will be suspect. The sample is very biased, yet the results are projected as if they came from the "average" patient.

The analysis and feedback processes appear to be based on a "two-point trend" analysis, where the results are studied in a vacuum, not in a process-oriented context. In addition, there is no evidence of any efforts to understand the processes that produced the results. The only action was to threaten groups who didn't meet expectations.

4b) Begin by constructing a run chart (Figure 7.20):

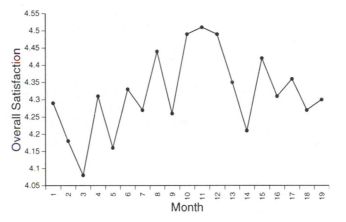

Check for **trends.** Since there are 20 or fewer data points, a trend is a sequence of six or more consecutive points all increasing or all decreasing. (Had there been more than 20 points, seven consecutive points all increasing or all decreasing would have been required.) The longest trend is four points, which occurs from months 11-14. No signs of a special cause.

Check for **alternation.** There is no series of 14 or more points alternating up and down. The longest sequence of alternating points is 9, from months 2 through 10. No special causes yet.

Next, find the median. Sort the data from smallest to largest, then count the total number of data points, N. In this case N = 19. Since N is odd, the median is the $\frac{19 + 1}{2}$ = 10th smallest number, or 4.31. Note that this is also the 10th largest number.

Month	Sorted Overall Satisfaction	Sorted Order
3	4.08	1st
5	4.16	2nd
2	4.18	3rd
14	4.21	4th
9	4.26	5th
7	4.27	6th
18	4.27	7th
1	4.29	8th
19	4.30	9th
4	4.31	10th
16	4.31	11th
6	4.33	12th
13	4.35	13th
17	4.36	14th
15	4.42	15th
8	4.44	16th
10	4.49	17th
12	4.49	18th
11	4.51	19th

Next, draw the median line on the plot and count the runs:

Note that two months had results exactly on the median. When identifying runs, these points do not break a run. A run is broken only when the line *crosses to the other side* of the median.

The next step is to check for **long runs**, i.e., length eight or greater. In this plot, the first five months comprise the longest run, length 4 because one month is on the median. Another run of 4 appears during months 10-13. This is not enough to declare a special cause.

Finally, count the **number of runs**. This plot contains 9 runs. Since there are two points exactly on the median, they are subtracted from the total number of data points for the purposes of counting runs and using Table 7.3. Thus we have 19 - 2 = 17 data points. Table 7.3 indicates we should expect between five and 13 runs. The runs analysis gives no indication of special causes.

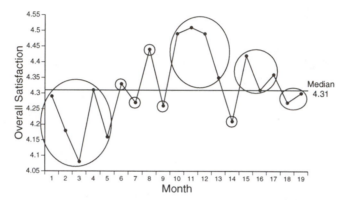

To summarize:

Test	Criterion	Result	Special Cause?
Trend	With more than 20 points, 7 consecutive increases or decreases	Longest was 4	No
Alternation	14 consecutive alternating up or down	Longest was 9	No
Long runs	8 consecutive on same side of median	Longest was 4	No
Number of runs	With 19-2=17 points, we expect 5-13	9 runs	No

There is no evidence of special causes. The performance seems to be stable.

4c) Table 7.11 describes the method for converting a run chart into a control chart. Since we've already done the runs analysis and found no special causes, we can begin with step 4, and compute the moving ranges.

Recall that the moving ranges are the absolute value of the difference between each point and the previous point. In other words, from each data point, subtract the previous value. (Note that the first data point has no associated moving range because there is no previous point.) If the difference is negative, drop the minus sign so that the difference becomes positive.

Month	Overall Satisfaction	MR	Sorted MR	Sorted Order
1	4.29	*		
2	4.18	0.11	0.02	1st
3	4.08	0.10	0.02	2nd
4	4.31	0.23	0.03	3rd
5	4.16	0.15	0.05	4th
6	4.33	0.17	0.06	5th
7	4.27	0.06	0.09	6th
8	4.44	0.17	0.10	7th
9	4.26	0.18	0.11	8th
10	4.49	0.23	0.11	9th
11	4.51	0.02	0.14	10th
12	4.49	0.02	0.14	11th
13	4.35	0.14	0.15	12th
14	4.21	0.14	0.17	13th
15	4.42	0.21	0.17	14th
16	4.31	0.11	0.18	15th
17	4.36	0.05	0.21	16th
18	4.27	0.09	0.23	17th
19	4.30	0.03	0.23	18th

To find the median, count the total number of data points, N. In this case N = 18. Recall that the number of moving ranges is one less than the total number of data points. Since N is even, the median is the average of the $\frac{18}{2} = 9$th smallest number and the next largest. These values are 0.11 and 0.14, respectively, making the MMR 0.125. Note that they are also the 9th and 10th largest numbers.

Next, calculate MRMax, the maximum difference between two consecutive months that would be expected from a common cause system. The calculation is MRMax = 3.865 x MMR = 3.865x0.125 = 0.48. Thus if any two consecutive months differ by more than 0.48, it is evidence of a special cause. In this case, no moving ranges exceeded the MMR.

4d) To calculate the common cause limits, use the following equations:

Upper Control Limit (UCL) = Average + (3.14 x MMR)
+2 sigma limit = Average + (2.1 x MMR)
-2 sigma limit = Average - (2.1 x MMR)
Lower Control Limit (LCL) = Average - (3.14 x MMR)

The average of all the data is 4.32, so the limits are:

UCL = 4.32 + (3.14 x 0.125) = 4.32 + 0.39 = 4.71
+2 sigma limit = 4.317 + (2.1 x 0.125) = 4.32 + 0.26 = 4.58
-2 sigma limit = 4.317 - (2.1 x 0.135) = 4.32 - 0.26 = 4.06
LCL = 4.32 - (3.14 x 0.135) = 4.32 - 0.39 = 3.93

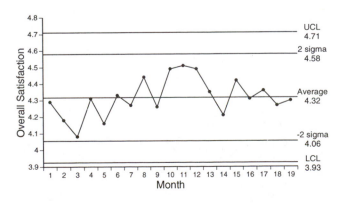

Conclusions:

- The common cause limits are 3.93 to 4.71.

- If nothing changes, 90-98% of the results will fall between 4.06 and 4.58.

The current process for using the data has not brought about significant improvement. It is similar to collecting data on "accidents." While accident data tell you the number of accidents, they don't really tell you how to improve. As a result, improvements are not likely to occur. A better idea would be to make focused, planned data collections with specific objectives. The current data process is too vague.

Since exhortation has always been part of the process, we are observing that it has also been absorbed as one of the inputs, since no progress has been observed. No answer was given to the logical question, What should I do differently from what I am doing now? This process is perfectly designed to give us the results we have been observing.

5. The Transcription Productivity Data

Note: The remaining solutions will be in "short form." We hope the detail of the previous solutions has helped you understand the methods for determining the presence of special causes using run and control charts.

5a)   The median is 11.2.

To summarize:

Test	Criterion	Result	Special Cause?
Trend	With more than 20 points, 7 consecutive increases or decreases	Longest was 4	No
Alternation	14 consecutive alternating up or down	Longest was 9	No
Long runs	8 consecutive on same side of median	Longest was 7	No
Number of runs	With 34-3=31 points, we expect 11-21	14 runs	No

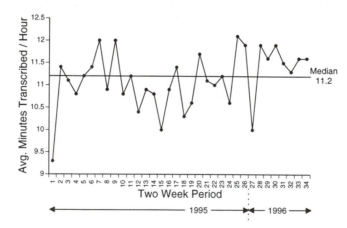

Thus these data pass all the runs rules. However, a few things look suspicious about the chart. For example, the first data point is quite low, and nine of the last 10 points are above the median. The period in that sequence that falls below the median appears to be a large drop. Comparing this to the MRMax will tell us whether it is a special cause.

5b) The MMR = 0.5 and MRMax = 3.865 x MMR = 3.865x0.5 = 1.9. Thus if any two consecutive periods differ by more than 1.9 minutes/hour, it is evidence of a special cause.

There are a couple of things to note. First, the moving range for period 2 (the difference between periods 1 and 2) exceeds MRMax. The difference between the first two periods was generated by a special cause of variation. At this stage, all we know is that it is the first period of the year.

Next, in your sorted sequence (not printed here), look at the 31st and 32nd largest sorted moving ranges. They are both 1.9, just at the edge of MRMax. *However, note that they are for consecutive two-week periods.* The moving ranges are both associated with period 27, which intuition tells is somewhat below the process toward the end of the chart. What might be unusual about period 27? *It is also the first two-week period of the year!* In other words, the first periods of 1995 and 1996 appear to be unusually low. A question to ask might be, Is there a good reason for the first period of the year to be low?

Let's reconsider the runs analysis in light of this new information. If period 27 is a special cause, perhaps it should be excluded from the runs analysis. If this is done, there is a run of 9 points at the end of the year - yet another special cause. The process average seems to have increased. Further investigation revealed that the department supervisor's office was moved away from the work area at the beginning of this sequence of 9. As a result, transcribers didn't leave their workstations as frequently to ask questions of her.

5c) Now that we know the process had two averages, it does not make sense to take an overall average of all the data points. It would represent nothing and would lead to poor decisions. To assess the current process performance, the average should be calculated based only on the current stable system: in this case, periods 25, 26, and 28-34. The common cause limits can be based on the median moving range of all the data as calculated in part b).

The average of the stable system is 11.71, so the limits are:

UCL = 11.71 + (3.14 x 0.5) = 11.71 + 1.57 = 13.28
+2 sigma Limit = 11.71 + (2.1 x 0.5) = 11.71 + 1.05 = 12.76
-2 sigma Limit = 11.71 - (2.1 x 0.5) = 11.71 - 1.05 = 10.66
LCL = 11.71 - (3.14 x 0.5) = 11.71 - 1.57 = 10.14

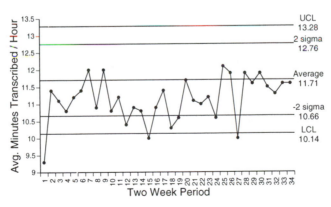

The previous system (periods 2-24) had an average of 11.03 minutes/hour. Thus the improvement has been 11.71 - 11.03 = 0.68 minutes/hour.

6.   The Overtime Data

6a) The median is 0.7 FTE and the run chart is:

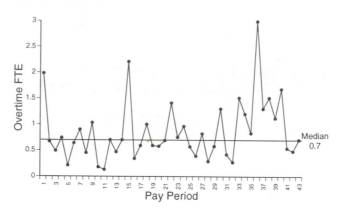

To summarize:

Test	Criterion	Result	Special Cause?
Trend	With more than 20 points, 7 consecutive increases or decreases	Longest was 3	No
Alternation	14 consecutive alternating up or down	Longest was 8	No
Long runs	8 consecutive on same side of median	Longest was 8	Yes
Number of runs	With 43-4=39 points, we expect 14-26	20 runs	No

There is evidence of a special cause of variation. It appears that the amount of overtime increased for a while near the end of the plot, although it may have come back down for the last three pay periods. There are also three points (periods 1, 15 and 36) which appear to be high outliers, but the run chart cannot detect them. Perhaps the moving ranges will give better insight.

6b) The MMR is 0.41, making MRMax = 3.865 x MMR = 3.865x0.41 = 1.58. Thus if any two consecutive pay periods differ by more than 1.58 FTE, it is evidence of a special cause.

In this case, three moving ranges exceed MRMax - the moving ranges associated with pay periods 16, 36, and 37. These account for two of the points that appeared to be outliers on the run chart.

6c) The pay periods with Monday holidays appear to be operating on a different system. The process also seemed to operate on another system when the receptionists quit. An overall average would be meaningless. This, however, is a different special cause. If the data are to be used to predict and forecast future overtime FTEs, we would likely overestimate the value. The system that functioned when the receptionists quit is not representative of the process and is likely to be a rare, one-time occurrence.

The issue of the Monday holidays is somewhat different, though. Is there a legitimate reason that Monday holidays have more overtime? If not, the reason for the overtime needs to be investigated. If it is reasonable to expect more overtime for the Monday holidays, they represent a system that is working in conjunction with the system that operates the rest of the year. Periods with Monday holidays may have to be plotted separately to see if behavior is stable and predictable.

6d) To evaluate the stability, plot a control chart with limits based on the MMR calculated in b). When calculating the average, omit the periods that contained special causes, i.e., 1, 15, and 33-40.

To calculate the common cause limits, use the following equations:

Upper Control Limit (UCL) = Average + (3.14 x MMR)
+2 sigma Limit = Average + (2.1 x MMR)
-2 sigma Limit = Average - (2.1 x MMR)
Lower Control Limit (LCL) = Average - (3.14 x MMR)

The average of all the "normal system" data is 0.62, so the limits are:

UCL = 0.62 + (3.14 x 0.41) = 0.62 + 1.29 = 1.91
+2 sigma Limit = 0.62 + (2.1 x 0.41) = 0.62 + 0.86 = 1.48
-2 sigma Limit = 0.62 - (2.1 x 0.41) = 0.62 - 0.86 = -0.24
LCL = 0.62 - (3.14 x 0.41) = 0.62 - 1.29 = -0.67

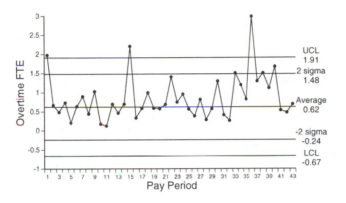

There are no indications of special causes aside from the issues mentioned in c), thus the process is consistent aside from those issues. The process is centered at 0.62 FTE per pay period, although in a particularly rough month, she could need as much as 1.91 FTE of overtime. However, 90-98% of the time the requirement will be less than 1.48.

6e) Given the current variation in the process, a pay period with 0 overtime is possible, but it would likely be due to common cause. She is not able to achieve 0 overtime consistently. Management "heat" does not seem to have made any difference because it couldn't.

6f) Management application of "heat" will maintain the status quo. The budgetary implications of this strategy are that the average will remain at 0.62 FTE. If pay periods with Monday holidays are legitimately different, forecasting can be based on an average of 0.62 overtime FTE for pay periods without Monday holidays, and with a higher average for pay periods with Monday holidays.

Both common and special cause strategies are appropriate. Special cause strategies apply to the Monday holiday pay periods. Are they appropriate? Should staff be reallocated during those time? Common cause strategies are more appropriate for the rest of the year. Some stratification options are reason, day of week, job function, person, etc.

6g) The reporting could be improved in a number of ways. A graphical approach would be a start. In this case, the year-to-date format is particularly misleading. Since the first pay period of this data set included a Monday holiday, the year-to-date number is high from the start. Periods reflecting normal variation that followed it do not have as much impact. Year-to-date numbers are extremely sensitive to variation at the beginning of the year and extremely insensitive to variation, even special cause, at the end of the year.

App.
C

7. The Utilization Management System

7a) Neither the table nor the combined bar/line plot are very insightful. Runs and control chart analyses would be more appropriate.

7b) The MMR is134.5, making MRMax = 519.8. Thus if any two consecutive months differ by more than 520 variance days, it is evidence of a special cause.

In this case, there are no points exceeding MRMax - no evidence of a special cause.

The average of all the data is 74, so the common cause limits are:

UCL = 74 + (3.14 x 134.5) = 74 + 422.3 = 496.3
+2 sigma Limit = 74 + (2.1 x 134.5) = 74 + 282.4 = 356.4
-2 sigma Limit = 74 - (2.1 x 134.5) = 74 - 282.4 = -208.4
LCL = 74 - (3.14 x 134.5) = 74 - 422.3 = -348.3

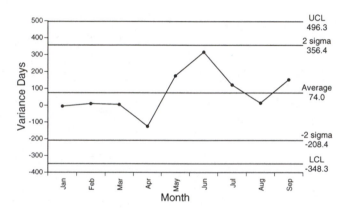

There is no evidence of special cause variation in this process.

7c) If the process is on budget, it should be centered at 0. An approach to evaluating this is to calculate the common cause limits around 0 instead of the actual average. If there are signs of special causes, it would indicate that the process is not centered at 0.

The limits would become:

UCL = 0 + (3.14 x 134.5) = 0 + 422.3 = 422.3
+2 sigma Limit = 0 + (2.1 x 134.5) = 0 + 282.4 = 282.4
-2 sigma Limit = 0 - (2.1 x 134.5) = 0 - 282.4 = -282.4
LCL = 0 - (3.14 x 134.5) = 0 - 422.3 = -422.3

The chart is:

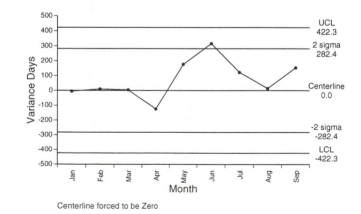

Centerline forced to be Zero

Clearly there are no special causes. The process could be on budget. Of course, that means that any given month has a 50% chance of being above budget.

7d) *On average*, the budgeting appears correct - the actual average of 74 is not distinguishable from an average of 0. About half the months are over budget and half are under. However, if the goal is for every month to come in under budget, the process will have to be improved. Since there are no special causes, a common cause strategy should be used. It will be fruitless to study only those months that are above budget. The data should be aggregated and studied as a whole. The behavior of the next three months, especially if they are also above 0, may indicate whether this process was indeed either on budget or above budget, and by how much.

7e) The common cause limits on the process are fairly wide. There could be a month with a variance close to 500 days! Chances are that this would not have been identified simply from the list of numbers and chart in the original presentation. Without knowledge of statistical theory, heads would most likely roll!

However, 90-98% of the time, the variance will be between -208 and 356 days.

Note that control charts of "Actual LOS" and Rate per 1000 could also be quite useful.

8. Patient Transfer Time Data

8a) The median is 28, and the run chart is:

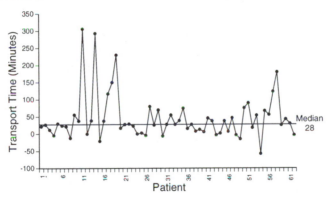

To summarize:

Test	Criterion	Result	Special Cause?
Trend	With more than 20 points, 7 consecutive increases or decreases	Longest was 5	No
Alternation	14 consecutive alternating up or down	Longest was 9	No
Long runs	8 consecutive on same side of median	Longest was 4	No
Number of runs	With 62-3=59 points, we expect 24-37	31 runs	No

The run chart gives no evidence of a special cause. However, some of the points e.g., 12 and 14 look quite high. Note also that some times are negative. These are cases where the data arrived at the non-critical care unit before the patient left the ICU.

8b) The MMR is 34, making MRMax = 3.865*34 = 131.4. Moving ranges on both sides of patients 11 and 14 exceed the MMR. The drops from patients 19 to 20 and from patients 58-59 also exceed the MMR. The two drops both follow what appear to be upward trends, albeit not statistically defined. Given the way the data are collected, one wonders whether several records were accumulated, then transferred from top to bottom all at the same time.

8c) The average of all the data is 45.0, so the limits are:

UCL = 45.0 + (3.14 x 34) = 45.0 + 106.8 = 151.8
+2 sigma = 45.0 + (2.1 x 34) = 45.0 + 71.4 = 116.4
-2 sigma = 45.0 - (2.1 x 34) = 45.0 - 71.4 = -26.4
LCL = 45.0 - (3.14 x 34) = 45.0 - 106.8 = -61.8

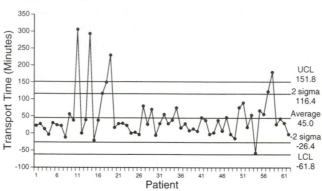

The outliers are confirmed. The current average is 45.0 with a typical (90-98%) range covering -26.4 - 116 minutes, approximately 30 minutes before the patient leaves the ICU until approximately 2 hours after the patient arrives at the new unit. However, the average is inflated because of the outliers.

8d) If patients 11, 14, 18, 19 , and 58 are removed from the calculation, the average becomes 28.6 minutes. The limits are then:

UCL = 28.6 + (3.14 x 34) = 28.6 + 106.8 = 135.3
+2 sigma Limit = 28.6 + (2.1 x 34) = 28.6 + 71.4 = 100.0
-2 sigma Limit = 28.6 - (2.1 x 34) = 28.6 - 71.4 = -42.8
LCL = 28.6 - (3.14 x 34) = 28.6 - 106.8 = -78.2

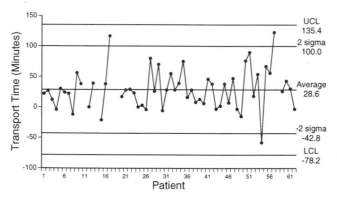

Patients' records typically arrive about 30 minutes after they leave the ICU. Ninety to 98% of the time, the records will arrive within 100 minutes. Note that there are three data points between the 2 sigma (-2 sigma) limit and the UCL (LCL). We would expect to see 2-10% in this range. Three times out of approximately 60 is 5%, i.e., what we should expect.

Could a wait of over one-and-a-half hours compromise patient care? Given the current system, it could even take as long as 135 minutes on rare occasions.

8e) Both strategies are appropriate. There are several special causes to investigate. Was workload particularly heavy in the ICU those days? Was the computer system down?

The remainder of the data follow a common cause process. What factors could contribute to transfer times? Are they a high priority with ICU staff? Is it easy to transfer the data? Is the location to which the data should be sent obvious for all patients? It would be appropriate to aggregate and stratify these data. Stratification possibilities include time of day, non-critical care location, diagnosis, etc. Particularly since the response of interest is time, another tool would be to cut new windows or disaggregate the data. The transfer of patients and their records is a process, and times could be measured along the way. It could also be desirable to reduce the range of inherent variation.

9. The Critical Pathway Data Problem

9a) Length of Stay

The median is 4 days, and the run chart is:

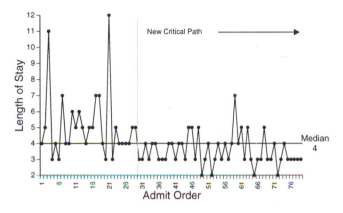

To summarize:

Test	Criterion	Result	Special Cause?
Trend	With more than 20 points, 7 consecutive increases or decreases	Longest was 3	No
Alternation	14 consecutive alternating up or down	Longest was 7	No
Long runs	8 consecutive on same side of median	Longest was 9	Yes
Number of runs	With 79-24=55 points, we expect 22-34	18 runs	Yes

There has been a change in the process. Evidently, the critical path change has had some effect.

Charges

The median is $10,714, and the run chart is:

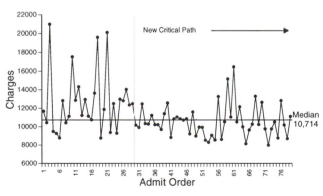

To summarize:

Test	Criterion	Result	Special Cause?
Trend	With more than 20 points, 7 consecutive increases or decreases	Longest was 4	No
Alternation	14 consecutive alternating up or down	Longest was 11	No
Long runs	8 consecutive on same side of median	Longest was 10	Yes
Number of runs	With 79-1=78 points, we expect 32-47	37 runs	No

The long run at the beginning of the chart indicates that the process has changed.

9b) The average for the pre-test period is $12,611 with a MMR of $3,007. None of the patient charges indicate any special causes, although the moving ranges associated with patient 3 come close to exceeding the MRMax of $11,622. Note that with 29 data points one would expect 1-3 (2-10%) between 2 sigma and UCL. This is in line with our observations.

The average for the post-test period is $10,550 with a MMR of $1,726. None of the moving ranges exceeds the MRMax of $6,671, but patient 61 indicates a special cause.

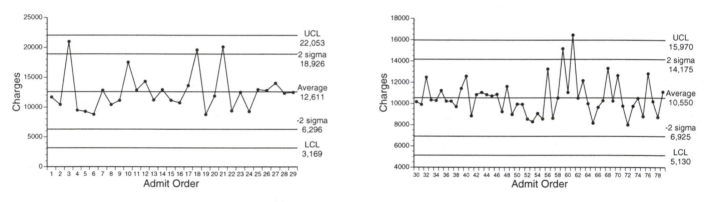

Removing patient 61 from the calculation of the average brings the typical charge to $10,429.

Thus the savings with the new critical path are $12,611 - $10,429 = $2,182 per patient.

Note also the reduction in charge variation with the new critical path. The common cause limits covered a range of ($22,053 - $3,169) = $18,884 under the old path; with the new their range is $10,840. Not only has the new critical path lowered the charges, it has lowered the variation by about 45%.

9c) The success of the new critical path is now somewhat mitigated by requirement of an explanation for any charges greater than $1,000 over the average. This is a goal that falls within the common cause limits, i.e., a special cause strategy being applied to a common cause process. The goal ($10,315 + $1,000 = $11,315) is contained well within the common cause limits, and will be exceeded almost half the time. A better approach would be to investigate charges greater than the UCL of $15,375, or when other evidence of a special cause is present.

A common cause strategy would be more appropriate. One could be to stratify the data by physician to see if anyone is outside the system. Or one could combine all the costs for the common cause patients and do a Pareto analysis of them by category, e.g., lab, x-ray, pharmacy, room, etc.

Chapter Eight Exercises

1. The PCTA Incidence Data

1a) The limits can be computed as follow:

The overall average is computed as the total number of incidences divided by the total number of PTCA. In this case it is $\frac{16}{336}$ = 0.476, or 4.76 percent. The three sigma limits are computed with the formula:

$$\text{Average} \pm 3 \times \sqrt{\frac{(\text{Average}) \times (1 - \text{Average})}{\text{Number of PTCA for that cardiologist}}}$$

Note that the only thing different when computing the limits for each cardiologist is the denominator. Thus for all cardiologists, the formula begins:

$$0.0476 \pm 3 \times \sqrt{\frac{(0.0476) \times (1 - 0.0476)}{\text{Number of PTCA for that cardiologist}}}$$

$$= 0.0476 \pm 3 \times \sqrt{\frac{0.0453}{\text{Number of PTCA for that cardiologist}}}$$

All that needs to be done is to substitute the appropriate number of PTCA. This results in the following limits:

Cardiologist	#Incidences/#PTCA	Upper limit	Lower limit
1	0.0278	0.1541	0
2	0.0755	0.1354	0
3	0.0506	0.1195	0
4	0.0344	0.1315	0
5	0.0455	0.1085	0

Recall that for proportions data, a lower limit less than 0 should be considered 0. In this case, they have all been plotted as 0. Note that the graph has the cardiologists sorted from smallest to largest incidence rate.

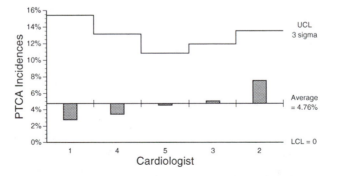

All the cardiologists seem to fall within the system. Neither of the two cardiologists with "above-average" rates can be considered a special cause. (After all, *someone* has to get the highest number!)

1b) A common cause strategy should be used.

1c) The current process treats common cause variation as special cause. Instead of studying the individual incidences, they should all be studied. Do they have anything in common? Can they be stratified?

To determine whether the current strategy is effective, a runs/control chart analysis of the aggregated departmental incidence rate would help.

1d) The more rigorous analysis did not make any difference.

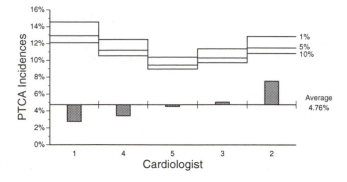

2. The 911 Signing Data

2a) The overall average is 19.87%, and the 3 sigma limits are listed below.

Medic	% Waivers Signed	Upper Limit	Lower Limit	Medic	% Waivers Signed	Upper Limit	Lower Limit
1	7.32	38.56	1.17	21	19.30	35.72	4.01
2	9.47	32.15	7.59	22	19.49	30.89	8.85
3	12.50	49.80	0.00	23	20.00	28.44	11.30
4	12.68	34.08	5.66	24	20.00	46.64	0.00
5	12.77	32.22	7.52	25	20.23	28.97	10.77
6	14.29	28.74	11.00	26	20.90	34.49	5.24
7	14.97	28.62	11.12	27	20.90	34.49	5.24
8	15.12	32.78	6.96	28	21.83	29.91	9.82
9	15.22	28.69	11.04	29	22.86	28.92	10.82
10	15.29	29.05	10.69	30	23.12	28.97	10.77
11	15.93	27.83	11.91	31	24.24	34.60	5.13
12	16.18	34.39	5.35	32	25.53	32.22	7.52
13	17.24	35.59	4.15	33	25.58	30.41	9.33
14	17.70	27.83	11.91	34	25.61	29.22	10.52
15	18.18	29.52	10.22	35	25.74	31.78	7.96
16	18.30	27.87	11.87	36	26.00	29.64	10.10
17	18.82	28.65	11.09	37	26.17	29.68	10.06
18	18.92	39.55	0.19	38	29.17	30.80	8.94
19	18.95	29.55	10.19	39	30.22	30.02	9.72
20	18.99	33.34	6.40	40	30.36	35.87	3.87

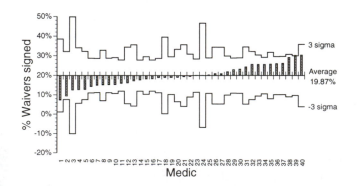

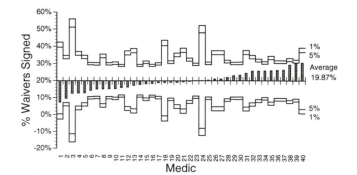

The only potential special cause from the 3 sigma limits is Medic 39, who is 0.2% over his upper common cause limit. Note that Medic 40, also at 30%, is well within his common cause range. With the statistically correct limits for 1% and 5%, even Medic 39 does not appear as a special cause.

2b) The fining policy is a special cause strategy (treating each deviation from the desired result as a unique occurrence). Chances are the problem is not related to differences in how the medics do their jobs. There is some knowledge lacking in the system: either in its overall design or lack of knowledge by the medics.

2c) A low aggressive strategy would be to stratify by other process inputs. For example, part of the city, time of day, and nature of the call would all be easy to collect from historical data. A potentially slightly higher but still low aggressive strategy would be to document the reasons for people not accepting treatment.

2d) If any fining is to be done in the current system, it should be for the people who designed it and continue to ignore common cause problems, i.e., the management!

3. The C-Section Data

3a) Analysis of Means could expose hidden special causes in the process. The system had been stable since February 1991, thus we know the data came from a common cause process. This gives us the right to "slice and dice" the data from this most recent stable period to identify these potentially hidden special causes.

3b)

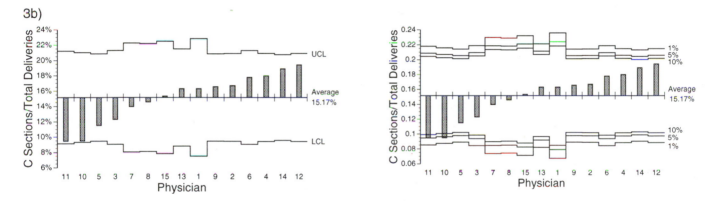

Physicians 10 and 11 may have a lower level of C-Sections. Note that with the approximate 3 sigma limits, all physicians appear to be from the same common cause system. When the more statistically rigorous limits from Table 8.1 are applied, physicians 10 and 11 fall outside the 5% line—if we declare them to be outside the system, we have less than a 5% chance of tampering. If indeed physicians 10 and 11 are operating with a different system, we can find out why, and if appropriate, their methodology can be adopted by the other physicians.

This exercise brings out the fact that things are not always "cut-and-dried" with statistical analysis. Different plots lend themselves to slightly different interpretations. Perhaps the moral of this portion of the analysis is that if something looks close with a 3 sigma approximation, it is best to replot the data using the values from Table 8.1.

3c) Adding the new data points to the control chart shows them to be all below the average. However, none fall outside the lower control limit. Adding 2 sigma limits would not cause us to declare a special cause, either. We could wait another month or two to determine whether the data presentation has had an impact or, we could try analysis of means (part d)).

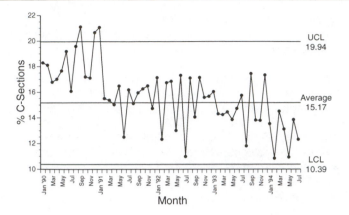

3d) The ANOM shows that the time periods were different–the second period has fewer C-section births than the first. The calculations are as follows:

Time	C-Sections	Births	% C-Sections
2/91-12/93	693	4568	15.17%
1/94-7/94	237	1861	12.74%
Total	930	6429	14.47%

The 1% limits are based on the equation:

$$0.1447 \pm 1.82 \times \sqrt{\frac{(0.1447) \times (1 - 0.1447)}{\text{Number of births during time period}}}$$

$$= 0.1447 \pm 1.82 \times \sqrt{\frac{0.1238}{\text{Number of births during time period}}}$$

The 5% percent results use the same equation but replace "1.82" with the value "1.39" from Table 8.1 Thus the results are:

Time	% C-sections	Upper 1%	Upper 5%	Lower 5%	Lower 1%
2/91-12/93	15.17%	15.41%	15.19%	13.74%	13.52%
1/94-7/94	12.74%	15.95%	15.60%	13.33%	12.98%

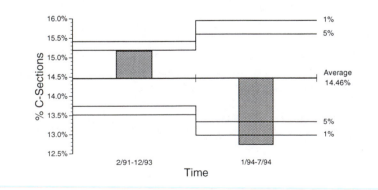

4. The Dictation Data

4a) The moving ranges appear in the tables along with their medians.

Time	MD 1	MR	MD 2	MR	MD 3	MR	MD 4	MR	MD 5	MR	MD 6	MR	MD 7	MR	MD 8	MR
1	32.7	*	39.2	*	35.0	*	37.0	*	30.7	*	33.0	*	32.8	*	31.7	*
2	31.7	1.0	31.7	7.5	18.3	16.7	26.4	10.6	37.5	6.8	23.7	9.3	37.9	5.1	24.8	6.9
3	31.5	0.2	37.2	5.5	33.1	14.8	31.7	5.3	38.2	0.7	24.3	0.6	38.1	0.2	34.8	10.0
4	43.5	12.0	32.5	4.7	33.6	0.5	24.3	7.4	34.1	4.1	33.7	9.4	32.7	5.4	32.6	2.2
5	27.2	16.3	27.0	5.5	35.6	2.0	32.6	8.3	31.3	2.8	20.8	12.9	31.3	1.4	31.9	0.7
6	27.4	0.2	36.8	9.8	31.7	3.9	31.5	1.1	32.1	0.8	30.0	9.2	37.3	6.0	28.0	3.9
7	35.0	7.6	23.3	13.5	25.8	5.9	33.7	2.2	32.3	0.2	31.3	1.3	37.7	0.4	22.9	5.1
Median		4.3		6.5		4.9		6.4		1.8		9.3		3.3		4.5

Combining all the moving ranges (the actual moving ranges, *not* their medians) into one group yields a *system* MMR of 5.1 The system standard deviation is $\frac{5.1}{0.954} = 5.34$. MRMax is 5.1 x 3.865 = 19.7. No moving range exceeds it.

So far, we're in a common cause system.

4b)

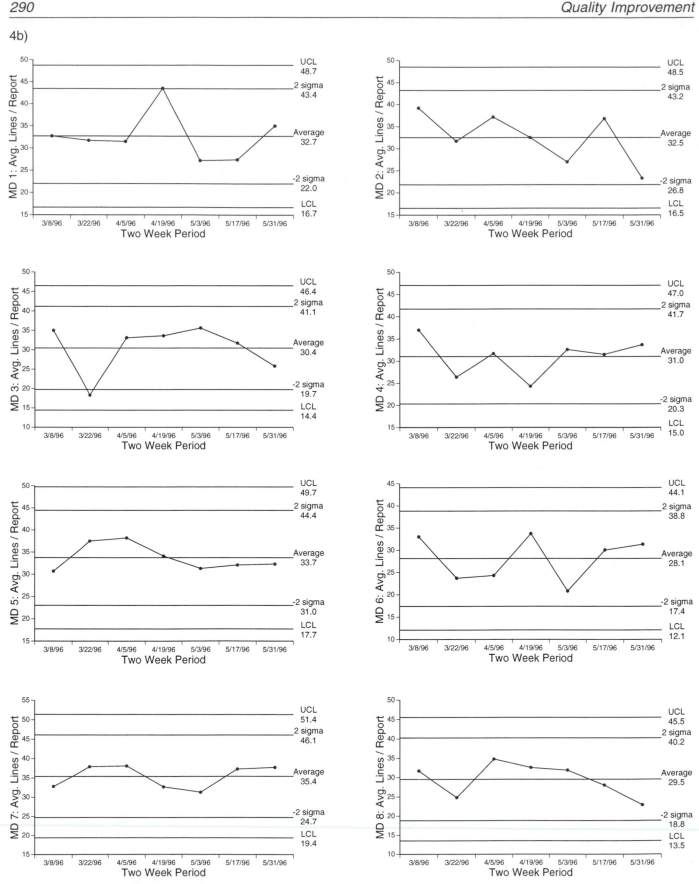

There are no outliers or other special causes. All of the doctors' reporting systems appear stable.

4c) Since there are no outliers, all the points can be included in the averages. Thus the averages can be taken directly from the control charts. They are:

MD	Average
1	32.7
2	32.5
3	30.4
4	31.0
5	33.7
6	28.1
7	35.4
8	29.5

The Analysis of Means limits are calculated from the system average and standard deviation. Because there are no special causes, the system average is calculated simply by taking the average of all the numbers. This value is 31.66. The system standard deviation was calculated in part a) as 5.34. The formula for the limits is:

$$\text{System Average} \pm 3 \times \frac{\text{System Standard Deviation}}{\sqrt{\text{Number of time periods per MD}}}$$

Since each MD had data for all 7 time periods, the equation becomes

$$31.66 \pm 3 \times \frac{5.34}{\sqrt{7}} = 31.66 \pm 6.05.$$

Thus the common cause limits for each MD's average are 25.61 - 37.71. The ANOM shows that all the MDs averages fall within the limits.

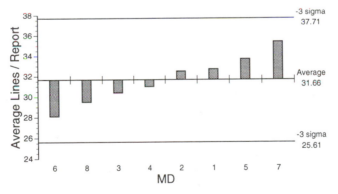

4d) There are no "hidden" opportunities among the MDs. As far as we can tell, they are all operating with the same system. (Note that this analysis does not, nor is it intended to, comment about the quality of the dictation or the information contained therein.)

4e) Control charts of the number of reports and number of lines both show no special causes. Thus, for a typical two-week period, we can predict the average of 171 reports and 5,103 lines.

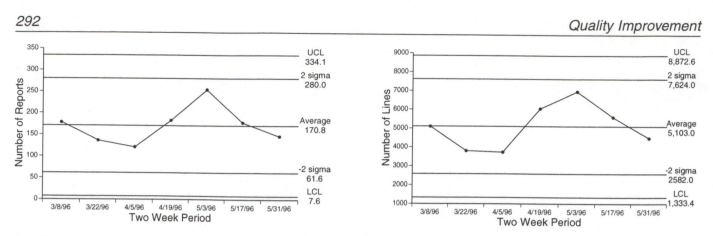

f) Everything seems to be stable, so the department can predict the budget for the entire year. Since there are 26 pay periods in each year, they simply have to multiply the control chart average by 26. This yields 170.8 x 26 = 4,441 reports, and 5,103 x 26 = 132,678 lines. If they continue to monitor the data and plot them against the common cause limits from part e), they will know to adjust the budget if they see evidence of a special cause.

For a typical two-week period, 90-98% of the time the workloads will fall between the -2 sigma and 2 sigma limits. This translates to 62 - 280 reports and 2,582 - 7,624 lines.

5.   The ER Lytic Data

5a) The median is 28, and the run chart is:

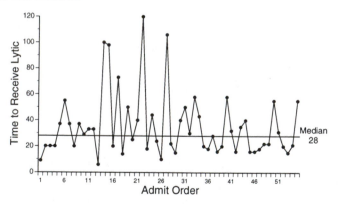

To summarize:

Test	Criterion	Result	Special Cause?
Trend	With more than 20 points, 7 consecutive increases or decreases	Longest was 4	No
Alternation	14 consecutive alternating up or down	Longest was 7	No
Long runs	8 consecutive on same side of median	Longest was 5	No
Number of runs	With 55-1=24 points, we expect 22-34	26 runs	No

There are no signs of special causes in the process.

5b) While there are no points outside the common cause limits, patients 14 and 15 fail the "two out of three" rule. The MMR is 17, making MRMax = 66. Moving ranges associated with patients 22 and 27 are greater than MRMax, making it likely that they are outliers, too. Thus the average should be recalculated with those points excluded.

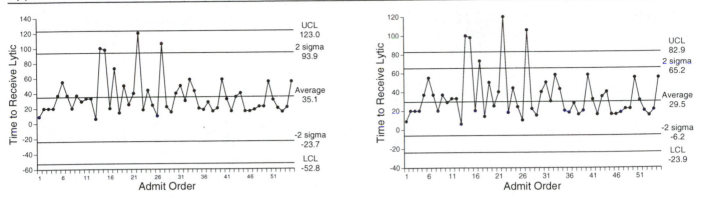

The average patient gets the drug in about 30 minutes but there's a fair amount of variation. Ninety to ninety-eight percent of the time, the patients receive the drug within about an hour (65 minutes). However, it is possible, given this system that it could take as long as 83 minutes.

5c) Both strategies will be useful. There are certainly outliers that should be investigated. The consecutive patients, 14 and 15, might lead one to check how busy the ER was that day. However, the common cause limits are wide, too, and a common cause strategy will lead to more longer-term improvements.

5d) The stratified histogram shows no difference between shifts.

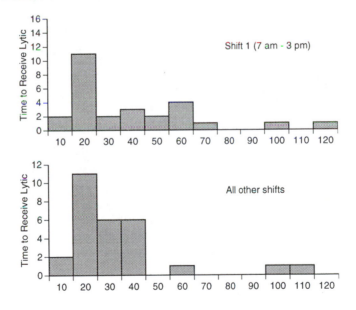

5e) The standard deviation used in the ANOM is $\frac{MMR}{0.954} = \frac{17}{0.954} = 17.8$. The overall average time is 29.5 minutes. Thus the limits for the ANOM are

$$29.5 \pm 3 \times \frac{17.8}{\sqrt{\text{Number of occurences on the shift}}}.$$

Excluding the outliers, there were 25 observations for the 7 AM to 3 PM shift and 26 observations for the other shifts combined. The limits for shift 1 are

$$29.5 \pm 3 \times \frac{17.8}{\sqrt{25}} = 29.5 \pm 10.7,$$

which yield a range of 18.8 - 40.2. The limits for shift 2 are

$$29.5 \pm 3 \times \frac{17.8}{\sqrt{26}} = 29.5 \pm 10.5,$$

for a range of 19.0 - 40.0. The ANOM plot confirms that there is no difference. Again, excluding outliers, the average of the shift 1 data is 32.0. The average of the shift 2 data is 27.2. Both fall well within the common cause range.

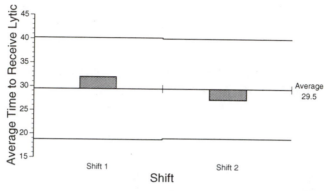

Technically, when comparing only two groups, the limits could be based on a factor of "2" instead of "3." The limits then change to a range of 22.4 - 36.6 for Shift 1, and 22.5 and 36.5 for Shift 2. Again, the averages fall well within the common cause limits. This provides further confirmation that the shifts are not different.

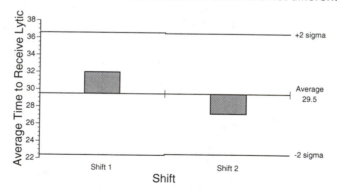

5f) The scatterplot shows no relationship between the number of RNs and the time to receive the lytic.

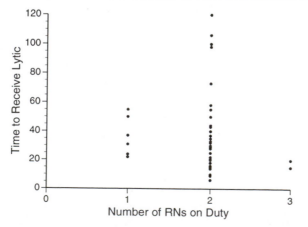

5g) Another possible way to study the current process might be to plot the time against the number of patients in the ER, or some operationally defined measure of activity level. The next data aggressiveness strategy (cutting new windows) could be employed by following the process the patient must go through to receive the lytic. If critical steps were listed, the time to pass through each of those steps could be studied and used to narrow in on the cause of the delays.

6. The DRG Analysis of Means Data (Part 1)

6a) For length of stay, the results are:

Test	Criterion	Result	Special Cause?
Trend	With more than 20 points, 7 consecutive increases or decreases	Longest was 4	No
Alternation	14 consecutive alternating up or down	Longest was 10	No
Long runs	8 consecutive on same side of median	Longest was 7	No
Number of runs	With 78-10=68 points, we expect 27-42	34 runs	Yes

The Charges results are:

Test	Criterion	Result	Special Cause?
Trend	With more than 20 points, 7 consecutive increases or decreases	Longest was 6	No
Alternation	14 consecutive alternating up or down	Longest was 9	No
Long runs	8 consecutive on same side of median	Longest was 4	No
Number of Runs	With 78-0=78 points, we expect 32-47	43 runs	No

There are no special causes identified in either LOS or charges with the run charts.

App.
C

6b) Since there are no special causes identified by the run charts, all the data can be used to create the control charts.

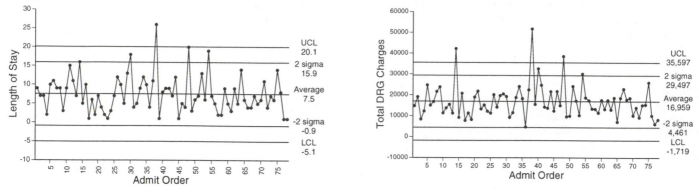

Both plots show evidence of "train wrecks," (outliers). The charts are redone with those points excluded.

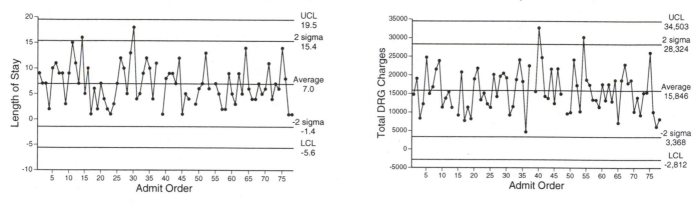

For LOS, 90-98% of the time, patients will stay no more than 15 days. The charges will not be higher than $28,000.

6c) While there are a few outlier special causes that need attention, the biggest improvements will come from a common cause strategy.

If insurers arbitrarily set a limit of $20,000, and demand explanations of charges above that goal, it would not help much. The current process will frequently produce charges that high. A goal of no more than 15 days LOS is also still within the common cause variation. One could possibly convince insurers to change the LOS threshold to 20 days (true special cause), but convincing them to change the charge threshold from $20,000 to $34,500 would be difficult. The system here allows prediction by considering each case as $15,846. Reacting to individual patient costs will only make things worse.

6d) One way to "slice-and-dice" the data would be to aggregate the non-outliers, and study them by physician.

7. The DRG Analysis of Means Data (Part 2)

7a) The common cause band is based on the formula:

$$\text{average} \pm 3 \times \frac{\text{Standard deviation}}{\sqrt{\text{Number of cases for this physician}}}$$

For LOS, the standard deviation is $\frac{3}{0.954} = 3.1$, and for charges it is $\frac{5,286.5}{0.954} = 5,541$.

The bands are as follows:

N	LOS Lower	LOS Upper	Charges Lower	Charges Upper
1	-2.3	16.3	-777	32,469
2	0.4	13.6	4,092	27,600
3	1.6	12.4	6,249	25,443
4	2.4	11.7	7,535	24,158
5	2.8	11.2	8,412	23,280
6	3.2	10.8	9,060	22,632
7	3.5	10.5	9,563	22,129

7b)

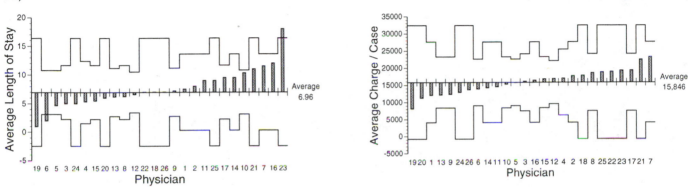

Physician 23's data point is a special cause, but it is based on only one case.

Physician 6's patients generally stay a shorter time. Perhaps Physician 6 has a different methodology that others could learn from. Some investigation may be warranted, but it can hardly be called a pattern.

There are no differences among the physicians when it comes to charges.

7c)   A common cause strategy would be appropriate.

Health Information Management: Medical Record Processes in Group Practice

by Lynn Kuehn, MS, RRA

This new, easy-to-use spiral bound text is essential for those who manage the medical records process in ambulatory care. The book presents critical information for the records manager who is new to the field of ambulatory care, or for those who want an up-to-date reference text. Practice administrators interested in the records management process will also use this important resource.

Key topics include:

- record systems
- storage/retrieval
- coding
- quality improvement
- computerization
- human resources
- legal issues
- transcription

JCAHO and AAAHC requirements are addressed. Evaluation techniques for major process areas are provided. CRAHCA demonstration site research applying quality improvement techniques to the records process in three small primary care group practices is described. Selected sample medical records forms from the research sponsor, Colwell Systems, Inc. are included. The book is endorsed by the American Health Information Management Association (AHIMA), the professional association for health information managers.

Item No. 4950 - $39.00 each for MGMA members, MGMA affiliates, and nonmembers plus shipping and handling.

Health Information Manager covers critical information for your practice

Chapter One: Overview of Key Issues
Chapter Two: Health Information Management - The Record
Chapter Three: Transcription
Chapter Four: Coding and Reimbursement Systems
Chapter Five: Legal Issues
Chapter Six: Computerization
Chapter Seven: Human Resources
Chapter Eight: Evaluating an Existing System
Chapter Nine: Systems Consolidation and Change
Chapter Ten: Future Directions in Computerized Patient Records

CENTER FOR RESEARCH
IN AMBULATORY
HEALTH CARE ADMINISTRATION

Source code: C10 981